AMERICAN JOURNAL of PUBLIC HEALTH
FEBRUARY 2025
Issue 2

AJPH

A PUBLICATION OF THE
AMERICAN PUBLIC HEALTH ASSOCIATION

REDLINING AND WHITENESS: COLORS OF RACISM

Racism and Firearm Violence, pp. 149 and 161
Whiteness and Rural Health, pp. 146 and 152

Also in this issue:

SNAP ACCESS
And Felony Drug Convictions, pp. 113 and 170

ABORTION MEDICATION
No-Test Telehealth Services in 21 US States, pp. 110 and 221

ARTIFICIAL INTELLIGENCE
Way Forward in Public Health, p. 123

NOTES FROM THE FIELD
Chronic Care Management, p. 133
Chinese American Community Health Workers, p. 138
Lead Poisoning, p. 142

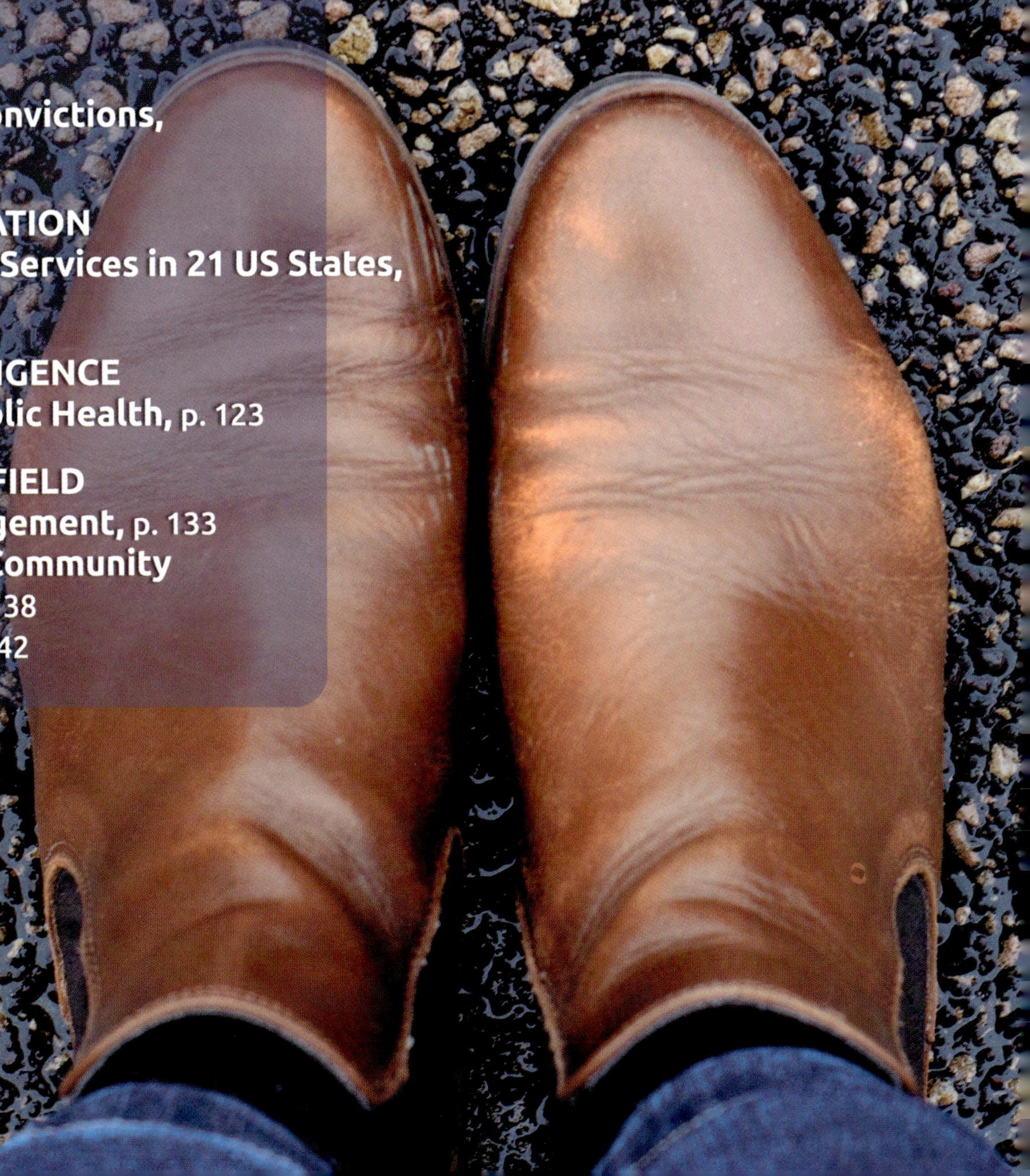

APHA
AMERICAN PUBLIC HEALTH ASSOCIATION
For science. For action. For health.

AJPH®, published monthly, is the official Journal of the American Public Health Association®, 800 I St NW, Washington, DC 20001-3710; (202) 777- APHA; TDD (202) 777-2500. APHA is a nongovernmental professional society founded in 1872, representing all disciplines and specialties in public health.

The *American Journal of Public Health*® (*AJPH*) (print ISSN: 0090-0036; electronic ISSN: 1541- 0048), first published in 1911, is the official journal of the American Public Health Association® (APHA). The oldest and largest organization of public health professionals in the world, APHA represents approximately 30 000 members from more than 50 occupations of public health.

Submissions: Visit www.editorialmanager.com/ajph or ajph.edmgr.com for online manuscript preparation and submission guidelines. Contributions of original unpublished research, social science analyses, scholarly essays, critical commentaries, departments, and letters to the editor are welcome. Questions? Write ajph.submissions@apha.org or call APHA at (202) 777-2469.

Print plus online subscriptions: Institutional price (print copy with online access for a single institution and all authorized users, regardless of geographic location) varies by size of organization and ranges from $993–$1445 for US organizations, and $1073–$1526 for international organizations (air delivery); multiple campuses not permitted without special arrangement. Details of the tiered pricing system at https://subscriptionoffice.com/pages/apha-landing-page. To order, write apha.subscriptions@apha.org.

Online-only subscriptions: Institutional price for one institution and its authorized users (regardless of geographic location) is $878–$1307. To order, write apha.subscriptions@apha.org. For academic consortia or multisite corporate subscriptions, contact apha.subscriptions@apha.org.

Print-only subscriptions: Institutional price is US $701, $782 international.

Back print issues: A limited number of print issues are for sale. Single copies are US $49, $55 international (air delivery). Shipping included; prepay only. To order, write apha.subscriptions@apha.org.

Reprints: For prices and ordering information on 50 or more reprints, check the Reprints section at www.ajph.org. To order smaller quantities of reprints (rush delivery), use the "Purchase Article" link on the article site itself.

Electronic access: Online articles more than 10 years old are available free for personal use at www.ajph.org. Recent articles are available through pay-per-view: single PDF article for $24, single issue access for 24 hours for $33, or entire site access for 24 hours for $38.

Postal information: Periodicals postage paid at Washington, DC, and additional mailing offices. Postmaster: Send address changes to American Journal of Public Health, 800 I St NW, Washington, DC 20001-3710.

Address changes: Send to AJPH, Membership Department (members) or AJPH Subscriptions (subscribers), APHA, 800 I St NW, Washington, DC 20001-3710. Or write to membership.mail@apha.org (members) or apha.subscriptions@apha.org (subscribers).

Indexes: Publications that index or abstract articles from *AJPH* include the following: Ageline, Assia (Applied Social Science Index and Abstracts), Biological Abstracts, Chemical Abstracts, CINAHL, Criminal Justice Abstracts, EMBASE, EMCare, Environmental Abstracts, e-psyche, ERIC, ETOH (Alcohol and Alcohol Problems Science Database), Excerpta Medica, Food Science and Technology, General Science Index, Grateful Med, Hospital Literature Index, Human Resources Abstracts, International Pharmaceutical Abstracts (IPA), Medline, Physical Education Index, Pollution Abstracts, Psychological Abstracts, PsychINFO, Safety Science Abstracts, Sage Family Studies Abstracts, Sage Human Resources Abstracts, Science Citation Index, SCOPUS, SIIC Data Bases, Social Work Research and Abstracts, and Statistical Reference Index (SRI)/LexisNexis.

AJPH
A PUBLICATION OF THE
AMERICAN PUBLIC HEALTH ASSOCIATION

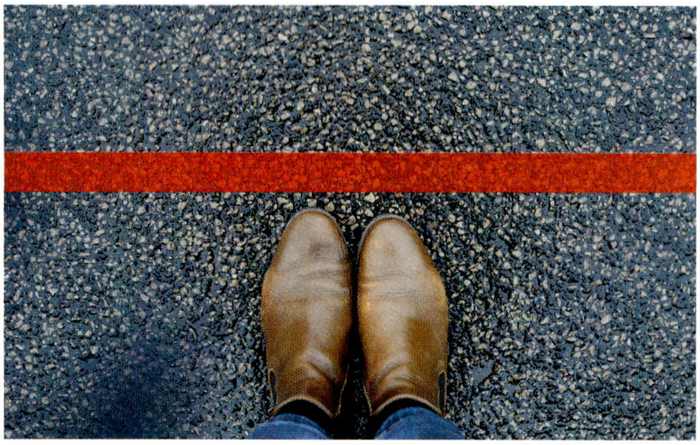

COVER: As a social determinant of health inequity, Whiteness is a fundamental yet often overlooked component of US racism. A critical examination of both racially minoritized and majoritized populations is essential to understanding US national population health. In this issue of *AJPH*, we delve deeply into this topic working to understand the context and the implications.

Cover concept and selection by Aleisha Kropf. Image by Berit Kessler via Adobe Stock. Printed with permission.

APHA
AMERICAN PUBLIC HEALTH ASSOCIATION
For science. For action. For health.

Promoting public health research, policy, practice, and education is the *AJPH* mission. As we widen our scope to embrace global issues, we also sharpen our focus to support the needs of public health practitioners. We invite contributions of original unpublished research, opinion and commentary, and letters to the editor.

The *Journal* is printed on acid-free recycled paper.

AJPH February 2025, Vol. 115, No. 2

OPEN ACCESS ONLINE ONLY PODCAST DATA SUPPLEMENT AVAILABLE

EDITOR'S CHOICE

108 Hank Aaron, Robert F. Kennedy Jr, and the Public's Health
A. Morabia

OPINIONS, IDEAS, & PRACTICE

EDITORIALS

110 Telehealth Is Necessary, But Not Sufficient, for Equitable Access to Quality Abortion Care
E. Janiak

113 The Supplemental Nutrition Assistance Program (SNAP) Ban and Perpetual Punishment for Justice-Affected Populations
K. R. Dong

116 Long-Acting Reversible Contraception (LARC) Removal and Birth Intendedness: Moving Beyond the Binary
D. G. Tsevat, G. A. Trompeter, and K. S. Arora

119 Street Trees and Public Health
A. Woodward and K. Wild

121 Moving From Invisibility to Inclusivity: A Better Way Forward for National Health Surveys
F. J. Dallo

PERSPECTIVES

123 The Way Forward to Embrace Artificial Intelligence in Public Health
G. Hattab, C. Irrgang, N. Körber, D. Kühnert, and K. Ladewig

129 A Research Agenda to Maximize the Health Equity Impacts of Paid Family and Medical Leave Policies
J. M. Goodman, A. Steeves-Reece, and D. M. Richardson

IMAGES OF HEALTH

132 The Public Health Implications of a Leaking Fire Backflow Preventer
O. B. Novoa and G. E. Ibañez

NOTES FROM THE FIELD

133 Evaluation of a Chronic Care Management Model for Improving Efficiency and Fiscal Sustainability
M. A. Kadree, P. Wiggins, L. Thompson, C. Warriner, and M. White

138 Development of Texas's First Chinese American Community Health Worker Certification for Family Health History-Based Cancer Prevention
Y-L. Yeh, Z. Zhang, D. Martinez, and L-S. Chen

142 A Public Health–Community Partnership to Address Lead Poisoning in King County, Washington
D. de Acosta, M. Ali, N. Hamidi, A. Anjaz, E. Mann, and E. Dawson-Hahn

WHITENESS AND REDLINING

146 A Critical Examination of Whiteness as a Fundamental Causal Determinant of US Health Inequities
J. A. Pearson

149 Redlining, Root Causes, and a Firearm Injury Scholarship of Consequence
J. Jay

RESEARCH & ANALYSIS

WHITENESS AND REDLINING

152 Whiteness: A Fundamental Determinant of the Health of Rural White Americans
C. R. Efird and D. M. Griffith

161 Legacy of Racism and Firearm Violence During the COVID-19 Pandemic in the United States
Z. Hans, D. B. Lee, M. A. Zimmerman, and D. J. Wiebe

LAW & ETHICS

170 Laws Limiting Access to SNAP Benefits for People With Felony Drug Convictions: A Policy-Mapping Study
H. Shah, A. D. McCourt, and S. Bandara

178 US State Recreational and Medical Cannabis Delivery Laws, 2024
T. Ebling, S. Azagba, M. Hall, and J. K. Jensen

191 Bills to Restrict Access to and Harm From Indoor Tanning Facilities in US State Legislatures, 1992–2023
D. B. Buller, J. Berteletti, C. Heckman, K. R. J. Schroth, A. C. Geller, J. L. Stapleton, I. Adjei, A. Mitarotondo, S. R. Guild, J. E. Gershenwald, R. Dellavalle, and S. Pagoto

OPEN-THEMED RESEARCH

201 Engaging Low-Wage Workers in Health and Well-Being Survey Research: Strategies From 5 Occupational Studies
E. L. Sabbath, M. Lovejoy, D. K. Schneider, Y. Diaz-Linhart, G. DeHorn, and S. E. Peters

209 Influenza Vaccination, Household Composition, and Race-Based Differences in Influenza Incidence: An Agent-Based Modeling Study
K. V. Williams, M. G. Krauland, L. H. Harrison, J. V. Williams, M. S. Roberts, and R. K. Zimmerman

217 HIV Trends in Metropolitan US Cities From 2014 to 2021: Baseline Data for the Ending the HIV Epidemic Initiative
R. Gupta and S. H. Vermund

221 No-Test Telehealth Medication Abortion Services Provided by US-Based Clinicians in 21 States and the District of Columbia, 2020–2022
E. M. Godfrey, A. E. Fiastro, E. K. Thayer, R. Gomperts, S. M. Orlando, and C. K. Myers

BACKMATTER

LETTERS & RESPONSES

232 From Taboo to Teaching: Transforming Menstrual Health in Schools
M. Stein

233 A School Nurse Perspective of Menstrual Health Equity
S. L. Brown

234 Bergen et al. Respond
S. Bergen, E. D. Maughan, K. E. Johnson, R. Cogan, M. Secor, and M. Sommer

ERRATA

235 Erratum In: "Health Care Delivery Site– and Patient-Level Factors Associated With COVID-19 Primary Vaccine Series Completion in a National Network of Community Health Centers"

OTHER DEPARTMENTS

240 Subscription Form

Hank Aaron, Robert F. Kennedy Jr, and the Public's Health

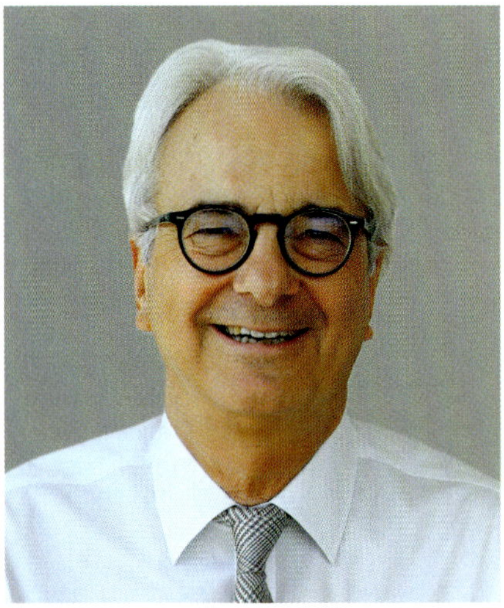

Alfredo Morabia, MD, PhD
Editor in Chief, *AJPH*

The tale of Hank Aaron, Robert F. Kennedy Jr, and the public's health highlights the vital importance of qualified leaders in public health institutions. As a public health historian and editor of a premier public health journal, I reflect on this recent history as we face a new administration.

On January 22, 2021, Henry Louis "Hank" Aaron—Baseball Hall of Famer and the man who broke Babe Ruth's all-time home-run record—passed away in his sleep at the age of 86 years. Just 2 weeks earlier, Aaron had been vaccinated against COVID-19 at a Morehouse School of Medicine clinic in Atlanta, Georgia.

Shortly afterward, Robert F. Kennedy Jr, chairman of Children's Health Defense and now being considered as secretary for the Department of Health and Human Services, claimed Aaron's death was "part of a wave of suspicious deaths among the elderly closely following administration of COVID vaccines" (https://bit.ly/4fET3iq).

THE PUBLIC HEALTH APPROACH TO AARON'S DEATH

Kennedy's claim, implying the vaccine caused Aaron's death, reflects a fundamental misunderstanding of how evidence-based public health operates. While it is impossible to determine counterfactuals—whether Aaron would have survived without vaccination—public health evaluates risks at the population level.

To assess this event properly, two key questions must be considered:

1. What was the likelihood of Hank Aaron dying the week he did if he had not been vaccinated?

   Aaron was 86 years old and likely experienced cardiac arrest or sudden death, a common occurrence at his age. By January 22, 2021, more than 11 million people aged 65 years and older in the United States had already received the vaccine. Among this group, thousands of cardiac arrests and sudden deaths would have been expected based solely on age-related mortality. Aaron's risk of death that week was high, irrespective of his vaccination status.

Continued on page 109...

HISTORY CORNER

2 YEARS AGO

Historic Redlining Practices and Contemporary Determinants of Health in the Detroit Metropolitan Area

The patterns identified through this study suggest variations in the distribution of widely used determinants of health, some 80 years after the HOLC [Home Owners' Loan Corporation] grading system was implemented. Our findings are consistent with existing studies that demonstrate that HOLC grades are associated with the contemporary distribution of risk and opportunity and that those distributions are associated with racial inequities in health. . . . Furthermore, our findings provide an example of the persistent effects of structural racism, or racist ideologies that are embedded in social policies. Neighborhoods with larger proportions of Black residents were more likely to be redlined; those neighborhoods remain disproportionately Black in contemporary Detroit. The contributions of those historical policies to differential patterns of investment, governance, and environmental exposures and to contemporary racial inequities in health offer one example of racism as a structural driver of health inequities.

From *AJPH*, Supplement 1 2023, pp. S54–S55, 144 words

AJPH February 2024, Vol. 115, No. 2

2. What was the likelihood the vaccine caused Aaron's death?

   Sudden deaths directly caused by the Moderna COVID-19 vaccine are exceedingly rare. A report from the National Academy of Medicine found the evidence insufficient to establish any causal relationship between COVID-19 vaccines and sudden cardiac events and rejected a causal link with myocardial infarction (https://bit.ly/4eGSEe3; p. 5).

Furthermore, the World Health Organization has highlighted the immense benefits of vaccination, particularly among older adults, estimating a 62% reduction in COVID-19 mortality in individuals aged 80 years or older (https://bit.ly/3ZM9cgo).

The timing of Aaron's death, though coincidental, does not support Kennedy's claim. His passing is better explained by age-related risks, whereas attributing it to the vaccine remains speculative and dangerous.

THE DANGER OF ANECDOTAL REASONING

Claims like Kennedy's undermine public trust in vaccines and endanger lives. During the COVID-19 pandemic, misinformation played a tragic role in vaccine hesitancy, leading to preventable deaths. Research by Woolf et al. published in *AJPH* demonstrated that excess mortality during the pandemic disproportionately occurred in states with Republican governors, where vaccine uptake was lower in people aged younger than 65 years (https://bit.ly/4gibwkW). The 10 states with the highest excess death rates were West Virginia, New Mexico, Mississippi, South Carolina, Wyoming, Louisiana, Arizona, Kentucky, Arkansas, and Alabama. Accurate, evidence-based communication about vaccines' life-saving effects is essential to prevent such outcomes.

The reasoning behind Kennedy's claim reflects a lack of familiarity with the population perspective—a foundational principle of public health. This approach, first pioneered in 1662 by John Graunt, uses data to identify patterns and relationships in health outcomes. It requires specialized training and is not something that can be improvised or based on anecdotal observations.

THE BROADER IMPLICATIONS OF FLAWED REASONING

The logic Kennedy applies to Aaron's death—extrapolating causality from single events—threatens to undermine well-established public health policies. For example, consider the causal link between smoking and lung cancer. While only about one in 10 heavy smokers develops lung cancer, the relationship is undeniable when comparing heavy smokers to nonsmokers: the risk of lung cancer is 20 times higher in smokers. Following Kennedy's reasoning, one might question the link between smoking and cancer simply because not all smokers are affected—a dangerous regression in understanding causality.

Such flawed reasoning has real-world consequences. Public health leaders must be equipped with the expertise to approach health issues systematically, relying on evidence rather than speculation.

THE VITAL NEED FOR PUBLIC HEALTH EXPERTISE

As I wrote at the beginning of this piece, the tale of Hank Aaron, Robert F. Kennedy Jr, and the public's health has profound implications for who should lead our public health institutions. The Department of Health and Human Services, the Centers for Disease Control and Prevention, the Food and Drug Administration, and the Environmental Protection Agency require leaders with specialized training in public health.

Public health is a science, grounded in rigorous data analysis and a population-based perspective. It cannot be improvised. Decisions affecting millions of lives demand expertise, not anecdotal reasoning or personal biases. As we enter a new administration, we must prioritize leadership that upholds these principles. AJPH

DOI: https://doi.org/10.2105/AJPH.2024.307945

Telehealth Is Necessary, But Not Sufficient, for Equitable Access to Quality Abortion Care

Elizabeth Janiak, ScD

ABOUT THE AUTHOR

Elizabeth Janiak is with Brigham and Women's Hospital, Harvard Medical School, and the Harvard T. H. Chan School of Public Health, Boston, MA.

See also Godfrey et al., p. 221.

AJPH February 2025, Vol. 115, No. 2

In the more than two years since the *Dobbs v Jackson Women's Health Organization* decision (*Dobbs*; https://bit.ly/48QT9B0) overturned *Roe v Wade* (*Roe*; https://bit.ly/4ezjnco) and eliminated the federal right to abortion, the landscape of abortion access has changed dramatically in the United States. Hundreds of thousands of individuals have crossed state lines to obtain in-person abortion care, while abortion provision via telehealth has grown increasingly common,[1] and the overall number of abortions appears to be up from prepandemic numbers, at 1 037 000 in 2023 versus 863 320 in 2017.[2,3]

Telehealth abortion usually involves the prescribing of an evidence-based two-drug regimen that includes misoprostol, a common drug in obstetric settings, and mifepristone, also known as the "abortion pill." Although this regimen can be used to self-manage an abortion without clinician involvement, it is more commonly prescribed in the formal health care system, both by providers affiliated with brick-and-mortar clinics and, increasingly, in "virtual clinics," such as the one described by Godfrey et al. in this issue of *AJPH* (p. 221). In their analysis, Godfrey et al. found that, before the *Dobbs* decision, residential distance to the nearest in-person abortion provider was correlated with an increased rate of fulfilled requests for telehealth medication abortion, even after controlling for area-level covariates that serve as proxy measures of barriers to abortion care. An increase of 100 miles in county-level distance to an abortion facility was associated with a 61% higher per capita rate of abortion utilization in this care model.

The findings of Godfrey et al. underscore the crucial role of telehealth abortion in providing access to individuals who do not live near an in-person abortion provider, a population whose numbers have dramatically increased in the context of new legal restrictions. Immediately after *Dobbs* was decided, an estimated 33% of pregnancy-capable people in the United States lived more than 60 minutes from an abortion facility, versus 15% before; more state bans and abortion clinic closures have occurred since.[4]

Robust evidence demonstrates that abortion via telehealth is safe and effective. Broadly, abortion care is a low-risk intervention, on par with common minor dental procedures, and has vastly lower mortality and morbidity rates than carrying a pregnancy to term.[5] Delivery of medication abortion via telehealth, although studied previously in academic trials, became widespread in practice out of necessity during the early, acute phase of the COVID-19 pandemic. The "no-touch" protocols developed in this era delineated that a fully remote model of care delivery is appropriate for individuals at low risk for ectopic pregnancy whose pregnancy can be dated without a physical exam or ultrasonography.[6]

British data from tens of thousands of individuals cared for using a hybrid model demonstrated that this no-touch method is safe and highly effective at scale. In this model, providers offered telehealth abortion to individuals whose pregnancy dating they were confident in and provided in-person care to those with uncertain pregnancy dating. The results showed that 98.8% of individuals completed the abortion without requiring surgical intervention.[7] The promulgation of telehealth for abortion, and the resulting data demonstrating the safety of this care delivery model, prompted the US Food and Drug Administration (FDA) to permanently lift a previous in-person dispensing requirement for mifepristone in January 2023, thereby opening the door to telehealth abortion as a routine practice. At this time, however, the FDA has left in place other onerous and medically unnecessary regulations on how mifepristone is prescribed and dispensed.

Although the safety and efficacy of telehealth medication abortion is clear, many aspects of the patient experience with telehealth abortion have yet to be robustly explored. In the present landscape, pregnant people choose telehealth medication abortion under conditions of legal restriction and high levels of social stigma. In these circumstances, they may find the telehealth model optimal; however, it is unknown how many of these individuals would prefer to receive in-person care in the absence of such barriers. It is clear that, as Godfrey et al. found, younger people seem to utilize telehealth abortion at higher rates. It remains unclear whether there are disparities in use according to race, ethnicity, socioeconomic status, and other sociodemographic factors. Future research on how people choose and experience different models of abortion care should focus in more depth on understanding preference alignment and satisfaction and how these factors vary by patient demographics and thereby contribute to health inequities.

Regardless of whether telehealth medication abortion is an ideal method of care delivery for all individuals, it is already clear it is not an appropriate method for some. Medication abortion using the standard mifepristone–misoprostol regimen is highly effective through at least 11 weeks of pregnancy, and most providers do not offer medication abortion at later stages of gestation.[8] Before the *Dobbs* decision, 12% of abortions in the United States were obtained at 12 weeks or later in gestation; individuals obtaining care at this stage are often the most socially disadvantaged and have been delayed by structural barriers.[9] As clinics close and care becomes more difficult to obtain, the number of people needing abortion at a gestational age when medication abortion is not routinely offered may increase. In addition, individuals in need of confidential care, such as minors without parental support and adults living with intimate partner violence, may find that procedural abortion better protects their privacy.

Moreover, physical abortion clinics are crucial safety net health care providers. Many of the clinics that provided in-person abortion care to millions of people in the *Roe* era offered additional benefits. These included access to medical translators, the ability to bill insurance for those with coverage, and connections to the larger health care and social service systems for patients needing further services. Many clinics also offered postabortion contraception and, in many cases, a wide array of other sexual and reproductive health services to those who were not pregnant.

The long-term future of abortion access in the United States is unclear. Since the *Dobbs* decision, large majorities of voters have generally voted in favor of state-level abortion rights expansions. At the same time, many legislators and advocates continue to favor a national abortion ban. To ensure the equitable access to the patient-centered, preference-aligned abortion care that every person deserves requires an array of policy changes. As data from Texas, which implemented its near-total abortion ban before any other state (September 2021), have made clear, abortion bans are killing pregnant people and must be lifted.[10] However, this change alone will not ensure access.

Evidence-based abortion policy would include the full decriminalization of self-managed abortion in every state as well as deregulation of mifepristone to allow routine dispensing in the same fashion as other medications.[11] Every person deserves a meaningful choice between procedural and medication abortion and, for those who choose medication abortion, the ability to access this care via telehealth if they prefer and are medically eligible. In a barrier-free world, it is likely many patients will choose telehealth because of its convenience. As abortion currently remains legal in more than half of US states and is becoming more accessible around the globe, a clearer landscape of truly patient-centered abortion care may emerge, even as restrictions increase elsewhere. Telehealth will surely continue to play a vital role in realizing this vision. AJPH

CORRESPONDENCE

Correspondence should be sent to Elizabeth Janiak, ScD, Dept of Obstetrics and Gynecology, Brigham and Women's Hospital, 75 Francis St, Boston, MA 02115 (e-mail: ejaniak@bwh.harvard.edu). Reprints can be ordered at https://www.ajph.org by clicking the "Reprints" link.

PUBLICATION INFORMATION

Full Citation: Janiak E. Telehealth is necessary, but not sufficient, for equitable access to quality abortion care. *Am J Public Health*. 2025;115(2): 110–112.

Acceptance Date: November 11, 2024.

DOI: https://doi.org/10.2105/AJPH.2024.307935

CONFLICTS OF INTEREST

The author has no conflicts of interest to declare.

REFERENCES

1. Society of Family Planning. #WeCount. October 22, 2024. Available at: https://societyfp.org/wp-content/uploads/2024/10/WeCount-Report-8-June-2024-data.pdf. Accessed November 5, 2024. https://doi.org/10.46621/728122kflzwf
2. Maddow-Zimet I, Gibson C. Despite bans, number of abortions in the United States increased in 2023. May 10, 2024. Available at: https://www.guttmacher.org/2024/03/despite-bans-number-abortions-united-states-increased-2023. Accessed November 5, 2024.
3. Jones RK, Kirstein M, Philbin J. Abortion incidence and service availability in the United States, 2020. *Perspect Sex Reprod Health*. 2022;54(4): 128–141. https://doi.org/10.1363/psrh.12215
4. Rader B, Upadhyay UD, Sehgal NKR, Reis BY, Brownstein JS, Hswen Y. Estimated travel time and spatial access to abortion facilities in the US before and after the *Dobbs v Jackson Women's Health* decision. *JAMA*. 2022;328(20):2041–2047. https://doi.org/10.1001/jama.2022.20424
5. National Academies of Sciences, Engineering, and Medicine. *The Safety and Quality of Abortion Care in the United States*. Washington, DC:

National Academies Press; 2018. https://doi.org/10.17226/24950

6. Raymond EG, Grossman D, Mark A, et al. Commentary: no-test medication abortion: a sample protocol for increasing access during a pandemic and beyond. *Contraception.* 2020;101(6):361–366. https://doi.org/10.1016/j.contraception.2020.04.005
7. Aiken A, Lohr PA, Lord J, Ghosh N, Starling J. Effectiveness, safety and acceptability of no-test medical abortion (termination of pregnancy) provided via telemedicine: a national cohort study. *BJOG.* 2021;128(9):1464–1474. https://doi.org/10.1111/1471-0528.16668
8. Kapp N, Eckersberger E, Lavelanet A, Rodriguez MI. Medical abortion in the late first trimester: a systematic review. *Contraception.* 2019;99(2):77–86. https://doi.org/10.1016/j.contraception.2018.11.002
9. Jones RK, Jerman J. Characteristics and circumstances of US women who obtain very early and second-trimester abortions. *PLoS One.* 2017;12(1):e0169969. https://doi.org/10.1371/journal.pone.0169969
10. Jaramillo C, Surana K. A woman died after being told it would be a "crime" to intervene in her miscarriage at a Texas hospital. October 30, 2024. Available at: https://www.propublica.org/article/josseli-barnica-death-miscarriage-texas-abortion-ban. Accessed November 5, 2024.
11. Schummers L, Darling EK, Elizabeth K. Abortion utilization and safety when mifepristone is available without regulations restricting practice? A population-based study using linked health administrative data from Ontario. *J Obstet Gynaecol Can.* 2021;43(5):671–672. https://doi.org/10.1016/j.jogc.2021.02.077

The Supplemental Nutrition Assistance Program (SNAP) Ban and Perpetual Punishment for Justice-Affected Populations

Kimberly R. Dong, DrPH, MS, RD

ABOUT THE AUTHOR

Kimberly R. Dong is with the Tufts University School of Medicine, Boston, MA.

See also Shah et al., p. 170.

In 1996, the Personal Responsibility and Work Opportunity Reconciliation Act (PRWORA) was enacted as a bipartisan measure that set time limits on receiving welfare benefits and imposed work requirements for many recipients.[1] The PRWORA included a lifetime ban on Supplemental Nutrition Assistance Program (SNAP) benefits for people with drug-related felony convictions—a ban subject to state modification. The PRWORA was implemented at a time when mass incarceration had skyrocketed because of the overcriminalization of drug use and possession, which contributed to approximately one million arrests annually[2] and sparked a public health crisis. About 58% of people incarcerated in prisons and 63% incarcerated in jails meet the *Diagnostic and Statistical Manual of Mental Disorders, Fourth Edition* (Washington, DC; American Psychiatric Association; 1994) criteria for drug dependance or abuse.[3]

At the end of 2022, about 1 in 48 adult US residents (2.1%) were under some form of correctional supervision, with approximately one third (1 827 600) incarcerated in prisons or jails and more than two thirds (3 668 800) on probation or parole.[4] Each year, an estimated 10 817 398 individuals are released from the carceral system; approximately 609 854 people were released from prison in 2019.[5] Given the large number of individuals released from the carceral system plus the number on community corrections, there are millions of individuals who need support to become successful community members.

In this issue of *AJPH*, Shah et al. (p. 170) mapped state SNAP bans for felony drug convictions between 2004 and 2021. As of 2021, all but one state has overturned the federal SNAP ban, and 23 states have enacted modified SNAP bans. Of states with modified bans, 13 require parole or probation compliance, 12 require drug treatment, 7 require drug testing, and 9 have limited eligibility for certain populations related to multiple drug felony convictions, higher-level felony drug convictions, or a temporary six-month ban for all individuals with a felony drug conviction. The restrictions of the modified bans continue to pose challenges to this population receiving SNAP benefits.

SNAP is intended to provide nutritious food and prevent food insecurity among low-income households. Food insecurity is pervasive among the justice-affected population. A study of people recently released from prison found that 91% experienced food insecurity.[6] Another study found that nearly 75% of people on probation experienced food insecurity, even with SNAP participation.[7] These studies highlight the disproportionate rates of food insecurity experienced by this population and the critical need for SNAP benefits above the current allotment provided. Food insecurity is associated with poor health outcomes, including an increased risk of developing chronic health illnesses, mental health conditions, and medication and resource shifting. This further exacerbates the adverse health conditions in justice-affected populations.

For most states, only those with drug felonies are subject to the SNAP ban.[1] Most individuals that enter the carceral system have substance use disorder. Because one state still has the full SNAP ban and many others have modified bans, these bans—which are not enacted for other felonies or health conditions—increase the barriers to participation in SNAP among people with substance use disorder. This further creates punitive policies among a group that perpetually faces stigma and discrimination. The sentence under correctional supervision is the punishment associated with the felony, but these punitive policies are biased against this population and extend punishment beyond the term of their original sentence. SNAP eligibility is meant to be based on income to assist with providing food and addressing food insecurity, which are critically needed for this population. The SNAP bans may preclude receiving SNAP benefits among a group that otherwise would be eligible based on low incomes, further contributing to their experiences of strikingly increased levels of health inequities.

Some of the stipulations of the modified bans continue to make it challenging for individuals with felony drug convictions to participate in SNAP. For example, participating in drug treatment programs can be extremely challenging because there are many barriers to participating in drug treatment, such as cost, access to insurance, ability to afford the program, geographic limitations, and placement availability. It is also likely that the cost to administer drug tests and treatment are higher than the cost of providing SNAP benefits.[8]

Some states with a modified SNAP ban require compliance with parole or probation. Community parole violations occur primarily because of new arrests, breaking curfews, failing to report to a parole officer, and failing drug tests. Many violations related to breaking curfew or failing to report to officers often relate to issues with transportation and jobs with inflexible work hours that prevent individuals from attending regular appointments with their parole officers.

Individuals with a history of felony convictions need support to be successful in the community, especially because they have more difficulty with employment. Jobs available for this population tend to provide lower wages and have less wage growth, which increase the risk of experiencing food insecurity. Food insecurity increases the risk of adverse health conditions, which can affect one's ability to stay employed and further compromise health and economic well-being.

The period within one year after release from incarceration is a time of high risk of recidivism. A study found that providing SNAP benefits to newly released drug offenders was associated with a 2.2% decrease in returning to prison within one year[9] and that the adoption of the SNAP ban was associated with a 9% increase in financially motivated recidivism.[10] In a qualitative study of people on probation supervision, individuals reported that they do not want to engage in drug sales or other felony activities, but if they are unable to become employed because of their felony convictions and need to provide for their family, they feel forced into these behaviors to survive.[11] Additionally, there are adverse consequences for intergenerational well-being. If someone is ineligible to participate in SNAP because of a felony drug conviction, the individual is not accounted for in the monthly benefits distributed to that household, leading to less money for the household and adjustments to their dietary intake based on the reduced amount of benefits.

Shah et al. report on the SNAP bans that are current in almost half of the states in our country. SNAP bans have not curbed the use or sales of drugs in our country. Additionally, Black/African American and Hispanic/Latino individuals are more likely to be convicted of drug felonies than are their White counterparts, even when drug use is the same.[12]

These bans make it difficult for people with felony drug convictions to participate in SNAP, which increases the risk of recidivism, food insecurity, and poor health outcomes in a population that experiences disproportionate levels of health disparities. It is critical to conduct research to further assess the impacts of these bans on this population. Proponents of the SNAP ban may challenge amendments to these policies as they argue in favor of welfare reform, combating drug use, and promoting community safety. Because these bans have not been effective at reducing drug use or sales, focus should be on policies that help people convicted of drug felonies with gainful employment and services to become successful community members. Because of the numerous inadequacies in accessing determinants of health in this population, policies should focus on improving access instead of contributing to longer-term punishments that affect individuals, their families, and communities. AJPH

CORRESPONDENCE

Correspondence should be sent to Kimberly R. Dong, Associate Professor, Tufts University School of Medicine, 136 Harrison Ave, Boston, MA 02111 (e-mail: kimberly.dong@tufts.edu). Reprints can be ordered at https://www.ajph.org by clicking the "Reprints" link.

PUBLICATION INFORMATION

Full Citation: Dong KR. The Supplemental Nutrition Assistance Program (SNAP) ban and perpetual punishment for justice-affected populations. *Am J Public Health*. 2025;115(2):113–115.

Acceptance Date: November 16, 2024.

DOI: https://doi.org/10.2105/AJPH.2024.307943

ORCID iD:

Kimberly R. Dong https://orcid.org/0000-0001-9941-2942

ACKNOWLEDGMENTS

The views expressed in this editorial are solely those of the author and do not necessarily reflect the views of Tufts University.

CONFLICTS OF INTEREST

The author has no conflicts of interest to disclose.

REFERENCES

1. Personal Responsibility and Work Opportunity Reconciliation Act, Pub L No. 104-193, §§ 115, 110 Stat 2105, 2180 (1996).

2. McGilton M, Adams W, Samuels J, Kelly J, Motivans M. Sentencing decisions for persons in federal prison for drug offenses, 2013–2018. July 2023. Available at: https://bjs.ojp.gov/document/sdpfpdo1318.pdf. Accessed October 22, 2024.
3. Bronson J, Stroop J, Zimmer S, Berzofsky M. Drug use, dependence, and abuse among state prisoners and jail inmates, 2007–2009. June 2017. Available at: https://bjs.ojp.gov/content/pub/pdf/dudaspji0709.pdf. Accessed October 22, 2024.
4. Buehler ED, Kluckow R. Correctional populations in the United States, 2022—statistical tables. May 2024. Available at: https://bjs.ojp.gov/document/cpus22st.pdf. Accessed October 22, 2024.
5. Carson EA, Kluckow R. Prisoners in 2022—statistical tables. November 2023. Available at: https://bjs.ojp.gov/document/p22st.pdf. Accessed October 22, 2024.
6. Wang EA, Zhu GA, Evans L, Carroll-Scott A, Desai R, Fiellin LE. A pilot study examining food insecurity and HIV risk behaviors among individuals recently released from prison. *AIDS Educ Prev.* 2013;25(2):112–123. https://doi.org/10.1521/aeap.2013.25.2.112
7. Dong KR, Tang AM, Stopka TJ, Beckwith CG, Must A. Food acquisition methods and correlates of food insecurity in adults on probation in Rhode Island. *PLoS One.* 2018;13(6):e0198598. https://doi.org/10.1371/journal.pone.0198598
8. Thompson D. Drug testing and public assistance. February 2019. Available at: https://www.clasp.org/wp-content/uploads/2022/01/2019_drug-testing-and-public-_0.pdf. Accessed October 30, 2024.
9. Yang CS. Does public assistance reduce recidivism? *Am Econ Rev.* 2017;107(5):551–555. https://doi.org/10.1257/aer.p20171001
10. Tuttle C. Snapping back: food stamp bans and criminal recidivism. *Am Econ J: Econ Policy.* 2019;11(2):301–327. https://doi.org/10.1257/pol.20170490
11. Dong KR, Must A, Tang AM, Beckwith CG, Stopka TJ. Competing priorities that rival health in adults on probation in Rhode Island: substance use recovery, employment, housing, and food intake. *BMC Public Health.* 2018;18(1):289. https://doi.org/10.1186/s12889-018-5201-7
12. Rosenberg A, Groves AK, Blankenship KM. Comparing Black and White drug offenders: implications for racial disparities in criminal justice and reentry policy and programming. *J Drug Issues.* 2017;47(1):132–142. https://doi.org/10.1177/0022042616678614

Long-Acting Reversible Contraception (LARC) Removal and Birth Intendedness: Moving Beyond the Binary

Danielle G. Tsevat, MD, Grace A. Trompeter, MD, MSPH, and Kavita S. Arora, MD, MBE, MS

ABOUT THE AUTHORS

All authors are with the Department of Obstetrics and Gynecology, University of North Carolina at Chapel Hill.

AJPH February 2025, Vol. 115, No. 2

Pregnancy planning and intention are constructs that have long been used to guide public health efforts and research.[1] Reducing the rate of unintended pregnancies has been a major motivation of contraception campaigns. Long-acting reversible contraception (LARC) has been favored for its high effectiveness and low failure rates, leading to its promotion by health organizations such as the American College of Obstetricians and Gynecologists.[2] Delaware, like many states, launched a statewide contraceptive access initiative from 2015 to 2020 known as DelCAN (Delaware Contraceptive Access Now) to improve access to all contraceptives, including LARC, with a primary goal of reducing unintended pregnancy.[3]

Targeted counseling, using a "tiered effectiveness" approach with LARCs as the preferred method, was a signature tenet of many of these campaigns. However, a recent shift to prioritizing patients' values, preferences, and lived experiences in contraceptive counseling and decision-making from solely efficacy-based counseling is now recommended.[4] This guidance along with studies exploring individual's preferences when selecting contraception and the complex attitudes toward contraception failure and pregnancy have led to the collective call for improved metrics in reproductive health research.

Following a trend away from research that focuses on LARC's usefulness in pregnancy prevention, Rendall et al. analyzed LARC's potential to increase "intended pregnancies and births," employing a valuable linked data set to reframe the metrics of success of Delaware's statewide contraceptive access initiative.[5] Using the Delaware Medicaid administrative database and the PRAMS (Pregnancy Risk Assessment Monitoring System), the authors modeled births and birth intendedness following Medicaid-covered LARC removals by using LARC removal as a proxy for pregnancy planning.

In showing that the proportion of intended births within three years of LARC removal was higher than the proportion of all Medicaid-covered births, particularly in women younger than 30 years, Rendall et al. concluded that LARC was used successfully to enable reproductive autonomy by enhancing an individual's ability to achieve birth at their chosen time. Furthermore, the authors found that despite a higher proportion of Delaware Medicaid LARC removals occurring at younger ages than those of privately insured women (41.6% vs 23.5% among aged < 25 years), more than 60% of births in the Delaware Medicaid group were intended, including 60.7% among those aged 15 to 20 years and 62.8% among those aged 21 to 24 years. Thus, the authors argue that the use and removal of LARC to ensure desired birth timing are important data to consider as we move away from conceptualizing LARC solely as a tool to prevent "unintended" pregnancies, especially among young people, and toward a personalized care model in which desired pregnancy timing is unique.

This analysis, however, continues to frame pregnancies in a dichotomous system of intended versus unintended, planned versus unplanned, good versus bad. Intendedness as an outcome measure is flawed both methodologically and conceptually. Methodologically, intendedness is a retrospective measure subject to recall bias.[6] Conceptually, intendedness lies in the assumption that birthing people view pregnancy as an event they can always or should plan although there is significant evidence regarding the complexities of people's values, experiences, and life circumstances.[7]

Furthermore, intendedness does not capture how someone may feel about a pregnancy once it occurs, including feelings of ambivalence, acceptance, or welcoming.[1,6,8] In the data of Rendall et al., it is difficult to state that simply because a LARC was removed a pregnancy was intended as both the goal and in the timing. The data also do not account for the fluidity in contraceptive decision-making separately from pregnancy intendedness.[9] Although the authors subsequently narrow the analysis to patients who responded positively to pregnancy intendedness survey questions, this approach continues to assume a binary and problematic dichotomization of intendedness.

Statewide initiatives, such as Delaware's DelCAN initiative, have been instrumental in improving statewide access to desired contraceptive care. However, as previously discussed and as Rendall et al. reference in the introduction, "LARC-first" efforts are often criticized for their potential to endanger reproductive autonomy by prioritizing public health goals of pregnancy prevention and reduction of unintended pregnancies over individual patient-centered goals. Some statewide programs had the primary goal of removing barriers to desired LARCs and thus did employ nuanced counseling tactics and use shared decision-making. However, the funding for many of these programs and the metrics of success still often centered on pregnancy prevention. This is especially true for those who are younger and of lower income, which sends a clear message regarding whose pregnancies are and are not societally valued.

LARC methods have also been criticized for threatening patients' contraceptive autonomy because of the inability to discontinue the method independently: without the added barrier of finding access to care for LARC removal. Unlike other contraceptive methods that patients can easily stop themselves, LARC methods require in-person clinician appointments for removal. LARC users may face many potential barriers to removal, including cost, lack or loss of insurance coverage, transportation, and inability to schedule an appointment.[10] Additionally, studies have demonstrated clinician barriers to removal, including clinician resistance to removal or attempts to persuade delaying early removal in patients who wish to discontinue their LARC.[11] These barriers may be even more pronounced in younger or lower-income patients who already face discrimination in reproductive health care.

Finally, the authors used a large health services data set to provide insight into statewide trends among a large sample. Although health services data can be very useful for providing big-picture trends and can allow well-powered analyses, using health services data as a proxy for reproductive health outcomes has its unique shortcomings. For example, there are several reasons patients desire LARC removal, including side effects, desire to change contraceptive methods, and even reproductive coercion and intimate partner violence. Simply using the Current Procedural Terminology code for device removal does not imply that the patient intended a subsequent pregnancy, but only that they underwent LARC removal. Conversely, lack of Current Procedural Terminology codes for removal does not equate to a patient not desiring pregnancy, as many patients who do desire pregnancy may face the aforementioned barriers to LARC removal despite pregnancy intention. In addition, other contraceptive methods that are independently stopped without requiring interaction with the health system or a Current Procedural Terminology code are difficult to capture and therefore compare with LARC removal.

Additionally, health services data include only those who interact with the health system, in this case, only those who had Medicaid insurance during the study period. Patients who did not have access to LARC removal, whether they lost previous Medicaid insurance or experienced other barriers, were not included in this data set. The exclusion of these patients from health services data not only skews the generalizability of these studies, but it also often ignores or flattens the experiences of those who are left out of the health care system. Consequently, health services study designs, such as those in this study, are more likely to exclude racial or ethnic minorities and low-income patients, who are subject to a higher rate of structural barriers to care. Thus, alternative metrics and study designs are needed to add additional context to the authors' findings, capture the complexity of reproductive decision-making, and increase inclusivity of the overall population.

In sum, Rendall et al. provide a unique analysis regarding LARC removal framed in the context of subsequent intended pregnancy. Such health services analyses are critical to assessing the impact of large statewide public health initiatives that reduce barriers to desired contraceptive care. For many patients, LARC can be a tool that contributes positively to reproductive autonomy and justice through ideal birth timing by allowing prevention of pregnancy when not desired and removal when pregnancy is desired. Yet, that is not the experience or goal for LARC use for all patients.

A tension exists, then, between desiring and pursuing the public health goals and clinical goals of reducing unintended pregnancies and reducing barriers to care, especially for those who are underserved—with the patient-centered goal of ensuring that contraceptive care is autonomous, nonbiased, and just. We must invest in contraceptive measures that better capture the subtleties of contraceptive desire and pregnancy goals—which exist across a continuum, rather than a binary framework—so that future large contraceptive initiatives and the resultant analyses of their impact situate results in frameworks that reflect patients' goals, experiences, and care. AJPH

CORRESPONDENCE

Correspondence should be sent to Kavita Shah Arora, MD, MBE, MS, Department of Obstetrics and Gynecology, University of North Carolina at Chapel Hill, 3031 Old Clinic Building CB #7570, Chapel Hill, NC 27599 (e-mail: kavita_arora@med.unc.edu). Reprints can be ordered at https://www.ajph.org by clicking the "Reprints" link.

PUBLICATION INFORMATION

Full Citation: Tsevat DG, Trompeter GA, Arora KS. Long-acting reversible contraception (LARC) removal and birth intendedness: moving beyond the binary. *Am J Public Health*. 2025;115(2):116–118.

Acceptance Date: November 5, 2024.

DOI: https://doi.org/10.2105/AJPH.2024.307923

ORCID iDs:

Grace A. Trompeter https://orcid.org/0000-0003-2539-7131

Kavita S. Arora https://orcid.org/0000-0002-9912-9466

CONTRIBUTORS

K. S. Arora supervised and provided the structure of the editorial. All authors conceptualized, drafted, revised, and reviewed the editorial and approved the final version.

CONFLICTS OF INTEREST

The authors have no conflicts of interest to disclose.

REFERENCES

1. Gomez AM, Arteaga S, Ingraham N, Arcara J, Villaseñor E. It's not planned, but is it okay? The acceptability of unplanned pregnancy among young people. *Womens Health Issues*. 2018;28(5):408–414. https://doi.org/10.1016/j.whi.2018.07.001
2. ACOG Committee opinion no. 450: Increasing use of contraceptive implants and intrauterine devices to reduce unintended pregnancy. *Obstet Gynecol*. 2009;114(6):1434–1438. https://doi.org/10.1097/AOG.0b013e3181c6f965
3. Choi YS, Rendall MS, Boudreaux M, Roby DH. Summary of the Delaware Contraceptive Access Now (DelCAN) initiative. 2020. Available at: https://popcenter.umd.edu/delcaneval/summary-init. Accessed November 9, 2024.
4. American College of Obstetricians and Gynecologists' Committee on Health Care for Underserved Women; Contraceptive Equity Expert Work Group; Committee on Ethics. Patient-centered contraceptive counseling: ACOG Committee statement number 1. *Obstet Gynecol*. 2022;139(2):350–353. https://doi.org/10.1097/AOG.0000000000004659
5. Rendall MS, Eeckhaut MCW, Gifford K, Hurtado-Acuna C. Long-acting reversible contraception (LARC) and early childbearing revisited: births and birth intendedness after LARC removal in a state Medicaid population (2012–2020). *Am J Public Health*. 2025;115(1):95–102. https://doi.org/10.2105/AJPH.2024.307844
6. Luker KC. A reminder that human behavior frequently refuses to conform to models created by researchers. *Fam Plann Perspect*. 1999;31(5):248–249.
7. Borrero S, Nikolajski C, Steinberg JR, et al. "It just happens": a qualitative study exploring low-income women's perspectives on pregnancy intention and planning. *Contraception*. 2015;91(2):150–156. https://doi.org/10.1016/j.contraception.2014.09.014
8. Cutler A, McNamara B, Qasba N, Kennedy HP, Lundsberg L, Gariepy A. "I just don't know": an exploration of women's ambivalence about a new pregnancy. *Womens Health Issues*. 2018;28(1):75–81. https://doi.org/10.1016/j.whi.2017.09.009
9. Viswanathan AV, Bullington BW, Berg KA, et al. Ongoing contraceptive goals of patients who did not achieve desired postpartum permanent contraception prior to hospital discharge. *Contraception*. [Epub June 28, 2004]. https://doi.org/10.1016/j.contraception.2024.110533
10. Petrie KA, McCoy EE, Benson LS. IUD self-removal: a randomized controlled trial of a self-removal guide in clinical and nonclinical settings. *Contraception*. 2024;135:110421. https://doi.org/10.1016/j.contraception.2024.110421
11. Amico JR, Bennett AH, Karasz A, Gold M. "She just told me to leave it": women's experiences discussing early elective IUD removal. *Contraception*. 2016;94(4):357–361. https://doi.org/10.1016/j.contraception.2016.04.012

Street Trees and Public Health

Alistair Woodward, PhD, MB, and Kirsty Wild, PhD

ABOUT THE AUTHORS

Alistair Woodward and Kirsty Wild are with the School of Population Health, University of Auckland, New Zealand.

Cities are generally healthier with trees than without. Two well-described benefits are reducing excess heat and mitigating psychological stress. Other benefits include better mental health (less anxiety and improved mood) and favorable effects on cardiovascular function.[1] Trees may also reduce air pollution, increase active living, and support social cohesion, but studies on these topics have less-clear-cut results.[2] There are likely to be health gains from carbon storage, reduced storm run-off, and increased biodiversity, but few studies yet have investigated these questions.

CITY TREES AND HEALTH

Positive effects are not guaranteed—if trees are diseased or stressed, or the species is not a good fit for the local environment, then the benefits for human health are likely to be much reduced. And there may be detrimental effects: trees may drop boughs, exacerbate allergies, block drains, disrupt footpaths, consume scarce water, reduce perceptions of safety, or, in various ways, worsen air pollution rather than improve it.

However, if well-chosen and well-maintained, city trees are an asset, and, unusually, this resource appreciates with age.[3] City streets provide a special opportunity to increase tree cover, because roads of all kinds occupy a large fraction of the urban footprint. One study estimated that more than one third of public green space in cities is typically road verge—the strips of grass and plantings between roads and sidewalks.[4]

THE HISTORY OF STREET TREES IN MANHATTAN

In *AJPH*, John Harris[5] wrote about street trees in Manhattan, New York City. It is a remarkable story, for two reasons, at least. One is the duration of the campaign to establish trees in Manhattan—it was more than 40 years before proposals were put into practice. And the other is that the push for trees on the street was based on an argument for better health, rather than aesthetic or spiritual improvement. The man at the center of the action was a New York surgeon, Stephen Smith, and he rested his case on the health risks of summer heat and the cooling effect of tree cover. A hundred years before anyone used the term "urban heat island," Smith understood that high temperatures were a particular problem in densely settled cities like New York, and he was unrelenting in his advocacy for more trees on city streets.

Smith's campaign began in 1872 and included two phases: (1) 30 years leading up to legislation that required the New York City Parks Department to take over management of street trees, in the cause of better public health, and (2) the struggle, that went on for another decade, to get the Parks Department to act on the legislation.

Why did it take so long? Partly, according to Harris, it was because the public health movement was lukewarm in its support. He argues that the reason for holding back was that greening the city did not fit with the burgeoning germ theory of disease. At the end of the 19th century, sanitation had moved on from unfocused environmental improvements to the detection and control of pathogenic microbes. Maybe the argument that trees would cool the city by providing shade and moisture and would also "clean the air" resembled, in some minds, old-fashioned miasma thinking. Harris writes that when "a laboratory-based biomedical model became public health's future,"[5(p68)] trees were left behind.

Despite his claim that street trees were justified primarily because they were good for health, Smith argued that responsibility should rest with Parks, not Health, and not the Department of Public Works. He believed the Parks administration was less affected by vested interests (he was thinking here of Health) and corruption (Public Works). Maybe he was right, but Smith's campaign was not carried along on the wave of late 19th-century public health legislation that mandated safe water, clean air, and the removal of many other nuisances.

RELEVANCE TO MODERN PUBLIC HEALTH

We agree with Harris that public health should be more energetic in its support for green cities. And, more broadly, the story reminds us that public health "can shape its destiny" if it thinks big, accepts a Health in All Policies view of the world, and participates fully in advocacy and politics. Harris also makes a compelling case for less laboratory work and more time in the field.

How might modern day supporters of street trees adopt or modify Smith's methods? Reducing heat probably remains the most compelling and unambiguous effect of increasing street tree cover, and with a warming climate, this benefit will be amplified. A recent health impact assessment estimated that increasing tree coverage to 30% would cool 93 European cities by an average of 0.4°C (0.72°F) during summertime (compared with conditions in 2015) and save about 2644 premature deaths a year.[6] Contemporary concerns with health equity and environmental racism have advanced debates about heat and trees, highlighting the need to focus on doubly disadvantaged lower-income neighborhoods, which lack both street trees and access to air conditioning.

Smith's successes with tree surveys and the power of visualization as a change-making tool in public health remain as relevant and important as ever. It is unlikely his binary treatment of the "healthy" and the "beautiful" would be embraced by all modern advocates. Harris argues that Smith saw street trees as central to a "managed City Healthy not a voluntary City Beautiful."[5(p69)] But the nascent body of research on the mental health benefits of trees suggests a role for aesthetic dimensions such as color, form, and sound. It is probable, Deng et al. argue, that "restorative potential and aesthetic preference may reinforce . . . one another."[7]

While biomedical research may not yet pin down the mechanisms involved, it would be surprising if humans were not attracted to and pleased and improved by street trees.[8] For most of the history of *Homo sapiens*, our ancestors were preoccupied with the task of identifying which tree provided the best conditions for health (food, shelter, and medicine), and humans have evolved vision that features an exquisite and perhaps unmatched capacity for distinguishing among shades of green.[9]

Smith was a pioneer in advocating street trees to promote health. A century later, as research in this field of environmental health picks up pace, we trust that Smith's story will motivate the next generation of arboreal enthusiasts. AJPH

CORRESPONDENCE

Correspondence should be sent to Professor Alistair Woodward, Department of Epidemiology and Biostatistics, University of Auckland, Private Bag 92019, Auckland 1010, New Zealand (e-mail: a.woodward@auckland.ac.nz). Reprints can be ordered at https://www.ajph.org by clicking the "Reprints" link.

PUBLICATION INFORMATION

Full Citation: Woodward A, Wild K. Street trees and public health. *Am J Public Health*. 2025; 115(2):119–120.

Acceptance Date: November 8, 2024.

DOI: https://doi.org/10.2105/AJPH.2024.307931

ORCID iDs:

Alistair Woodward https://orcid.org/0000-0001-5425-6018

Kirsty Wild https://orcid.org/0000-0002-3875-038X

CONTRIBUTORS

A. Woodward wrote the first draft of the article. Both authors contributed to writing the final version.

CONFLICTS OF INTEREST

The authors have no conflicts of interest to declare from funding or affiliation-related activities.

REFERENCES

1. Nieuwenhuijsen MJ. Green infrastructure and health. *Annu Rev Public Health*. 2021;42(1): 317–328. https://doi.org/10.1146/annurev-publhealth-090419-102511
2. Wolf KL, Lam ST, McKeen JK, Richardson GRA, van den Bosch M, Bardekjian AC. Urban trees and human health: a scoping review. *Int J Environ Res Public Health*. 2020;17(12):4371. https://doi.org/10.3390/ijerph17124371
3. Woodward A, Hinwood A, Bennett D, et al. Trees, climate change, and health: an urban planning, greening and implementation perspective. *Int J Environ Res Public Health*. 2023;20(18):6798. https://doi.org/10.3390/ijerph20186798
4. Marshall AJ, Grose MJ, Williams NSG. From little things: more than a third of public green space is road verge. *Urban For Urban Green*. 2019;44: 126423. https://doi.org/10.1016/j.ufug.2019.126423
5. Harris JM Jr. Manhattan's street trees: an unfinished public health story. *Am J Public Health*. 2025;115(1):66–74. https://doi.org/10.2105/AJPH.2024.307856
6. Iungman T, Cirach M, Marando F, et al. Cooling cities through urban green infrastructure: a health impact assessment of European cities. *Lancet*. 2023;401(10376):577–589. https://doi.org/10.1016/S0140-6736(22)02585-5
7. Deng L, Luo H, Ma J, et al. Effects of integration between visual stimuli and auditory stimuli on restorative potential and aesthetic preference in urban green spaces. *Urban For Urban Green*. 2020;53:126702. https://doi.org/10.1016/j.ufug.2020.126702
8. Frumkin H. Beyond toxicity. *Am J Prev Med*. 2001;20(3):234–240. https://doi.org/10.1016/S0749-3797(00)00317-2
9. Lucas PW, Dominy NJ, Riba-Hernandez P, et al. Evolution and function of routine trichromatic vision in primates. *Evolution*. 2003;57(11): 2636–2643. https://doi.org/10.1111/j.0014-3820.2003.tb01506.x

Moving From Invisibility to Inclusivity: A Better Way Forward for National Health Surveys

Florence J. Dallo, PhD, MPH

ABOUT THE AUTHOR

Florence J. Dallo is with the School of Health Sciences, Oakland University, Rochester, MI.

Health outcomes are affected by many factors. One important consideration is the influence of immigration status and policies on health outcomes. These are the issues tackled in the analytic essay by Marouf et al., "Adding Nativity, Citizenship, and Immigration Status to Health Monitoring and Survey Data."[1] The authors recognize that national health surveys do not include detailed information about immigration status, which renders many groups largely invisible. Being invisible and disadvantaged has been the case for the Middle Eastern and North African (MENA) population in the United States for more than 200 years, which is when major waves of MENA individuals began immigrating to the United States.[2] Even though they have been in the United States for all these years, they have been "missing" from federal and state data. To overcome this, one way the federal government made MENA communities more visible was to add an "ancestry" question in 1980 to the American Community Survey. However, this question was limited in its sampling strategy and sample sizes.

For example, the ancestry question may not have captured important information such as that approximately 60% of MENA are immigrants. According to the Migration Policy Institute, the MENA immigrant population has more than doubled between 1980 and 2022. In addition, MENA immigrants have outpaced the growth of the total US immigrant population.[2]

Marouf et al. discuss the negative effects that missing immigration information has on the health of communities and populations. These effects of exclusion are magnified and exacerbated in MENA communities because not only are these crucial questions about immigration not asked in surveys but there also has never been a MENA option within the race and ethnicity question in these surveys.

REVISION TO STATISTICAL POLICY DIRECTIVE NO. 15

After several decades of convenings, political will, data collection, and content testing, a major change took place in March 2024: the Office of Management and Budget's Revisions to Statistical Policy Directive No. 15, which sets the standards for maintaining, collecting, and presenting federal data on race and ethnicity, added a MENA option to the race and ethnicity question.[3] This means that the US Census and all federal surveys, state forms, and others will be required to use the new race and ethnicity question. However, if questions about nativity, citizenship, and immigration status are limited or missing in national and state surveys, the goal to better understand and improve the health of immigrant populations is threatened. Therefore, incorporating and taking a lead on the recommendations made in the essay by Marouf et al. will help provide a more comprehensive profile of how immigration status affects health outcomes.

Having such data will help ensure that resources, budget allocations, and necessary services can be appropriately invested and distributed among MENA communities across the country. This new focus and effort will improve public health, alleviate health disparities, and result in important policy changes. For example, when researchers, clinicians, and policymakers can identify where MENA communities live and work, access to and use of public health services that are culturally and linguistically relevant may be made readily available. Clinics, hospitals, community health centers, and similar organizations will be required to change their policies and include MENA as a race response option. This way, these organizations will better understand their patient population with respect to burden of disease, risk factors, and other variables. With valid and reliable baseline data, resources will be allocated to design, implement, and evaluate tailored programs and interventions that will be effective in improving health, reducing risk factors, and modifying health behaviors.

As the US Census moves forward with incorporating the MENA category in the race and ethnicity question, there are several surveys to use as models to learn how to ask about immigration. These are the National Agricultural Workers Survey,[4] the Kaiser Family Foundation/Los Angeles Times Survey of Immigrants,[5] the Hispanic Community Health Study/Study of Latinos,[6] and the Los Angeles Family and Neighborhood Survey.[7] These surveys provided the strong support needed to counter the objections raised by opponents of such data collection.

In addition to these example surveys, another strategy to improve and enhance the questions asked in federal surveys to capture immigrant status, nativity, and citizenship is to work with the Centers for Disease Control and Prevention's (CDC's) Division of Global Migration Health.[8] They are tasked with providing specific and technical instructions for all physicians performing overseas—and US-based medical screening examinations for immigrants and refugees. The purpose of the medical examination is to examine and collect health information from individuals to ensure that communicable diseases, for example, are identified and treated before immigration. Collaborations with the CDC could be useful when adding new questions to federal health surveys.

INCLUSIVITY VERSUS INVISIBILITY

We now have convincing evidence from the past and promising examples for the future so that we choose inclusivity versus invisibility when assessing and determining what questions to ask in national surveys to ensure that every individual in the United States is heard. This practice will ameliorate the shame and stigma that has for so long been attached to being "othered" for one's immigration status, mental health condition, sexual orientation, and other factors. The United States spends $451 billion and $1377 per person on excess medical care, lost labor market productivity, and premature deaths because of health disparities.[9] If the United States is truly dedicated and committed to reducing racial, ethnic, and other health disparities, the first step must be to remain curious and ask the questions that for so long were associated with fear and negative consequences. Who emigrates, when they emigrate, and how they emigrate from their country of origin to the United States is a life-changing decision that is not made haphazardly and has implications for generations to come. It is time the United States aligns itself with the experiences of immigrants by capturing all the richness, diversity, and depth that comes with this transformative journey. AJPH

CORRESPONDENCE

Correspondence should be sent to Florence J. Dallo, PhD, MPH, 433 Meadow Brook Rd, Rochester, MI 48309-4452 (e-mail: dallo@oakland.edu). Reprints can be ordered at https://www.ajph.org by clicking the "Reprints" link.

PUBLICATION INFORMATION

Full Citation: Dallo FJ. Moving from invisibility to inclusivity: a better way forward for national health surveys. *Am J Public Health*. 2025;115(2): 121–122.

Acceptance Date: November 8, 2024.

DOI: https://doi.org/10.2105/AJPH.2024.307932

ORCID iD:
Florence J. Dallo https://orcid.org/0000-0003-0093-1289

CONFLICTS OF INTEREST

The author reports no conflicts of interest.

REFERENCES

1. Marouf FE, Perreira KM, Pham H. Adding nativity, citizenship, and immigration status to health monitoring and survey data. *Am J Public Health*. 2025; 115(1):75–82. https://doi.org/10.2105/AJPH.2024.307867
2. Marrow B, Batalova J. Middle Eastern and North African immigrants in the United States. June 12, 2024. Migration Policy Institute. Available at: https://www.migrationpolicy.org/article/middle-eastern-and-north-african-immigrants-united-states. Accessed October 11, 2024.
3. Revisions to OMB's Statistical Policy Directive No. 15: Standards for Maintaining, Collecting, and Presenting Federal Data on Race and Ethnicity. *Federal Register*. March 29, 2024. Available at: https://www.federalregister.gov/documents/2024/03/29/2024-06469/revisions-to-ombs-statistical-policy-directive-no-15-standards-for-maintaining-collecting-and. Accessed September 29, 2024.
4. US Department of Labor. National Agricultural Workers Survey. Available at: https://www.dol.gov/agencies/eta/national-agricultural-workers-survey. Accessed October 11, 2024.
5. Kaiser Family Foundation/Los Angeles Times Survey of Immigrants. Available at: https://www.kff.org/report-section/health-and-health-care-experiences-of-immigrants-the-2023-kff-la-times-survey-of-immigrants-methodology. Accessed October 11, 2024.
6. National Heart, Lung, and Blood Institute. Hispanic Community Health Study/Study of Latinos. Available at: https://www.nhlbi.nih.gov/science/hispanic-community-health-studystudy-latinos-hchssol. Accessed October 11, 2024.
7. Los Angeles Family and Neighborhood Survey. Available at: https://lasurvey.rand.org. Accessed October 11, 2024.
8. Centers for Disease Control and Prevention. Immigrant and refugee health. Available at: https://www.cdc.gov/immigrant-refugee-health/index.html. Accessed September 29. 2024.
9. LaVeist TA, Pérez-Stable EJ, Richard P, et al. The economic burden of racial, ethnic, and educational health inequities in the US. *JAMA*. 2023;329(19): 1682–1692. https://doi.org/10.1001/jama.2023.5965

The Way Forward to Embrace Artificial Intelligence in Public Health

Georges Hattab, PhD, Habil, Christopher Irrgang, PhD, Nils Körber, PhD, Denise Kühnert, PhD, and Katharina Ladewig, PhD

ABOUT THE AUTHORS

Georges Hattab, Christopher Irrgang, Nils Körber, Denise Kühnert, and Katharina Ladewig are with the Center for Artificial Intelligence in Public Health Research, Robert Koch Institute, Berlin, Germany. Georges Hattab is also with the Department of Mathematics and Computer Science, Freie Universität Berlin, Berlin, Germany.

The promise of revolutionizing disease surveillance, health service delivery, and medical research through the integration of artificial intelligence (AI) is real.[1] The capabilities of AI, from predictive analytics to automated decision-making, have been aptly explored in medical research and health care delivery in recent years, but the unparalleled opportunities to improve public health outcomes have yet to be harnessed to the same extent. AI-powered predictive analytics can be used to analyze large data sets, identify risk factors for disease, detect patterns, and predict outbreaks.[2] However, the path to realizing the full potential of AI in public health is fraught with challenges that must be carefully navigated.[3]

The impetus for exploring AI readiness in public health stems from the urgent need to address the escalating complexity of global health challenges.[4] Rising health care costs, the emergence of novel pathogens, and the growing prevalence of chronic diseases are pushing the boundaries of traditional public health strategies.[5] AI is poised to augment human efforts by analyzing big data, identifying patterns, and predicting public health crises. However, realizing its potential will require overcoming key challenges in AI readiness, adoption by practitioners, and integration into public health systems.[6]

KEY CHALLENGES FOR AI INTEGRATION

This article examines five key challenges impeding AI's integration in public health, despite its immense potential, and offers insights to overcome these barriers for effective implementation:

1. Improve transparency and applicability for professionals to enable trust and effective use of AI in health care;
2. Address data bias and quality issues to improve AI development and practical application;
3. Establish standardized protocols and dual-use controls to facilitate the use of AI in production;
4. Implement human-in-the-loop approaches to improve the accuracy and reliability of AI systems; and
5. Develop a robust AI infrastructure to ensure readiness for integration into public health practice.

This article synthesizes the evidence on AI in public health, highlights key challenges, and proposes a structured approach to address them. It advocates for interdisciplinary collaboration, high-quality data, dual-use controls, continuous human feedback, and investment in AI-enabled infrastructure. By addressing these critical issues, the article aims to catalyze transformative thinking and advance AI readiness in the vital field of public health.

Challenge 1: Transparency and Acceptance

The opacity of AI techniques is a significant barrier to their integration into public health, fostering skepticism and unrealistic expectations among professionals. To overcome this challenge, it's critical to develop and implement clear guidelines that address ethical considerations, transparency, accountability, and interpretability.[7] These measures will ensure that AI systems provide transparent rationales for their decisions, thereby fostering trust and facilitating effective collaboration between AI and public health professionals.

The COVID-19 pandemic highlighted the transformative potential of AI in public health through effective virus tracking and hotspot prediction, and underscored the need for transparency and expert trust. These lessons might have helped inform the European Union's (EU) AI Act, which sets ethical guidelines for AI use. It emphasizes the importance of human oversight and responsible use.[8] In medical diagnosis, AI systems must not only make recommendations, but also provide transparent and understandable explanations of their reasoning.[9] By integrating Explainable AI with interdisciplinary collaboration, we can foster trust among health care professionals and ensure responsible AI implementation. Prioritizing transparency, ethical standards, and interpretability will help overcome skepticism and enable AI to improve patient outcomes and health care efficiency.

Challenge 2: Data Bias and Data Quality

When AI is applied to public health, data quality faces significant challenges, including regulatory restrictions, compatibility issues, and data gaps. These barriers impede the development and implementation of AI. In addition, privacy concerns and biases, such as underrepresentation of minorities, can compromise data reliability. Overcoming these barriers requires robust data-centric frameworks that facilitate the secure sharing of high-quality, unbiased data, which is essential for effective AI use in public health.[10]

Google DeepMind's collaboration with Moorfields Eye Hospital demonstrated the potential of AI to detect eye disease through anonymized scans, but it faced challenges with low-resolution images and lighting variations. This example highlights the critical importance of robust, data-centric frameworks for AI applications in public health. Such frameworks, such as the European Health Data Space, are essential for integrating diverse data sources—including electronic health records and social determinants of health—to create accurate predictive models and targeted interventions.[11] By prioritizing comprehensive data-centric approaches that address quality, bias, and integrity concerns, public health institutions can foster an environment conducive to AI readiness and ensure that systems remain effective and equitable in real-world health care settings.[12,13]

Challenge 3: Standards and Dual-Use Controls

The lack of standardized protocols for the dual use of AI in public health significantly hinders its seamless integration into health systems, despite AI's proven capabilities in data processing and analysis. Establishing such standards is critical to ensuring the effective use of AI for both public health and administrative functions, thereby unlocking its full potential in health care.

Integrating AI into health care diagnosis and treatment planning requires a comprehensive approach centered on the nested model for AI design and validation.[14] This model, along with standardized data formats and interoperability protocols,[15] aims to streamline the integration of AI into existing health care systems while maintaining dual-use capabilities for public health and administrative functions. The EU AI Act seeks to regulate these systems based on their potential impact, balancing innovation with necessary safeguards. However, challenges remain, as exemplified by AI-assisted mental health screening using social media and social network data. This underscores the urgent need for robust regulatory frameworks to protect privacy and mitigate bias, and highlights the delicate balance between technological advancement and ethical considerations in health care AI applications.[16,17]

Challenge 4: Accuracy and Reliability

The integration of human-in-the-loop mechanisms is critical to improving the accuracy and trustworthiness of AI applications in public health. Although AI excels at processing medical data, its generalizability remains limited. Continuous human feedback enables error identification and correction, refining AI-generated insights and improving the reliability of AI-driven recommendations.[18] This human-in-the-loop approach ensures that human expertise consistently validates and improves AI systems, ultimately leading to more trustworthy and accurate public health decisions.

In medical AI applications, continuous human feedback is critical for identifying and correcting inaccuracies or biases in AI-generated recommendations. This iterative process of human oversight and AI refinement enhances system reliability, mitigates errors, and builds trustworthiness, ultimately maximizing AI transparency and acceptance among health care professionals. A study has found that large language models in medical settings can produce inaccurate cancer treatment advice, underscoring the critical need for human expertise to validate AI recommendations.[19] This highlights the importance of proper training and resources for health care professionals to effectively collaborate with AI systems to ensure patient safety and optimal care.

Challenge 5: Compatible Infrastructure

Integrating AI into public health requires an AI-enabled infrastructure for building, testing, training, and deploying applications. This requires significant investment in secure, scalable systems that can support AI while protecting personal data from breaches and unauthorized access. Prioritizing the development of robust infrastructure mitigates the risks associated with AI integration and fosters an environment that protects privacy and maintains data integrity and security in public health systems.

The COVID-19 pandemic's use of AI in contact-tracing applications has illustrated both the potential and the challenges of AI in public health, particularly in terms of infrastructure, privacy, and security.[20] This experience underscores the need for a resilient and secure infrastructure capable of processing large amounts of data while adhering to strict privacy protocols. The development of these applications demonstrated the delicate balance required between leveraging AI for public health benefits and protecting individual privacy. By prioritizing investments in secure, scalable infrastructure and clear privacy policies, we can foster trust in AI-driven technologies while maintaining the high standards necessary for the responsible use of health data in an AI-enabled landscape.

THE WAY FORWARD TO EMBRACE AI IN PUBLIC HEALTH

To successfully integrate AI into public health, a proactive and collaborative approach is essential to address associated challenges and limitations. We propose a five-step validation board, outlined in Box 1, to guide stakeholders through the process of fostering AI readiness in public health with transparency. This multifaceted approach, with each step highlighting two key points, aims to navigate the complexities of AI integration while maintaining integrity and effectiveness in public health applications. We also provide a hierarchical mind map for AI preparedness in public health (see Supplemental Figure A, available as a supplement to the online version of this article at http://www.ajph.org).

Step 1: Promoting Transparency

The adoption of AI in public health requires transparency and comprehensibility for health care professionals and experts. This fosters trust, acceptance, and effective collaboration between AI developers and domain experts, leading to more impactful solutions. The objective of step 1 is to ensure that AI solutions are transparent and understandable to health care professionals and public health experts.

Explainable AI models are critical to fostering trust and understanding of AI decisions among health care professionals. Tjoa and Guan's study highlights how explainability increases the acceptability of AI in sensitive health applications,[21] as exemplified by DeepMind's Streams app for risk assessment of kidney injury, which prioritizes transparency through detailed information disclosure and independent review.[22] At the same time, Wilson and Daugherty's article highlights the importance of collaboration between AI developers and health care professionals, and how this synergy leads to more impactful, tailored AI solutions.[23] Mayo Clinic's AI for radiology illustrates this approach, providing extensive documentation and training for radiologists to foster collaborative intelligence and effective AI adoption.

Step 2: Advocating for High-Quality, Unbiased Data

High-quality, unbiased data are the foundation for AI systems to make accurate predictions and equitably address public health challenges. The objective of step 2 is to highlight

BOX 1— Validation Board to Help Stakeholders Navigate Through a Plan to Promote Artificial Intelligence (AI) Readiness in Public Health With Transparency

Steps	1. Promoting Transparency in AI Adoption	2. Advocating for High-Quality, Unbiased Data	3. Implementing Standards and Dual-Use Controls	4. Enhancing AI Reliability With Human Feedback	5. Building Robust Infrastructure for AI Model Training and Testing
1st key point	Health care professionals must try to understand how AI decisions are made to gain trust and acceptance.	Quality data are crucial for accurate predictions and equitable management of public health challenges.	Dual-use implications of AI require controls to limit misuse and ensure safe applications.	Human oversight ensures ethical, fair, and accountable decisions in AI applications.	Robust AI infrastructure is essential for effective implementation of AI solutions in public health.
2nd key point	Collaboration between AI developers and health experts enhances solution effectiveness.	Addressing data bias is essential to prevent skewed outcomes affecting specific populations.	Standards for dual-use controls prevent harmful uses and promote positive outcomes.	Integrating human expertise supports trust and reliability in AI-driven public health initiatives.	Adequate infrastructure includes technical components and organizational capacity.

the importance of unbiased data in AI-driven public health decision-making.

For AI systems to make accurate predictions and address public health challenges equitably, high-quality data are paramount. As highlighted by Habehh and Gohel[24] and Olawade et al.,[25] reliable health care and public health outcomes depend on high-quality data inputs. Without clean, representative data sets, AI models run the risk of producing flawed predictions, potentially leading to ineffective or harmful decisions. Therefore, rigorous data collection, cleaning, and validation processes are prerequisites for realizing the potential of AI in public health.

Equally important is addressing data bias to prevent skewed AI-driven outcomes that may disproportionately affect certain populations. Vokinger et al. outline various strategies to identify and mitigate bias, including adjusting for confounding variables, employing debiasing algorithms, and ensuring diverse and representative training data.[26] Failure to address these biases can exacerbate existing health care disparities, undermining AI's potential to promote health equity. Examples of initiatives addressing these challenges include IBM Watson Health's Oncology Data Initiative, which is working with cancer institutes to create diverse data sets,[27] and the National Institute of Health's All of Us Research Program, which aims to collect health data from underrepresented populations in the United States.[28]

Step 3: Implementing Standard Dual-Use Controls

AI technologies in public health have dual-use implications, offering the potential for both beneficial applications, such as disease outbreak prediction, and harmful applications, such as the creation of bioweapons. To protect public health and ensure the responsible use of AI, it is imperative to implement standardized dual-use controls. The objective of step 3 is to implement standard controls to ensure that potential uses are accounted for and that misuse is limited.

The dual-use nature of AI technologies in public health necessitates robust controls to prevent misuse while ensuring safe applications. Research by Urbina et al. highlighted the importance of safeguards in AI-driven drug discovery,[29] and the Defense Advanced Research Projects Agency's Explainable AI program aims to create interpretable AI systems for sensitive applications. Whittlestone et al. provided a framework for developing dual-use control standards, addressing ethical and societal implications of AI.[30] Recent work by Ning et al. focused on ethical considerations for generative AI in health care.[31] Practical implementations—such as OpenAI's strict use policy for Generative Pre-trained Transformer 3 (GPT-3), which limits the generation of harmful content—demonstrate how clear policies can mitigate dual-use risks.

Step 4: Enhancing AI Reliability

Human oversight of AI applications, particularly in public health, is crucial to ensure ethical, fair, and accountable decision-making. The objective of step 4 is to improve AI reliability in public health through continuous human feedback.

Integrating human expertise into AI systems is critical to maintaining trust and reliability in public health initiatives. As highlighted by Díaz-Rodríguez et al., human oversight ensures ethical and responsible decision-making in AI.[32] For example, Google's breast cancer screening AI incorporates feedback from radiologists to improve accuracy, exemplifying a human-in-the-loop approach. Ongoing human input is essential for refining AI systems to address complex public health challenges. Human experts provide essential context, domain knowledge, and oversight that AI alone cannot, ensuring ethical, fair, and accountable decisions.[33] Although integrating human feedback requires careful design and resources, it is critical to building trust. Microsoft's AI for Accessibility program illustrates this approach, using human input to improve tools such as the Seeing AI app for visually impaired users.

Step 5: Building Infrastructure for AI Models

A robust AI infrastructure is a critical prerequisite for implementing AI solutions in public health. It includes not only the technical hardware and software, but also the organizational capacity to maintain, update, and manage AI systems. Without adequate infrastructure, even the most advanced AI algorithms cannot be used effectively to address public health challenges. The objective of step 5 is to build robust infrastructure for AI model training and testing.

Building a robust AI infrastructure for public health requires two key components: a strong technical foundation and organizational capacity. The technical foundation includes powerful computing resources, data management systems, and software frameworks for model training and deployment, as highlighted by Zhang et al.[34] Organizational capacity includes skilled personnel, governance structures, and processes for data security and privacy, as discussed by Shimonski[35] and Dixon and Grannis.[36] This comprehensive infrastructure is critical for the effective implementation of AI solutions in public health, enabling secure model training and testing while protecting data privacy, and ultimately improving population health outcomes and intervention efficiency.

CONCLUSION

Although it is impractical to address all key challenges simultaneously, a structured approach enables stakeholders to transparently advance AI readiness in public health, address critical issues sequentially, and ensure successful AI integration for improved health outcomes and system efficiency.

The symbiosis of AI and public health is a multifaceted endeavor that requires a concerted effort to address the challenges discussed here. By fostering collaboration, implementing strong data governance, ensuring dual-use standards, integrating continuous human feedback, and investing in AI infrastructure, we can make AI a standard and transformative force in public health. This article not only addresses current challenges, but also puts forth a future where AI and public health professionals work together to improve health outcomes and enhance the delivery of health services. AJPH

CORRESPONDENCE

Correspondence should be sent to Georges Hattab, Nordufer 20, Berlin, 13353, Berlin, Germany (e-mail: hattabg@rki.de, georges.hattab@fu-berlin.de). Reprints can be ordered at https://www.ajph.org by clicking the "Reprints" link.

PUBLICATION INFORMATION

Full Citation: Hattab G, Irrgang C, Körber N, Kühnert D, Ladewig K. The way forward to embrace artificial intelligence in public health. *Am J Public Health*. 2025;115(2):123–128.

Acceptance Date: September 27, 2024.

DOI: https://doi.org/10.2105/AJPH.2024.307888

ORCID iDs:

Georges Hattab https://orcid.org/0000-0003-4168-8254

Christopher Irrgang https://orcid.org/0000-0001-8274-1678

Katharina Ladewig https://orcid.org/0000-0003-3397-1308

CONTRIBUTORS

G. Hattab conceptualized the editorial, wrote the entire piece, reviewed and edited for technical accuracy, ensured that all claims were substantiated, and articulated the five key steps, the validation board, and the hierarchical mind map. C. Irrgang edited the editorial for clarity and coherence and ensured that complex ideas were accessible. N. Körber edited the editorial for clarity and provided specific case studies to illustrate key points in the editorial. D. Kühnert offered critical feedback on the draft. K. Ladewig provided critical feedback on the draft and suggested additional references.

CONFLICTS OF INTEREST

The authors declare no competing interests.

REFERENCES

1. Anderson B, Sutherland E. *Collective Action for Responsible AI in Health.* Paris, France: OECD Publishing; 2024. OECD Artificial Intelligence Papers No. 10.
2. Bauer GR, Lizotte DJ. Artificial intelligence, intersectionality, and the future of public health. *Am J Public Health.* 2021;111(1):98–100. https://doi.org/10.2105/AJPH.2020.306006
3. Zhu L, Chen P, Dong D, Wang Z. Can artificial intelligence enable the government to respond more effectively to major public health emergencies? Taking the prevention and control of Covid-19 in China as an example. *Socioecon Plann Sci.* 2021;80:101029. https://doi.org/10.1016/j.seps.2021.101029
4. Olorunsogo TO, Anyanwu A, Abrahams TO, Olorunsogo T, Ehimuan B, Reis O. Emerging technologies in public health campaigns: artificial intelligence and big data. *Int J Sci Res Arch.* 2024;11(1):478–487. https://doi.org/10.30574/ijsra.2024.11.1.0060
5. Farlow A, Hoffmann A, Tadesse GA, et al. Rethinking global digital health and AI-for-health innovation challenges. *PLOS Glob Public Health.* 2023;3(4):e0001844. https://doi.org/10.1371/journal.pgph.0001844
6. Fehr J, Citro B, Malpani R, Lippert C, Madai VI. A trustworthy AI reality-check: the lack of transparency of artificial intelligence products in healthcare. *Front Digit Health.* 2024:6:1267290. https://doi.org/10.3389/fdgth.2024.1267290
7. Tiribelli S, Monnot A, Shah SF, Arora A, Toong PJ, Kong S. Ethics principles for artificial intelligence–based telemedicine for public health. *Am J Public Health.* 2023;113(5):577–584. https://doi.org/10.2105/AJPH.2023.307225
8. Masel J, Petrie JIM, Bay J, et al. Combatting SARS-CoV-2 with digital contact tracing and notification: navigating six points of failure. *JMIR Public Health Surveill.* 2023;9:e49560. https://doi.org/10.2196/49560
9. Liao QV, Gruen D, Miller S. Questioning the AI: informing design practices for explainable AI user experiences. In: *Proceedings of the 2020 CHI Conference on Human Factors in Computing Systems.* New York, NY: Association for Computing Machinery; 2020:1–15. https://doi.org/10.1145/3313831.3376590
10. Mittermaier M, Raza MM, Kvedar JC. Bias in AI-based models for medical applications: challenges and mitigation strategies. *NPJ Digit Med.* 2023;6(1):113. https://doi.org/10.1038/s41746-023-00858-z
11. Norori N, Hu Q, Aellen FM, Faraci FD, Tzovara A. Addressing bias in big data and AI for health care: a call for open science. *Patterns.* 2021;2(10):100347. https://doi.org/10.1016/j.patter.2021.100347
12. Heaven WD. Google's medical AI was super accurate in a lab. Real life was a different story. *MITS Technol Rev.* 2020;4:27. Available at: https://www.technologyreview.com/2020/04/27/1000658/google-medical-ai-accurate-lab-real-life-clinic-covid-diabetes-retina-disease/. Accessed November 15, 2024.
13. Li J, Carayon P. Health Care 4.0: a vision for smart and connected health care. *IISE Trans Healthc Syst Eng.* 2021;11(3):171–180. https://doi.org/10.1080/24725579.2021.1884627
14. Dubey A, Yang Z, Hattab G. A nested model for AI design and validation. *iScience.* 2024;27(9):110603. https://doi.org/10.1016/j.isci.2024.110603
15. Baumgart DC. An intriguing vision for transatlantic collaborative health data use and artificial intelligence development. *NPJ Digit Med.* 2024;7(1):19. https://doi.org/10.1038/s41746-024-01005-y
16. Couture V, Roy MC, Dez E, Laperle S, Bélisle-Pipon JC. Ethical implications of artificial intelligence in population health and the public's role in its governance: perspectives from a citizen and expert panel. *J Med Internet Res.* 2023;25:e44357. https://doi.org/10.2196/44357
17. Bommasani R, Hudson DA, Adeli E, Altman R, Arora S, von Arx S, et al. On the opportunities and risks of foundation models. arXiv e-prints. 2021:arXiv-2108.
18. Shneiderman B. Human-centered artificial intelligence: three fresh ideas. *AIS Trans Hum-Comput Interact.* 2020;12(3):109–124. https://doi.org/10.17705/1thci.00131
19. Chen S, Kann BH, Foote MB, et al. Use of artificial intelligence chatbots for cancer treatment information. *JAMA Oncol.* 2023;9(10):1459–1462. https://doi.org/10.1001/jamaoncol.2023.2954
20. Harborth D, Pape S. A privacy calculus model for contact tracing apps: analyzing the use behavior of the German Corona-Warn-App with a longitudinal user study. *Comput Secur.* 2023;132:103338. https://doi.org/10.1016/j.cose.2023.103338
21. Tjoa E, Guan C. A survey on explainable artificial intelligence (XAI): toward medical XAI. *IEEE Trans Neural Netw Learn Syst.* 2021;32(11):4793–4813. https://doi.org/10.1109/TNNLS.2020.3027314
22. Powles J, Hodson H. Google DeepMind and healthcare in an age of algorithms. *Health Technol (Berl).* 2017;7(4):351–367. https://doi.org/10.1007/s12553-017-0179-1

23. Wilson HJ, Daugherty PR. Collaborative intelligence: humans and AI are joining forces. *Harv Bus Rev.* 2018;96(4):114–123.
24. Habehh H, Gohel S. Machine learning in healthcare. *Curr Genomics.* 2021;22(4):291–300. https://doi.org/10.2174/1389202922666210705124359
25. Olawade DB, Wada OJ, David-Olawade AC, Kunonga E, Abaire O, Ling J. Using artificial intelligence to improve public health: a narrative review. *Front Public Health.* 2023;11:1196397. https://doi.org/10.3389/fpubh.2023.1196397
26. Vokinger KN, Feuerriegel S, Kesselheim AS. Mitigating bias in machine learning for medicine. *Commun Med.* 2021;1(1):25. https://doi.org/10.1038/s43856-021-00028-w
27. Strickland E. IBM Watson, heal thyself: how IBM overpromised and underdelivered on AI health care. *IEEE Spectr.* 2019;56(4):24–31. https://doi.org/10.1109/MSPEC.2019.8678513
28. All of Us Research Program Investigators. The "All of Us" research program. *N Engl J Med.* 2019;381(7):668–676. https://doi.org/10.1056/NEJMsr1809937
29. Urbina F, Lentzos F, Invernizzi C, Ekins S. Dual use of artificial-intelligence-powered drug discovery. *Nat Mach Intell.* 2022;4(3):189–191. https://doi.org/10.1038/s42256-022-00465-9
30. Whittlestone J, Nyrup R, Alexandrova A, Dihal K, Cave S. *Ethical and Societal Implications of Algorithms, Data, and Artificial Intelligence: A Roadmap for Research.* London, UK: Nuffield Foundation; 2019.
31. Ning Y, Teixayavong S, Shang Y, et al. Generative artificial intelligence in healthcare: ethical considerations and assessment checklist. arXiv. Preprint posted online November 3, 2023. https://doi.org/10.48550/arXiv.2311.02107
32. Díaz-Rodríguez N, Del Ser J, Coeckelbergh M, de Prado ML, Herrera-Viedma E, Herrera F. Connecting the dots in trustworthy artificial intelligence: from AI principles, ethics, and key requirements to responsible AI systems and regulation. *Inf Fusion.* 2023;99:101896. https://doi.org/10.1016/j.inffus.2023.101896
33. Xin D, Ma L, Liu J, Macke S, Song S, Parameswaran A. Accelerating human-in-the-loop machine learning: challenges and opportunities. In: Proceedings of the Second Workshop on Data Management for End-to-End Machine Learning. June 2018:1–4. https://doi.org/10.1145/3209889.3209897
34. Zhang JJ, Liu K, Khalid F, et al. Building robust machine learning systems: current progress, research challenges, and opportunities. In: *Proceedings of the 56th Annual Design Automation Conference 2019.* New York, NY: Association for Computing Machinery; 2019:1–4. https://doi.org/10.1145/3316781.3323472
35. Shimonski R. *AI in Healthcare: How Artificial Intelligence Is Changing IT Operations and Infrastructure Services.* New York, NY: John Wiley & Sons; 2020.
36. Dixon BE, Grannis SJ. Information infrastructure to support public health. In: Magnuson J, Dixon B, eds. *Public Health Informatics and Information Systems.* Cham, Switzerland: Springer; 2020:83–104.

A Research Agenda to Maximize the Health Equity Impacts of Paid Family and Medical Leave Policies

Julia M. Goodman, PhD, MPH, Anna Steeves-Reece, PhD, MPH, MA, and Dawn M. Richardson, DrPH, MPH

ABOUT THE AUTHORS

Julia M. Goodman and Dawn M. Richardson are with the School of Public Health, Oregon Health & Science University–Portland State University, Portland, OR. Anna Steeves-Reece is with OCHIN, Inc., Portland, OR.

Access to paid family and medical leave is an important structural determinant of health. In the face of major life events that affect our health, such as the birth of a child or a medical emergency, the ability to access paid time away from work to focus on caregiving and healing without endangering economic security is vital. A robust and growing body of evidence underscores that the inability to access paid time away from work to concentrate on major life events negatively affects public health.[1,2]

Paid family and medical leave (PFML) policies entitle workers to receive wage replacement, and sometimes job security, while they take time off work for qualifying reasons. The United States is the only high-income country without a national PFML policy. This leaves most workers dependent on their employers to voluntarily offer PFML, resulting in 73% of nonfederal workers without any paid leave through their jobs.[3] Given how racism, patriarchy, and socioeconomic oppression challenge equitable access to employment opportunities where access to PFML is more likely, reliance on employer-based policies only reifies entrenched and pervasive inequities.[4]

Over the course of the past two decades, 13 states and the District of Columbia have moved to address these inequities by passing their own state-level PFML policies. The adoption of PFML policies by a growing number of states has allowed public health researchers to evaluate policy impacts and develop critical insights into how the introduction of PFML policies can improve health and well-being at the population level, particularly for birthing parents.

We draw from our research experience and ongoing conversations with multisectoral collaborators to highlight two broad areas of PFML research needed to further advance health equity: (1) expanding the research focus to populations newly affected by more inclusive PFML policies, and (2) using principles and tools from the fields of policy dissemination and implementation science.

EXPANDING THE RESEARCH FOCUS

There is now a vast body of research focusing on the public health effects of leave taken around the time of childbirth. Much of this research focuses on infant and child health, with a smaller body of research on the health of birthing people.[1,2] Understanding the health consequences of PFML policies during this critical period remains imperative; however, PFML policies are relevant for nearly everyone in society across the lifespan.

Each of the existing state PFML policies covers leave for bonding (which can be used to welcome a new child through adoption or fostering in addition to childbirth), to address one's own serious medical condition, and to care for a loved one with a serious medical condition. Some states' PFML policies also cover leave for situations such as a servicemember's deployment; being a victim of domestic violence, stalking, sexual assault, or abuse; and serving as an organ or bone marrow donor.[5]

Furthermore, the definition of a family member for caregiving purposes has expanded greatly over time. Although the earliest PFML policies covered only children, parents, spouses, and domestic partners, most current policies now include grandparents, grandchildren, siblings, and, increasingly, chosen family. These policy expansions have made PFML policies accessible to a broader range of individuals, including multigenerational households that often form due to caregiving needs, particularly among lower-income households. They also benefit members of the LGBTQ+ (lesbian, gay, bisexual, transgender/-sexual, queer or questioning, and all subsects) community, who are more likely to adopt or

AJPH February 2025, Vol. 115, No. 2

foster children rather than add to their family through birth and whose support networks, because of homophobia and transphobia, are more likely to be based on found family.[6–8]

The expansion of PFML policies to cover more leave types calls for a corresponding expansion in research to understand the experiences of diverse individuals taking leave. A recent review highlighted a need for more research on PFML policies in regard to workers who need leave to care for older children, adult family members, and older adult relatives.[2] In addition, we call for more research into the experiences of multigenerational households and LGBTQ+ people and families. Understanding the varied and complex needs people have with respect to PFML will allow us as public health researchers to build strong theories on how PFML policies affect people's health and well-being.

GUIDING PRINCIPLES AND RESOURCES

Public health policy research—including the PFML studies we have referenced—often uses state-level policy variation to examine whether the existence of a policy affects population-level health. However, our own and others' research demonstrates that, even in states with PFML policies, workers may face significant barriers to using policy benefits, potentially limiting their public health effects.[9,10]

Relatively little research has focused on how differences in policy administration and implementation affect health equity or how to effectively engage and communicate with multisector partners, including policymakers, to design and update PFML policies based on current, rigorous evidence. As public health researchers have asserted time and time again, our field must work proactively to coordinate our research initiatives with policymakers and administrators.

To address these gaps and advance public health research, we can draw on principles and messages in the fields of policy dissemination science, policy implementation science, and community-based participatory research. Policy dissemination science "seeks to understand how research evidence can be most effectively communicated to policymakers and integrated into policymaking processes."[11(pS180)] In Oregon, we have put this into practice with a monthly "paid leave working group" that brings together researchers, advocates, and representatives from the state's Paid Leave Oregon program to share updates, ask questions, and discuss potential collaborations. Other examples include daylong or multiday convenings, such as Next Generation PFML, that have brought together researchers, advocates, and program administrators from across the country to learn from each other's experiences designing, implementing, and studying their state's paid leave programs.[12]

Policy implementation science "seeks to understand how the roll out of policies can be optimized to maximize health benefits."[11(S180)] In policy implementation science, it is essential to pay attention to policy design elements, such as eligibility, included benefits, and the application process. To offer another example from our work in Oregon, we have learned from our state partners that, as we had anticipated based on research from other states, low-wage earners submit paid leave claims at much lower rates than do high-wage earners. This awareness has validated our current approach to focus research efforts on low-wage workers and those with precarious employment. It has also been beneficial for us to be aware of ongoing efforts by the state to reach these workers so that we can tailor our research to better understand the effect of those efforts and then communicate our findings back to our state partners.

Although we do not characterize this work as community-based participatory research, our efforts are informed by this body of work, emphasizing broad community engagement and drawing from conceptual models that highlight the importance of trusting partnerships, engagement of affected communities, and strong relationships with supportive policymakers.[13] Engaged approaches are essential for equity-focused policy change owing to the highly cyclical nature of policy dissemination and policy implementation. Working with partners in government and other sectors can inform and validate the research questions in the beginning stages of a research project; later, communicating the results to those partners will be more effective if they were engaged in the research process from the onset.[14]

CONCLUSIONS

Access to paid time away from work to respond to major life events is an important structural determinant of health, as demonstrated by a large body of evidence. We have argued that to maximize the societal health benefits of PFML policies, we must place greater emphasis on understanding how a wider range of populations uses these policies. We also need to study how variations in policy implementation and administration affect access to policy benefits and to foster multisector partnerships to ensure that research findings are effectively translated to changes in how PFML policies are developed and modified over time.

The future of public health needs to focus on the importance of social policies in driving changes in health outcomes and equity at the population level.[15] Given the potential for increased state uptake and the possibility of national adoption of a PFML policy, we as public health researchers are in an ideal position to take advantage of this policy research window. Although our recommendations focus on PFML policies, the principles should be pertinent to a wide range of policies that broadly affect population health. AJPH

CORRESPONDENCE

Correspondence should be sent to Julia M. Goodman, OHSU-PSU School of Public Health—Vanport Building, 1810 SW 5th Ave, Suite 510, Portland, OR 97201 (e-mail: goodmanj@ohsu.edu). Reprints can be ordered at https://www.ajph.org by clicking the "Reprints" link.

PUBLICATION INFORMATION

Full Citation: Goodman JM, Steeves-Reece A, Richardson DM. A research agenda to maximize the health equity impacts of paid family and medical leave policies. *Am J Public Health*. 2025;115(2):129–131.

Acceptance Date: November 7, 2024.

DOI: https://doi.org/10.2105/AJPH.2024.307929

ORCID iDs:

Julia M. Goodman https://orcid.org/0000-0002-9296-8697

Anna Steeves-Reece https://orcid.org/0000-0001-9740-5079

CONTRIBUTORS

The authors contributed equally to writing this editorial.

ACKNOWLEDGMENTS

We are grateful to Lindsey Smith, PhD, MPP, for her comments on an earlier draft of this editorial.

CONFLICTS OF INTEREST

The authors do not have any conflicts of interest to report.

REFERENCES

1. Heshmati A, Honkaniemi H, Juárez SP. The effect of parental leave on parents' mental health: a systematic review. *Lancet Public Health*. 2023;8(1):e57–e75. https://doi.org/10.1016/S2468-2667(22)00311-5
2. Bartel A, Rossin-Slater M, Ruhm C, Slopen M, Waldfogel J. The impacts of paid family and medical leave on worker health, family well-being, and employer outcomes. *Annu Rev Public Health*. 2023;44:429–443. https://doi.org/10.1146/annurev-publhealth-071521-025257
3. US Bureau of Labor Statistics. National Compensation Survey: employee benefits in the United States, March 2022. Available at: https://www.bls.gov/ncs/ebs/benefits/2022/home.htm#overview. Accessed November 28, 2022.
4. Goodman JM, Richardson DM, Dow WH. Racial and ethnic inequities in paid family and medical leave, United States 2011 and 2017–18. *Am J Public Health*. 2022;112(7):1050–1058. https://doi.org/10.2105/AJPH.2022.306825
5. National Partnership for Women & Families. State paid family and medical leave insurance laws. 2024. Available at: https://nationalpartnership.org/wp-content/uploads/2023/02/state-paid-family-leave-laws.pdf. Accessed August 8, 2024.
6. Cohn D, Horowitz JM, Minkin R, Fry R, Hurst K. Financial issues top the list of reasons US adults live in multigenerational homes. March 24, 2022. Available at: https://www.pewresearch.org/social-trends/2022/03/24/financial-issues-top-the-list-of-reasons-u-s-adults-live-in-multigenerational-homes. Accessed August 8, 2024.
7. Jackson Levin N, Kattari SK, Piellusch EK, Watson E. "We just take care of each other": navigating "chosen family" in the context of health, illness, and the mutual provision of care amongst queer and transgender young adults. *Int J Environ Res Public Health*. 2020;17(19):7346. https://doi.org/10.3390/ijerph17197346
8. Wilson B, Bouton L. LGBTQ parenting in the US. 2024. Available at: https://williamsinstitute.law.ucla.edu/publications/lgbt-parenting-us. Accessed August 8, 2024.
9. Setty S, Skinner C, Wilson-Simmons R. Bonding time: low-income mothers and New Jersey's family leave insurance program. *Community Work Fam*. 2020;23(2):141–161. https://doi.org/10.1080/13668803.2018.1501551
10. Goodman JM, Elser H, Dow WH. Among low-income women in San Francisco, low awareness of paid parental leave benefits inhibits take-up. *Health Aff (Millwood)*. 2020;39(7):1157–1165. https://doi.org/10.1377/hlthaff.2020.00157
11. Shelton RC, Brownson RC. Enhancing impact: a call to action for equitable implementation science. *Prev Sci*. 2024;25(suppl 1):174–189. https://doi.org/10.1007/s11121-023-01589-z
12. Abrahamson-Richards T, Sterling A, Sandfort J, Aronowitz K. Building the next generation of state paid leave programs. 2023. Available at: https://evans.uw.edu/community-engagement/epic/paid-family-medical-leave. Accessed August 8, 2024.
13. Cacari-Stone L, Wallerstein N, Garcia AP, Minkler M. The promise of community-based participatory research for health equity: a conceptual model for bridging evidence with policy. *Am J Public Health*. 2014;104(9):1615–1623. https://doi.org/10.2105/AJPH.2014.301961
14. Freudenberg N, Tsui E. Evidence, power, and policy change in community-based participatory research. *Am J Public Health*. 2014;104(1):11–14. https://doi.org/10.2105/AJPH.2013.301471
15. Ray R, Lantz PM, Williams D. Upstream policy changes to improve population health and health equity: a priority agenda. *Milbank Q*. 2023;101(suppl 1):20–35. https://doi.org/10.1111/1468-0009.12640

The Public Health Implications of a Leaking Fire Backflow Preventer

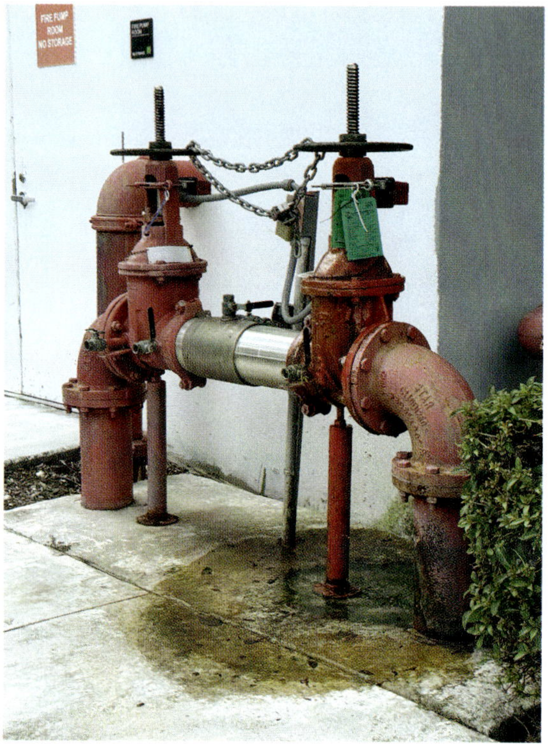

Osmari B. Novoa, MPH, and Gladys E. Ibañez, PhD

Fire backflow preventers are critical to a building's fire protection system and its main water supply. This device is designed to ensure that the water inside of a building's fire sprinkler system flows in only one direction: from the main water source to the systems pipes.[1] This process is absolutely necessary to prevent any possibility of cross-contamination that can occur when water from the fire sprinkler system flows backward into the main water supply, potentially carrying hazardous contamination into the public drinking water supply.[1,2]

A leaking fire backflow preventer can be a public health threat and risk to the main water supply.[2–4] There are many health risks associated with backflow contamination, such as gastrointestinal issues, dehydration, long-term harmful health effects, immediate illnesses, and exposure to human waste. In addition, leaks in the backflow preventer cause mold, mildew, water damage, and odors that can exacerbate health and structural issues.[2–5]

Signs of a defective backflow preventer include cloudy or discolored water, slow drainage, and a rising water level in the bathtub when the sink is running. Even if there are no signs of a leak, the backflow preventer should be checked regularly. Leaks may be caused by a variety of factors, such as, a rubber part that is cracked or has shifted, dirt, shifts in water pressure, chlorine and rust, and thermal expansion.[6] If any of these signs are present, it is imperative to call a licensed plumber or report the signs to the city immediately.[5,7,8] AJPH

ABOUT THE AUTHORS

Osmari B. Novoa is a PhD candidate at the Department of Health Promotion and Disease Prevention, Robert Stempel College of Public Health & Social Work, Florida International University, Miami. Gladys E. Ibañez is an associate professor and graduate program director in the Department of Epidemiology, Robert Stempel College of Public Health & Social Work.

CORRESPONDENCE

Correspondence should be sent to Osmari B. Novoa, 10010 NW 44th Terrace, APT 303, Doral, FL 33178 (e-mail: onovoa@fiu.edu). Reprints can be ordered at https://www.ajph.org by clicking the "Reprints" link.

PUBLICATION INFORMATION

Full Citation: Novoa OB, Ibañez GE. The public health implications of a leaking fire backflow preventer. *Am J Public Health*. 2025;115(2):132–132.

Acceptance Date: October 24, 2024.

DOI: https://doi.org/10.2105/AJPH.2024.307907

ORCID iDs:

Osmari B. Novoa https://orcid.org/0000-0002-8240-9090

Gladys E. Ibañez https://orcid.org/0000-0002-1626-0881

CONFLICTS OF INTEREST

The authors do not have any potential or actual conflicts of interest from funding or affiliation-related activities to report.

REFERENCES

1. Koorsen Fire & Security. Backflow preventers—a critical component in fire protection systems. July 21, 2022. Available at: https://blog.koorsen.com/backflow-preventers-a-critical-component-in-fire-protection-systems. Accessed November 12, 2024.
2. Woolf Plumbing & Gas. What is backflow prevention? July 4, 2024. Available at: https://woolfplumbing.com.au/blog/backflow-prevention-water-supply. Accessed November 12, 2024.
3. King Heating & Cooling. The importance of backflow prevention. May 15, 2024. Available at: https://www.kingheating.com/blog/the-importance-of-backflow-prevention. Accessed November 12, 2024.
4. Backflow Direct. Fact or fiction: a closer look at backflow preventers. June 27, 2022. Available at: https://backflowdirect.com/blog/fact-or-fiction-a-closer-look-at-backflow-preventers. Accessed November 12, 2024.
5. Backflow Direct. Common issues with backflow preventer devices. December 8, 2021. Available at: https://backflowdirect.com/blog/common-issues-with-backflow-preventer-devices. Accessed November 12, 2024.
6. Backflow Direct. Signs your backflow preventer needs repair. August 24, 2022. Available at: https://backflowdirect.com/blog/signs-your-backflow-preventer-needs-repair. Accessed November 12, 2024.
7. WM Henderson. 3 types of backflow preventer valves & signs of issues. February 6, 2023. Available at: https://www.wmhendersoninc.com/blog/what-is-a-backflow-prevention-device. Accessed November 12, 2024.
8. Plumbers 911. How professionals fix a backflow preventer leaking in the sprinkler system. December 8, 2020. Available at: https://plumbers911.com/backflow-preventer-leaking. Accessed November 12, 2024.

Evaluation of a Chronic Care Management Model for Improving Efficiency and Fiscal Sustainability

Margaret A. Kadree, MD, Patrick Wiggins, MPH, Lura Thompson, PharmD, Cynthia Warriner, BS, and Michelle White, MSW

Chronic care management is effective. Barriers to program durability include dependence on the provider–nurse duo to carry out labor-intensive services and the lack of a fiscally sustainable model. Between January and October 2022, an expanded chronic care management team—consisting of a provider, nurse, community health worker, and pharmacist—conducted a four-month intervention in an ambulatory setting. This intervention, using a convenience sample of 134 Medicare patients with uncontrolled type 2 diabetes or hypertension, demonstrated statistically significant improvements in controlling type 2 diabetes ($P < .01$) and blood pressure ($P < .001$). Direct provider workload decreased, and the Medicare reimbursement rate was 85.5%. (*Am J Public Health*. 2025;115(2):133–137. https://doi.org/10.2105/AJPH.2024.307886)

AJPH February 2025, Vol. 115, No. 2

In the United States, more than half of the current population[1,2] has at least one chronic disease. Of the more than $4 trillion annual health care costs, 90% is attributable to chronic disease. Heart disease is the leading cause of death in this country,[3] with hypertension and diabetes being two leading predisposing chronic diseases.[3] Almost 15 million children are obese.[4] Obesity predisposes people to type 2 diabetes and hypertension, so in the absence of effective control measures, the burden of type 2 diabetes, hypertension, and heart disease can be predicted to increase imminently. Currently, there is a shortage of primary care physicians. According to the 2021 American Association of Medical Colleges' projections of physician shortages in 2019 to 2034, it is predicted that by 2034, we will have a shortage of 17 800 to 48 000 primary care physicians.[5] Exacerbating this situation is population growth. These statistics underscore the dire circumstances related to chronic diseases and our current primary health care infrastructure.

Chronic care management (CCM) as a mechanism to enhance chronic disease care was introduced to the United States in 1996.[6] Yet 28 years later despite CCM being repeatedly demonstrated as an effective model for managing chronic diseases, the US health care system is still struggling to successfully implement and sustain it.[7–9] Major barriers include the absence of provider-led integrated clinical teams and inadequate financial support.[10,11]

In 2014, Medicare introduced reimbursement for CCM[12]; however, this source of funding has been underused because of the intensity of services needed to qualify for reimbursement.

The traditional model of the physician–nurse team as the core for providing all clinical services to the patient is no longer effective. The intensity of services and concomitant documentation demands, exacerbated by clinical staffing shortages and provider burnout, exceed what this duo can carry out readily. The provider and nurse are standard, salaried members of the clinical team. Adding a pharmacist and a community health worker (CHW) requires a new funding stream. We consider these facts in terms of creating an extended clinical team with the appropriate skill set to support the provider while using Medicare CCM reimbursement as a dependable funding stream to support the remuneration of the pharmacist and CHW.

INTERVENTION AND IMPLEMENTATION

We sought to increase the efficiency of CCM by extending the CCM clinical team to include a pharmacist and a

CHW in addition to the provider–nurse duo and to create fiscal sustainability of CCM through Medicare reimbursement.

The goals of this intervention were (1) to increase the proportion of patients with type 2 diabetes who, starting with an A1c above 7%, achieve a subsequent reduction of at least 0.5%; (2) to increase the number of patients with hypertension who reach a final blood pressure reading below 140 over 90; (3) to decrease direct provider workload by distributing certain tasks to an extended clinical team; and (4) to secure CCM reimbursement at levels sufficient to cover the added costs associated with employing a team pharmacist and a full-time CHW.

We defined uncontrolled type 2 diabetes as a hemoglobin A1c of greater than 7 and uncontrolled hypertension as blood pressure of higher than 140 over 90. We identified Medicare patients with both type 2 diabetes and hypertension from a central Virginia ambulatory clinic's database, and we extracted those with uncontrolled disease; 256 patients met our criteria for uncontrolled type 2 diabetes or hypertension. We established the integrated CCM team of provider, nurse, pharmacist, and CHW and created a team workflow. The CHW reached out to patients to educate them and offer them participation in the CCM program; they conducted social determinant of health assessments with consenting patients using the Protocol for Responding to and Assessing Patients' Assets, Risks and Experiences.[13] Pharmacists conducted comprehensive medication reviews and medication follow-ups, and nurses created care plans. Providers reviewed all notes, wrote orders, and submitted claims monthly. Team members met on a weekly basis.

PLACE, TIME, AND PERSONS

Between January and November 2022, using the CCM eligible list of the central Virginia clinic, we obtained a convenience sample by reaching out to patients, educating them about the CCM program, and assessing their willingness to participate in the intervention. We selected controls from the group who declined CCM.

The CCM team provided enrollees with standard type 2 diabetes and hypertension treatment tracking, comprehensive medication reviews, social determinant of health assessments,[13] and monthly care plans.

PURPOSE

We sought to address the two major barriers to implementing durable CCM programs, namely provider overload and fiscal sustainability.

EVALUATION AND ADVERSE EFFECTS

The overall cohort consisted of 134 patients (84 enrolled in CCM; 50 controls); 61 of 84 of the CCM patients completed the protocol. All 61 CCM patients had type 2 diabetes, and 29 of the 61 had both type 2 diabetes and hypertension. All 50 controls had type 2 diabetes, and 10 of the 50 had both type 2 diabetes and hypertension.

There were no missing values in the data set we used to compare pre- and postintervention results. Tests for differences included the *t* test for continuous variables and the χ^2 test for categorical variables. We used a 2-sided $P<.05$ for all analyses. We conducted analyses in Jamovi version 2.3.19 (https:\\www.jamovi.org).

Among the CCM type 2 diabetes cohort, 41% demonstrated significantly improved A1c levels compared to 12% of controls ($P<.01$; Table 1).

There were 39 patients in the hypertension group: 29 in the CCM group and 10 controls. There were no statistically significant differences in initial systolic and diastolic pressures between the two groups; however, unlike the controls, the CCM group attained statistically significant decreases in both systolic and diastolic pressures ($P<.001$). For the CCM hypertension group, the average systolic blood pressure decreased 17 points: from 155.8 to 138.8; the average diastolic blood pressure decreased 9 points: from 86.4 to 77.8; both decreases were statistically significant ($P<.001$). For the CCM hypertension group, 25 of 29 (86%) demonstrated improvement in systolic blood pressure. For the control group, 4 of 10 (40%) demonstrated improvement. A study limitation was the size of the hypertension groups (Table 2).

In the medication reviews, 71 of 84 enrollees received a comprehensive medication review using the Blue Bag Initiative program.[14] We identified at least one potential adverse drug event in 57 of 71 (80.3%) patients in the CCM group and a total of 366 potential adverse drug events.

All 61 patients who completed the protocol had two or more social determinants of health assessments. Except among five patients (three with food issues, one with housing issues, and one with a behavioral health problem), we did not identify any issues.

TABLE 1— Characteristics and Outcome Measures for Patients With Type 2 Diabetes: United States, January–October 2022

Demographics	Overall	Chronic Care Management Group (n = 61)	Control Group (n = 50)	P
Age, y, mean	71.0	69.6	72.8	< .05
Sex, no. (%)				< .05
Male	36 (32.7)	21 (35.0)	15 (30.0)	
Female	74 (67.3)	39 (65.0)	35 (70.0)	
Laboratory values, mean ±SD				< .01
Baseline hemoglobin A1c	8.1 ±2.0	8.6 ±2.1	7.5 ±1.8	
Remeasurement hemoglobin A1c	7.9 ±1.9	8.1 ±1.7	7.7 ±2.1	
Outcome measure, no. (%)				< .01
Improvement (i.e., decrease of ≤ 0.5 hemoglobin A1c between baseline and remeasurement)	31 (27.9)	25 (41.0)	6 (12.0)	
Worsening (i.e., increase of ≤ 0.5 hemoglobin A1c between baseline and remeasurement)	24 (21.6)	12 (19.7)	12 (24.0)	
No change (i.e., change of < 0.5 hemoglobin A1c between baseline and remeasurement)	56 (50.5)	24 (39.3)	32 (64.0)	

Note. Tests for differences included the *t* test for continuous variables and the χ^2 test for categorical variables. We used a 2-sided $P < .05$ for all analyses.

Our financials analyses showed that the Medicare reimbursement rate for submitted claims was 85.5%. Reimbursements were decreased by copays, low negotiated reimbursement rates, and a 10.8% denial rate owing to incorrect coding or late filing. Using the prospective pay system rate and the 85.5% reimbursement rate, we extrapolated that if a CHW carries a minimum patient load of 100 per month for 12 months, the remuneration will be approximately $78 000, sufficient to support a CHW median annual salary of $50 000,[15] with the remaining $28 000

TABLE 2— Characteristics and Outcome Measures for Patients With Hypertension: United States, January–October 2022

Demographics	Overall	Chronic Care Management Group (n = 29)	Control Group (n = 10)	P
Age, y, mean	72.3	70.6	77.4	< .05
Sex, no. (%)				< .05
Male	11 (28.2)	7 (24.0)	4 (40.0)	
Female	28 (71.8)	22 (76.0)	6 (60.0)	
Vitals and laboratory values, mean				< .01
Baseline systolic pressure	155.0	155.8	152.8	
Baseline diastolic pressure	83.9	82.9	86.6	
Remeasurement systolic pressure	143.0	139.0	156.0	
Remeasurement diastolic pressure	78.3	77.8	76.9	
Outcome measure, no. (%)				< .01
Improvement (i.e., remeasurement systolic pressure < baseline systolic pressure)	29 (74.4)	25 (86.2)	4 (40.0)	
No improvement (i.e., remeasurement systolic pressure ≥ baseline systolic pressure)	10 (25.6)	4 (13.8)	6 (60.0)	

Note. Tests for differences included the *t* test for continuous variables and the χ^2 test for categorical variables. We used a 2-sided $P < .05$ for all analyses.

available to support 467 hours of pharmacist time (with a median salary of $80 000/year)[15] to conduct comprehensive medication reviews.

Using a convenience sample affected the generalizability of the outcome and created selection and other biases; however, we felt this approach was permissible in this instance, as the evaluation was exploratory. It attempted to rapidly generate insight into our hypotheses that (1) adding a pharmacist and CHW to the standard provider–nurse duo CCM clinical team could substantially free up the provider–nurse duo to enroll more patients in CCM, and (2) revenues obtained through Medicare CCM reimbursement could fund the added costs of the pharmacist and CHW. Our project budget and time were also constrained. We felt that this preliminary information was critical to planning a full-scale research project.

SUSTAINABILITY

Traditionally, the provider–nurse duo has shouldered the demanding responsibility of reimbursable care management. In traditional CCM protocols, the following functions are the responsibility of the provider–nurse duo: assessing the patient's medical, functional, and psychosocial needs; ensuring patient receipt of timely recommended preventive services; reviewing the patient's medications and potential adverse drug events; and overseeing the patient's medication self-management and coordinating care with home- and community-based clinical service providers. Performing all of these functions often exceeds the workload bandwidth of the provider–nurse duo and has contributed substantially to the underuse of CCM.

To address this, our model integrated a CHW and pharmacist into the team. The pharmacist directly decreased the provider workload while optimizing pharmaceutical care and decreasing potential adverse drug events. The CHW was also invaluable, spending more time with the patient, doing outreach and patient education and referral and care transition retention activities, conducting social determinant of health assessments, and building trust-based relationships.

CCM is a salaried provider–nurse duo responsibility, whereas the pharmacist and CHW are adjunctive; therefore, their remuneration needs to be funded. Our model demonstrates that Medicare CCM payments can be a reliable, sustainable funding source.

Medicare CCM reimbursement covers more than 15 chronic diseases. Thus, this model, properly implemented, can potentially improve the health-related quality of life for people with chronic diseases, help to lower health care costs, and allow redirection of funds to health promotion.

Implementing this model requires a CCM preparedness assessment to ensure that staffing, patient workflows, patient tracking, outreach mapping, and billing mechanisms are in place—before enrolling patients. A clinical driver is needed to oversee workflow aspects, patient identification, enrollment, and retention. In addition, proper documentation and coding, along with timely, accurate claims filing, are crucial for successful reimbursement.

PUBLIC HEALTH SIGNIFICANCE

The continued upsurge in chronic disease amplifies the need to redesign health care delivery systems to incorporate effective, fiscally sound CCM models. Our evaluation reaffirms the effectiveness of CCM in enhancing outcomes for patients with type 2 diabetes and hypertension. Additionally, it highlights the model's potential ability to reduce overall provider overload while providing financial support for the extended team. By design, the model can be engineered to fit into any health care setting. However, further large-scale studies, using probability sampling, are needed to establish its general applicability. AJPH

ABOUT THE AUTHORS

Margaret A. Kadree is with the Johnson Federally Qualified Health Center, Lynchburg, VA. Margaret A. Kadree and Patrick Wiggins are with the Division of Prevention and Health Promotion, Virginia Department of Health, Richmond. Lura Thompson is with Care Connexion Rx Richmond, Richmond. Cynthia Warriner and Michelle White are with Health Quality Innovators, Richmond.

CORRESPONDENCE

Correspondence should be sent to Margaret Kadree, MD, Clinical Specialist, Office of Family Health Services, Division of Prevention and Health Promotion, Virginia Department of Health, 109 Governor St, Richmond, VA 23219 (e-mail: margaret.kadree@vdh.virginia.gov). Reprints can be ordered at https://www.ajph.org by clicking the "Reprints" link.

PUBLICATION INFORMATION

Full Citation: Kadree MA, Wiggins P, Thompson L, Warriner C, White M. Evaluation of a chronic care management model for improving efficiency and fiscal sustainability. *Am J Public Health*. 2025; 115(2):133–137.

Acceptance Date: September 25, 2024.

DOI: https://doi.org/10.2105/AJPH.2024.307886

ORCID iDs:

Margaret A. Kadree https://orcid.org/0009-0005-3211-2909

Patrick Wiggins https://orcid.org/0009-0009-7235-9219

Cynthia Warriner https://orcid.org/0009-0001-4435-3102

Michelle White https://orcid.org/0009-0003-3069-4269

CONTRIBUTORS

M. A. Kadree designed the new chronic care management model and the clinical assessment protocol, implemented and supervised clinic protocol, collected data, and wrote the article. P. Wiggins identified and added local partners to form the intervention team. L. Thompson provided the pharmacy support and template to assess the comprehensive medication and pharmacy reviews. C. Warriner contributed the tool used to identify and assess potential adverse drug events based on pharmacist-collected data. M. White conducted the statistical analyses and created the tables.

ACKNOWLEDGMENTS

This project was funded by the Virginia Department of Health (VDH; Centers for Disease Control and Prevention cooperative agreement NU58DP006620).

We thank the following for their steadfast help in supporting this intervention: Gary Campbell, chief executive officer, Nicole Williamson, certified professional coder, and Kimberly Dyke-Harsley, certified community health worker, with the Johnson Health Center, Christopher Nye, community health specialist with the Virginia Department of Health, and Karen Winslow, grants supervisor with the Virginia Pharmacists Association.

CONFLICTS OF INTEREST

At the time of the evaluation, Margaret Kadree was the chief medical officer at the Johnson Health Center and a clinical information specialist in the VDH's Chronic Disease Division. Lura Thompson was the chief pharmacist on the study, and two additional consulting pharmacists were obtained from her company Care Connections Rx.

HUMAN PARTICIPANT PROTECTION

The VDH institutional review board approved this study.

REFERENCES

1. Centers for Disease Control and Prevention. Chronic diseases. Available at: https://www.cdc.gov/chronic-disease/?CDC_AAref_Val=https://www.cdc.gov/chronicdisease/about/index.htm. Accessed October 29, 2024.
2. US Census Bureau. Population and housing units estimates. Available at: https://www.census.gov/programs-surveys/popest.html. Accessed October 29, 2024.
3. Centers for Disease Control and Prevention. Heart disease facts. Available at: https://www.cdc.gov/heart-disease/data-research/facts-stats/index.html. Accessed October 29, 2024.
4. Centers for Disease Control and Prevention. Childhood obesity facts. Available at: https://www.cdc.gov/obesity/childhood-obesity-facts/childhood-obesity-facts.html?CDC_AAref_Val=https://www.cdc.gov/obesity/data/childhood.html. Accessed October 29, 2024.
5. Association of American Medical Colleges. *The Complexities of Physician Supply and Demand: Projections From 2019 to 2034*. June 2021. Available at: https://digirepo.nlm.nih.gov/master/borndig/9918417887306676/9918417887306676.pdf. Accessed October 29, 2024.
6. Wagner EH, Austin BT, von Korff M. Organizing Care for patients with Chronic Illness. Group Health Cooperative, Puget Sound Seattle. *Published by Blackwell* 238 Main Street, Cambridge, MA 02142, USA, and Oxford OX4 1JF, UK.; Available at: https://www.researchgate.net/figure/The-chronic-care-model-CCM-Wagner-1998-Reproduced-with-permission-from-the-American_fig1_43518759. Accessed October 29, 2024.
7. Si D, Bailie R, Weeramanthri T. Effectiveness of chronic care model–oriented interventions to improve quality of diabetes care: a systematic review; *Prim Health Care Res Dev.* 2008;9(1):25–40. https://doi.org/10.1017/S1463423607000473
8. Bodenheimer T, Wagner EH, Grumbach K. Improving primary care for patients with chronic illness. *JAMA.* 2002;288(14):1775–1779. https://doi.org/10.1001/jama.288.14.1775
9. Goh LH, Siah CJR, Tam WWS, Tai ES, Young DYL. Effectiveness of the chronic care model for adults with type 2 diabetes in primary care: a systematic review and meta-analysis. *Syst. Rev.* 2022;11(1):273. https://doi.org/10.1186/s13643-022-02117-w
10. Coleman K, Austin BT, Brach C, Wagner EH. Evidence on the chronic care model in the new millennium. *Health Aff (Millwood).* 2009;28(1):75–85. https://doi.org/10.1377/hlthaff.28.1.75
11. Mattke S, Seid M, Ma S. Evidence for the effect of disease management: is $1 billion a year a good investment? *Am J Manag Care.* 2007;13(12):670–676.
12. Centers for Medicare & Medicaid Services. Chronic care management services. Available at: https://www.cms.gov/outreach-and-education/medicare-learning-network-mln/mlnproducts/downloads/chroniccaremanagement.pdf. Accessed October 29, 2024.
13. National Association of Community Health Centers. Protocol for responding to and assessing patients' assets risk and experiences (PRAPARE). 2022. Available at: https://prapare.org/#:~:text=The%20Protocol%20for%20Responding%20to%20and%20Assessing%20Patients'%20Assets%2C%20Risks,patients'%20social%20determinants%20of%20health. Accessed October 29, 2024.
14. Fernández EV, Warriner CL, David T, Gordan E, Twigg G, Carroll NV. Potential cost savings by prevention of adverse drug events with a novel medication review program. *J Am Pharm Assoc (2003).* 2020;60(3):462–469.e4. https://doi.org/10.1016/j.japh.2019.12.004
15. Indeed.com. Discover your earning potential. Available at: https://www.indeed.com/career/salaries. Accessed October 29, 2024.

Development of Texas's First Chinese American Community Health Worker Certification for Family Health History-Based Cancer Prevention

Yu-Lyu Yeh, PhD, Zihan Zhang, MS, Denise Martinez, MPH, and Lei-Shih Chen, PhD, MS

To address leading health organizations' calls for public health professionals to adopt family health history (FHH) into their practice, we developed the first community health worker Texas state-certification program focusing on FHH-based cancer prevention for Chinese Americans, for whom cancer is the leading cause of death. The 160-hour program trained 46 Chinese American CHWs to provide FHH-based cancer prevention services for 1129 Chinese Americans. Our program contributes to the establishment of a public health workforce with FHH-based competence and reduces cancer disparities. (*Am J Public Health*. 2025;115(2): 138–141. https://doi.org/10.2105/AJPH.2024.307895)

AJPH February 2025, Vol. 115, No. 2

Cancer is the leading cause of death for Chinese Americans, of whom 62% are immigrants and 43% have limited English-language fluency.[1,2] Family health history (FHH)–based education and prevention is an evidence-based approach for preventing cancer.[3] Clients receiving FHH-based cancer prevention and education services can understand their FHH and cancer risk, adopt a better lifestyle, undergo screening, and utilize genetic services if necessary. Leading health organizations (e.g., National Institutes of Health,[4] Centers for Disease Control and Prevention,[5] and American Public Health Association[6]), have urged public health professionals to adopt FHH into their practice.

Training community health workers (CHWs) in FHH-based cancer prevention has been a successful, evidence-based model for serving Latinx and Black communities.[7] CHWs can educate clients on the importance of FHH and assist them in creating FHH trees, and offer suggestions and resources based on the clients' FHH.[7] Texas has an official CHW certification program regulated by the Texas Department of State Health Services (TDSHS).[7] Texas residents aged 16 years or older can become CHWs by completing a 160-hour CHW certification training that addresses eight core competencies.[7]

Among the existing CHW certification programs in Texas, none are provided in Mandarin.[8] Among the nearly 4000 TDSHS-certified CHWs, moreover, only 11 (0.28%) are Chinese Americans.[9] As Texas has the third-largest Chinese American population in the United States,[10] the small number of certified Chinese American CHWs may contribute to cancer disparities for this underserved community. Research has shown that Chinese Americans lack knowledge and face cultural and health care system barriers in FHH use.[11] Therefore, training more Chinese American CHWs with FHH-based cancer prevention competencies is crucial to reducing health disparities and responding to the calls from leading health agencies.

INTERVENTION AND IMPLEMENTATION

We developed and implemented the first TDSHS-certified CHW certification program in Mandarin focused on FHH-based cancer prevention for Chinese Americans. The program fees were waived, and participants received $75 once the program was completed.

An advisory board consisting of administrators from TDSHS-certified CHW training centers, leaders from Chinese American community organizations, and researchers with expertise in Chinese American health was formed to advise the program. Partnering with the TDSHS-certified National Community Health Worker Training Center (NCHWTC), our team—consisting of three CHW instructors with expertise in public health genomics, health promotion, psychology, nutrition, and CHW training, along with one researcher who is a public health genomics expert, a CHW, and a certified health education specialist—developed a 160-hour CHW certification program that included online training, assignments, internship, mentoring sections, and an in-person group workshop. The program curriculum was reviewed by six Chinese American CHWs, three Chinese American CHW instructors, and four Chinese American community members. Revisions were made based on their feedback. The final curriculum was approved by the TDSHS.

Online Training

The online training included one overview introductory module, 20 modules addressing the eight CHW core competencies required by the TDSHS, and six modules targeting the delivery of FHH-based cancer prevention with a focus on five common cancers experienced by Chinese Americans—breast, colorectal, gastric, liver, and lung cancer. Each module addressed specific learning objectives (Table A, available as a supplement to the online version of this article at https://www.ajph.org).[12] The 4MAT model was adopted to address different learning styles of CHW trainees (Table B, available as a supplement to the online version of this article at https://www.ajph.org).[13]

Assignments

Trainees were asked to complete assignments that were created to address the learning objectives of the training. The assignments aimed to help the trainees better understand the training content and possess the skills and knowledge necessary to incorporate what they have learned into practice.

Internship

The TDSHS requested CHWs to participate in a supervised internship to gain experience on how to serve their community. Our program collaborated with hospitals and Chinese American communities for trainees to complete a 12-hour internship related to cancer prevention. Trainees were asked to turn in documentation that included the date, time, tasks, the CHW core competencies they applied for, and supervisor signatures.

Mentoring Section

A mentoring component was integrated into the program to provide guidance for trainees. Two trained Chinese American CHW instructors and a Chinese American CHW provided a personalized 30-minute weekly mentoring phone call for each trainee. Trainees could use this opportunity to ask questions about the training and discuss challenges. Mentors were able to solve problems, share their experiences, and encourage trainees to complete the program.

In-Person Group Workshop

Trainees were asked to participate in an eight-hour in-person hands-on workshop after they completed the online training, assignments, and internship. The workshop included a review of the program, role play, and CHW certification form completion. It connected the trainees for future collaboration. Trainees were asked to deliver FHH-based cancer prevention education and services for Chinese Americans within three months of program completion. We provided relevant materials and tips on how to effectively deliver services to Chinese Americans.

PLACE, TIME, AND PERSONS

Between 2018 and 2022, we developed and implemented the Chinese American CHW certification program and recruited trainees across Texas.

Ninety-nine Chinese Americans applied for the CHW certification program. After interviewing, 55 Chinese Americans were selected based on our screening criteria: trainees must be Texas residents, be fluent in Mandarin, be willing to provide cancer prevention services for Chinese Americans, possess basic computer skills, and have experience in Chinese American community-related services or have worked or volunteered in health-related fields. Forty-six (83.6%) trainees completed the program and obtained TDSHS-approved CHW certification. Among them, 83.9% were female (mean age 47.7 ± 14.9 years), and 76.8% had earned a college degree or above. All were born outside of the United States with a mean length of residence in the United States of 16.9 ± 9.8 years. Nine trainees did not complete the program because they were unable to finish the online training and assignments within the required timeline of three months.

PURPOSE

The limited number of Chinese American CHWs in Texas has precluded Chinese Americans, for whom cancer is the leading cause of death,[14] from receiving FHH-based cancer prevention education and services. We developed, implemented, and evaluated a CHW certification program focusing on FHH-based cancer prevention for Chinese Americans.

EVALUATION AND ADVERSE EFFECTS

We used an online posttraining survey to obtain trainees' feedback on the training. Overall, trainees reported that the online training achieved the learning objectives well or extremely well (Table A). Trainees were satisfied with training videos (95.7%), examples (97.8%), handouts (95.7%), the structure (97.8%), content (95.7%), duration (97.8%), organization (100%), difficulty level (97.8%), and ordering of concepts that were presented (95.7%) of the online training. All the trainees reported that the online training content was important and very helpful and included up-to-date materials on cancer prevention and community health.

Each module had an average of five multiple-choice questions, each with five response options. Trainees were asked to complete the pretraining quizzes before each module and retook the same quizzes after finishing each module. The paired *t* test showed that trainees significantly improved their knowledge scores at posttraining compared with their pretraining scores for all modules (Table A).

After receiving the CHW certification from the TDSHS, trainees were encouraged to provide FHH-based cancer prevention services to Chinese Americans. Within three months of the conclusion of the training program, 1129 Chinese Americans in Texas had been provided FHH-related cancer prevention services. Based on the three-month follow-up survey completed by 76.1% of trainees, offering these services gave them a sense of accomplishment and allowed them to help others and apply what they had learned from training into practice. Yet, some trainees reported challenges while delivering services, such as a lack of time, the impact of the COVID-19 pandemic, clients' reluctance to share FHH, and clients' lack of interest because of their engagement in other cancer prevention activities. Moreover, 60.0% of survey respondents had searched for and learned more about FHH-based cancer prevention information, and 91.4% had recommended our program to a total of more than 400 Texas Chinese Americans.

We are not aware of any adverse training effects, nor were any reported to us. Nevertheless, we received feedback on the program, including concerns about having too many assignments, a preference for an alternative face-to-face format, and the need for more interactions among trainees.

SUSTAINABILITY

The NCHWTC is a financially stable organization with nearly 20 years of experience in training CHWs. This infrastructure facilitates the continued availability of our training. The NCHWTC continues to offer the CHW certificate program at no cost. The trained CHWs continue providing FHH-based cancer prevention education and services to Chinese Americans in Texas. Because more states either already have CHW certification programs or are in the process of developing them,[15] our curriculum could be adopted nationwide. Public health organizations can benefit from our program by adopting our curriculum for their employees.

PUBLIC HEALTH SIGNIFICANCE

CHWs are the link between health care systems and their communities.[7] Aligning with leading health agencies that advocate for public health professionals to provide FHH-based education and services to communities,[4–6] we developed a CHW certification program for Texas Chinese Americans. Forty-six Chinese Americans were trained, which more than quadrupled the existing number of Chinese American CHWs available to serve Texans. These trained CHWs later served many Chinese Americans within three months of program completion. Accordingly, our program has helped establish a strengthened public health workforce with FHH-based competencies. The work of our trained CHWs has helped and will continue to help reduce cancer disparities in an underserved Chinese American population in Texas. AJPH

ABOUT THE AUTHORS

Yu-Lyu Yeh is with the Department of Healthcare Administration, Asia University, Taichung, Taiwan. Zihan Zhang, Denise Martinez, and Lei-Shih Chen are with the Department of Health Behavior, Texas A&M University, College Station, TX.

CORRESPONDENCE

Correspondence should be sent to Lei-Shih Chen, Department of Health Behavior, Texas A&M University, 367H SPH Administration Bldg, 212 Adriance Lab Rd, College Station, TX 77843-1266 (e-mail: lacechen@tamu.edu). Reprints can be ordered at https://www.ajph.org by clicking the "Reprints" link.

PUBLICATION INFORMATION

Full Citation: Yeh Yu-Lyu, Zhang Z, Martinez D, Chen Lei-Shih. Development of Texas's first Chinese American community health worker certification for family health history-based cancer prevention. *Am J Public Health*. 2025;115(2):138–141.

Acceptance Date: September 30, 2024.

DOI: https://doi.org/10.2105/AJPH.2024.307895

ORCID iDs:

Zihan Zhang https://orcid.org/0000-0001-8960-7121

Denise Martinez https://orcid.org/0000-0003-2359-9741

CONTRIBUTORS

All authors were involved in the Chinese American CHW certification program conceptualization and design and contributed to program development and data collection. Y. L. Yeh led the data analysis. The initial draft of the article was completed by Y. L. Yeh, Z. Zhang, and L. S. Chen. All authors reviewed and approved the final version of the article.

ACKNOWLEDGMENTS

This project is funded by the Cancer Prevention and Research Institute of Texas (grant PP180110).

CONFLICTS OF INTEREST

The authors have no conflicts of interest to declare related to the conduct of this project.

HUMAN PARTICIPANT PROTECTION

This study was exempt from institutional review board oversight at Texas A&M University because it is an education and training study.

REFERENCES

1. Mao W, Wu B, Yang W, Chi I. Factors of dental care utilization in foreign-born older Chinese Americans. *J Dent Res*. 2023;102(8):895–900. https://doi.org/10.1177/00220345231170845
2. Budiman A. Chinese in the US fact sheet. Pew Research Center. April 29, 2021. Available at: https://www.pewresearch.org/social-trends/fact-sheet/asian-americans-chinese-in-the-u-s. Accessed June 24, 2024.
3. Li M, Zhao S, Young CM, et al. Family health history-based interventions: a systematic review of the literature. *Am J Prev Med*. 2021;61(3):445–454. https://doi.org/10.1016/j.amepre.2021.03.022
4. National Human Genome Research Institute. Family health history. November 10, 2021. Available at: https://www.genome.gov/For-Patients-and-Families/Family-Health-History. Accessed June 24, 2024.
5. Centers for Disease Control and Prevention. Family health history. May 15, 2024. Available at: https://www.cdc.gov/family-health-history/about/index.html. Accessed June 24, 2024.
6. American Public Health Association. Advancing cancer genomics in public health. November 5, 2013. Available at: https://www.apha.org/policies-and-advocacy/public-health-policy-statements/policy-database/2014/07/23/10/25/advancing-cancer-genomics-in-public-health. Accessed June 24, 2024.
7. Chen LS, Zhao S, Stelzig D, et al. Development and evaluation of a genomics training program for community health workers in Texas. *Genet Med*. 2018;20(9):1030–1037. https://doi.org/10.1038/gim.2017.236
8. Texas Department of State Health Services. CHW and instructor training. Available at: https://www.dshs.texas.gov/community-health-worker-or-promotora-training-certification-program/chw-instructor-training. Accessed June 24, 2024.
9. Promotor(a) or Community Health Worker Training and Certification Advisory Committee. 2018 Annual Report. April 2019. Available at: https://www.dshs.texas.gov/sites/default/files/legislative/2019-Reports/CommunityHealthWorkerAnnualReport2018.pdf. Accessed June 24, 2024.
10. US Census Bureau. Asian alone or in any combination by selected groups. Available at: https://data.census.gov/table?q=B02018&g=010XX00US$0400000&y=2022. Accessed November 9, 2024.
11. Chen LS, Li M, Talwar D, Xu L, Zhao M. Chinese Americans' views and use of family health history: a qualitative study. *PLoS One*. 2016;11(9):e0162706. https://doi.org/10.1371/journal.pone.0162706
12. Sharma N, Tridimas A, Fitzsimmons PR. A readability assessment of online stroke information. *J Stroke Cerebrovasc Dis*. 2014;23(6):1362–1367. https://doi.org/10.1016/j.jstrokecerebrovasdis.2013.11.017
13. Spatz TS. Improving breast self-examination training by using the 4MAT instructional model. *J Cancer Educ*. 1991;6(3):179–183. https://doi.org/10.1080/08858199109528116
14. Lei F, Zheng Y, Lee E. Interventions for cancer screening among Chinese Americans: a systematic review and meta-analysis. *PLoS ONE*. 2022;17(3):e0265201. https://doi.org/10.1371/journal.pone.0265201
15. Association of State and Territorial Health Officials. State approaches to community health worker certification. March 19, 2024. Available at: https://www.astho.org/topic/brief/state-approaches-to-community-health-worker-certification. Accessed September 21, 2024.

A Public Health–Community Partnership to Address Lead Poisoning in King County, Washington

Diego de Acosta, PhD, Mohamed Ali, MPH, Navid Hamidi, BA, Ariana Anjaz, BA, Erin Mann, MPH, and Elizabeth Dawson-Hahn, MD, MPH

To strengthen lead poisoning prevention efforts among Afghan children, King County, Washington's Hazardous Waste Management Program partnered with Afghan Health Initiative, a community-based organization. The partnership arranged culturally tailored home visits and follow-ups, in which a health environment investigator and a community health advocate identified lead exposure risks and offered parents guidance. The involvement of an Afghan-led organization significantly increased community responsiveness and case management opportunities, demonstrating how public health–community collaborations can address health challenges disproportionately affecting refugees and immigrants. (*Am J Public Health*. 2025;115(2):142–145. https://doi.org/10.2105/AJPH.2024.307905)

AJPH February 2025, Vol. 115, No. 2

Refugee children resettled in the United States have higher average blood lead levels (BLLs) than US-born children.[1–4] This disparity stems from pre- and postmigration circumstances. BLLs of newly arrived refugee children strongly correlate with country of origin or last residence,[1–4] reflecting known global variance in childhood lead exposure.[5] After arrival, refugee children may face further exposure risks if they are resettled into older housing with lead-based paint or plumbing, or if their families unintentionally use lead-contaminated imports like cookware, jewelry, cosmetics, traditional remedies, spices, and toys.[1,6]

Primary prevention—reducing exposure to environmental lead hazards—is essential to avoid the harmful developmental effects of lead toxicity.[7] Secondary prevention—identifying and managing elevated BLL cases—protects lead-exposed children from serious complications.[7] Both strategies require sustained collaboration between public health and community stakeholders.[4]

INTERVENTION AND IMPLEMENTATION

The Hazardous Waste Management Program (HWMP) is a regional coalition in King County that works to prevent exposure to hazardous materials, including lead. HWMP is formed by Public Health–Seattle and King County, together with King County Solid Waste Division, King County Water and Land Resources Division, Seattle Public Utilities, and Sound Cities Association. HWMP provides services and education to limit toxic material exposures in homes and workplaces.

Since 2018, HWMP has funded a partnership with Afghan Health Initiative (AHI) to prevent childhood lead poisoning through culturally tailored home visits and follow-ups. AHI is an Afghan led nonprofit offering community-based interventions to improve access to health, education, and economic self-sufficiency. AHI is based in south King County, where most of King County's new Afghan arrivals live, and has reached more than 8000 families through its programs.[8]

Home visits unfold in three stages, with an AHI Community Health Advocate and an HWMP Health Environment Investigator (hereafter "advocate" and "investigator") playing key roles:

- Before the visit: The Washington Department of Health informs HWMP of children in King County with elevated BLLs, reporting more than 300 cases annually. For each case in an Afghan family, HWMP securely relays contact details to AHI. An AHI advocate calls the parents to establish rapport, notify them of the child's condition, educate them about lead poisoning, describe

HWMP's role, and explain how home visits protect children from further lead exposures. This conversation takes place in Dari or Pashto. If the parents consent, a home visit is scheduled.

- During the visit: An HWMP investigator and an AHI advocate visit the home together, with the advocate interpreting and acting as a cultural broker. The investigator brings translated educational materials for the family and collects small samples from household items that may contain lead (e.g., paint, spices, cosmetics) for later testing. These samples will be analyzed in an accredited laboratory using inductively coupled plasma mass spectrometry. The investigator uses a portable x-ray fluorescence analyzer to detect lead in other items (e.g., dishes, cookware, jewelry) on site, in the home.
- After the visit: HWMP creates recommendations for the family based on the visit and sample analysis. Guidance may range from nutritional advice to suggestions to exchange or discard lead-contaminated items. An AHI advocate communicates these recommendations to the family in a culturally sensitive manner and continues to serve as a liaison for follow-up questions and referrals as needed. After sharing recommendations, the HWMP–AHI partnership checks in with the family for periodic retesting and, if necessary, reevaluation of household lead exposure sources. HWMP closes the case when the child's BLL remains below five micrograms per deciliter (μg/dL) for at least three months.

After HWMP and AHI began collaborating, a team of local scientists found that traditional Afghan cookware brought by Afghan families—or even purchased in the United States—could be a significant lead exposure hazard.[9] HWMP therefore started inviting families to exchange lead-contaminated pots for lead-free Instant Pots or stainless-steel cookware, at no cost, in their postvisit recommendations. To raise community awareness, AHI produced videos promoting Instant Pots in Dari and Pashto.

PLACE, TIME, AND PERSONS

HWMP and AHI's tailored intervention prioritized the rapidly growing Afghan population in King County. According to US Census 5-year estimates, there were 752 county residents reporting Afghan ancestry in 2017, increasing to 3648 in 2020 and 4793 in 2022.[10] The Afghan languages most commonly spoken in King County are Dari and Pashto.

Although HWMP and AHI's collaboration is ongoing, the work described here occurred between July 2018 and July 2024.

PURPOSE

In Washington State, Afghan arrivals are disproportionately affected by lead exposure. Among newly arrived children from Afghanistan (n = 2690) screened between 2018 and 2022, 26% had BLLs of five to nine μg/dL and 5% had more than 10 μg/dL. The corresponding values for children in Washington State from all countries (n = 5030) were 15% and 3%, respectively.[11] Of the childhood elevated BLL cases reported to HWMP between January 2021 and July 2024, 91% were Afghan children.

The HWMP–AHI partnership emerged when HWMP recognized a complementary set of challenges and opportunities to prevent lead poisoning among Afghan children. Before collaborating with AHI, HWMP experienced difficulties communicating with Afghan families because of linguistic, cultural, and health literacy factors. Specifically, HWMP encountered a landscape where there was little awareness of lead as a health hazard, sources of lead exposure, or the purpose of home environment investigations. Phone calls and messages to Afghan families about lead-exposed children often went unanswered, and many cases had to be closed after three months without a response, with no opportunity for intervention.

Meanwhile, Washington's governor's office issued a directive instructing state agencies and partners to address potential lead sources.[12] HWMP created a racial equity strategic plan that acknowledged the disproportionate burden of hazardous material exposures on communities of color and prioritized better engagement through community partnerships.[13] It was in this context that HWMP requested proposals to address lead poisoning among Afghan children. HWMP selected AHI to support home health investigations through cultural brokering by a female, Dari- and Pashto-speaking community health advocate.

EVALUATION AND ADVERSE EFFECTS

Participation in the home-visit program grew dramatically through the HWMP–AHI partnership. Before AHI's involvement, few Afghan families (< 5% monthly average) responded to calls from HWMP. After the partnership, response rates increased and remained around a 20% monthly average. The number of home visits similarly climbed from three to five households monthly to more than 20 households. These households have four children on average, so the program now touches more than 80 children per month. Finally, more than 200 families participated in the cookware exchange program. Once HWMP and AHI refined their strategy to communicate the health risks of lead exposure and the importance of secondary prevention, news of the home visits and cookware exchange spread widely. Indeed, even Afghan families without affected children began to inquire about participating.

The local Afghan community's awareness of lead exposure risks and trust in the home visit program increased through the partnership. According to feedback gathered by AHI, parents who received home visits initially expressed unfamiliarity with lead exposure risks, concern about being found at fault, and some hesitation to part with culturally significant items like cookware and cosmetics. Afterward, they expressed gratitude to the community health advocate for information and guidance. Over time, AHI has observed local Afghan families becoming more aware of lead poisoning and more familiar with possible household sources of lead.

The home-visit program had no known adverse effects.

SUSTAINABILITY

HWMP and AHI developed a successful partnership based on mutual respect, rapport, and shared goals, and their collaboration has been extremely effective. Members of both organizations interviewed for this article each cited the other's attentiveness, deep commitment, and flexibility as key ingredients of their working relationship (Box 1).

Both partners are eager to keep collaborating and expect their work to continue with newly resettled Afghans, as well as Indian, Pakistani, Middle Eastern, and East African immigrants. Lead poisoning prevention remains largely unfamiliar among recent arrivals, who therefore benefit from the partnership's proven outreach, home visits, and follow-up. Even so—especially after the surge of Afghan arrivals in 2021—both partners recognize that lead poisoning prevention must be part of a comprehensive approach to supporting families navigating the many hardships of resettlement.

PUBLIC HEALTH SIGNIFICANCE

The Public Health 3.0 framework urges public health departments to build and guide strategic multisector partnerships, including local partnerships grounded in community networks.[14] When HWMP requested proposals from potential partners, most applicants were well-established health systems that communicate with Afghan clients through a staff interpreter. Although AHI was a newer organization, HWMP recognized that this Afghan-led and public health–minded nonprofit was uniquely poised to reach the Afghan community and build its own capacity in the process.

Indeed, partnerships that strengthen community-led, culturally and linguistically concordant preventive interventions

BOX 1— Perspectives on the Working Relationship Between the Hazardous Waste Management Program (HWMP) and Afghan Health Initiative (AHI): King County, WA, July 2018–July 2024

"When a community-based organization is able to give feedback that they think is the best for the community, and they see that it is being implemented and is actually being listened to by County . . . that was a huge confidence-booster for AHI as a whole, that if we do advocate on behalf of our community, there's a seat at the table for us." —AHI leader

"Our approach to power-sharing involves integrating community health issues into our work plan when they are brought to our attention. However, historically, if these issues were not already part of our work plan, we tended to overlook them. This was mainly due to our team's heavy workload and existing priorities in public health." —HWMP program manager

"What we've heard is . . . that County has been able to take the information we give and also adapt it to a lot of other departments, that AHI can provide some support and some guidance on how best to reach the community and what are some equitable practices they can take away and also implement for other refugee communities." —AHI leader

"That is the potential we saw in [AHI] when we gave them our first funding four or five years ago. . . . Government doesn't allow you to waste money, so it is hard to bet on someone who has no track record. But [we] agreed that this is where our dollars will be better spent, because they are from the community, they speak the languages, and we need them. . . . That is something, building the capacity of the partner, which is the community-based organization. Now they are able to provide services. Even if we move on, if we stop funding, they will continue." —HWMP program manager

"It was not very prescriptive—'This is what we want'—but like, 'How can we work together?' . . . I think that was one of the biggest pieces with capacity, giving us essentially our first shot at working with County and them showing us the ropes, and then, in addition to that, giving us a platform and a voice." —AHI leader are vital to address structural and community-derived barriers among refugees and immigrants.[15] After a few years of dedicated funding from HWMP, AHI grew from a fledgling organization to an experienced leader in local public health efforts with a broader platform for community advocacy. Meanwhile, with AHI's crucial support, HWMP revitalized and strengthened its approach to lead poisoning prevention. Both partners benefited from critical information about traditional Afghan cookware,[9] a culturally specific risk factor along with imported cosmetics, glazed ceramics, and spices. Overall, the HWMP–AHI partnership highlights the unique ways a public health–community collaboration can galvanize health professionals and community members to take coordinated action and enhance their collective impact. AJPH

ABOUT THE AUTHORS

Diego de Acosta and Erin Mann are with the National Resource Center for Refugees, Immigrants, and Migrants (NRC-RIM), University of Minnesota, Minneapolis. Mohamed Ali is with Public Health–Seattle and King County, WA. Navid Hamidi and Ariana Anjaz are with Afghan Health Initiative, Kent, WA. Elizabeth Dawson-Hahn is with the Department of Pediatrics, University of Washington, Seattle.

CORRESPONDENCE

Correspondence should be sent to Diego de Acosta, PhD, Mayo Bldg, Suite C311, 420 Delaware St SE, Minneapolis, MN 55455 (e-mail: deaco011@umn.edu). Reprints can be ordered at https://www.ajph.org by clicking the "Reprints" link.

PUBLICATION INFORMATION

Full Citation: Acosta DD, Ali M, Hamidi N, Anjaz A, Mann E, Dawson-Hahn E. A public health–community partnership to address lead poisoning in King County, Washington. *Am J Public Health*. 2025;115(2):142–145.

Acceptance Date: October 18, 2024.

DOI: https://doi.org/10.2105/AJPH.2024.307905

ORCID iD:

Diego de Acosta https://orcid.org/0000-0002-2885-5639

CONTRIBUTORS

D. de Acosta led the writing and analyses. M. Ali, N. Hamidi, and A. Anjaz co-coordinated the interventions and data gathering and assisted with the writing. E. Mann assisted with the writing and conceptualization of the study. E. Dawson-Hahn was team lead and assisted with the writing.

ACKNOWLEDGMENTS

This work was performed under NRC-RIM, which is funded by the US Centers for Disease Control and Prevention and the International Organization for Migration (award CK000495-03-00/ES1874).

We thank Steve Whittaker, Katie Fellows, Linda Van Hooser, Fanaye Amsalu, Ashley Bullock, and Hena Parveen from Public Health–Seattle and King County's Hazardous Waste Program for their dedicated work on lead poisoning prevention. We express special gratitude to Sharon Cohen, Matt Wilson, and Roda Mohamed, the home environment investigators from the Hazardous Waste Management Program, and Nilu Pedram, the community health advocate from Afghan Health Initiative, who performed the home visits. We sincerely thank the many families that participated in the home visit program. Finally, we express our appreciation to the members of the Qualitative Collaborative at NRC-RIM who reviewed these Notes From the Field.

CONFLICTS OF INTEREST

The authors have no conflicts of interest to declare.

HUMAN PARTICIPANT PROTECTION

The University of Minnesota institutional review board determined that the findings from these interviews with King County's Hazardous Waste Management Program and Afghan Health Initiative were not human participant research.

REFERENCES

1. Pezzi C, Lee D, Kennedy L, et al. Blood lead levels among resettled refugee children in select US states, 2010–2014. *Pediatrics*. 2019;143(5):e20182591. https://doi.org/10.1542/peds.2018-2591
2. Balza JS, Bikomeye JC, Beyer KMM, Rublee C, Flynn KE. Elevated blood lead levels of refugee children in the United States: a systematic review of recent literature (2011–2021). *Rev Environ Health*. 2023;38(2):361–383. https://doi.org/10.1515/reveh-2022-0015
3. Yun K, Matheson J, Payton C, et al. Health profiles of newly arrived refugee children in the United States, 2006–2012. *Am J Public Health*. 2016;106(1):128–135. https://doi.org/10.2105/AJPH.2015.302873
4. Anil L, Ma Z, Nambiar A, Watkins SM. Blood lead level testing and retesting among newly arriving refugee children, Pennsylvania, 2015–2019. *Am J Public Health*. 2022;112(suppl 7):S706–S714. https://doi.org/10.2105/AJPH.2022.306856
5. Rees N, Fuller R. *The Toxic Truth: Children's Exposure to Lead Pollution Undermines a Generation of Future Potential*. UNICEF. 2020. Available at: https://www.unicef.org/reports/toxic-truth-childrens-exposure-to-lead-pollution-2020. Accessed November 8, 2024.
6. Centers for Disease Control and Prevention. Lead screening guidelines. Domestic guidelines. June 16, 2022. Available at: https://www.cdc.gov/immigrantrefugeehealth/guidelines/lead-guidelines.html. Accessed November 3, 2023.
7. Ettinger AS, Leonard ML, Mason J. CDC's Lead Poisoning Prevention Program: a long-standing responsibility and commitment to protect children from lead exposure. *J Public Health Manag Pract*. 2019;25(1):S5–S12. https://doi.org/10.1097/PHH.0000000000000868
8. National Association of County and City Health Officials. Site spotlight: Afghan Health Initiative. June 27, 2024. Available at: https://www.naccho.org/blog/articles/site-spotlight-afghan-health-initiative. Accessed August 8, 2024.
9. Fellows KM, Samy S, Rodriguez Y, Whittaker SG. Investigating aluminum cookpots as a source of lead exposure in Afghan refugee children resettled in the United States. *J Expo Sci Environ Epidemiol*. 2022;32(3):451–460. https://doi.org/10.1038/s41370-022-00431-y
10. US Census Bureau. B04006. People reporting ancestry. Available at: https://data.census.gov/table/ACSDT1Y2018.B04006?t=Ancestry&g=050XX00US53033. Accessed October 24, 2023.
11. *Annual Refugee Health Screening Report, Washington State, FFY 2022*. Olympia, WA: Refugee and Immigrant Health Program, Washington State Department of Health; 2023.
12. *Governor's Directive on Lead 16-06 Lead Service Line and Component Survey Summary of Findings*. Olympia, WA: Washington State Department of Health; 2017.
13. Local Hazardous Waste Management Program in King County. *Racial Equity Strategic Plan Summary*. 2018. Available at: https://kingcountyhazwastewa.gov/-/media/hazwaste/lhwmp-documents/program-plans/esj-equity-strategic-plan-summary.pdf. Accessed January 8, 2024.
14. DeSalvo KB, Wang YC, Harris A, Auerbach J, Koo D, O'Carroll P. Public health 3.0: a call to action for public health to meet the challenges of the 21st century. *Prev Chronic Dis*. 2017;14:E78. https://doi.org/10.5888/pcd14.170017
15. Abdi N, Ebengho S, Mohamed N, et al. Early pandemic access to COVID-19 testing in the Somali community in King County, Washington, USA: a mixed-methods evaluation. *J Racial Ethn Health Disparities*. 2023;10(6):2930–2943. https://doi.org/10.1007/s40615-022-01470-9

A Critical Examination of Whiteness as a Fundamental Causal Determinant of US Health Inequities

Jay A. Pearson, PhD, MPH

ABOUT THE AUTHOR

Jay A. Pearson is with the Sanford School of Public Policy, Duke University, Durham, NC.

See also Whiteness and Redlining, pp. 149–169.

Population and public health researchers increasingly implicate racism as a fundamental causal social determinant of racialized health inequities in the United States.[1] Such work focuses almost exclusively on the disadvantaged health status of racially minoritized populations of color. A few notable recent examples addressing COVID-19 and life expectancy notwithstanding,[2,3] considerably less research addresses the health status of majoritized ethnic White Americans.

In the current issue of *AJPH*, Efird and Griffith (p. 152) define Whiteness as "a dynamic system that typically upholds White Americans' social supremacy." The authors go on to integrate rurality into the theoretical framework on Whiteness of Malat et al. (https://bit.ly/4i1RGfr) to produce a multilevel, multidimensional model explicating how Whiteness is a social determinant of rural White health. This analytic essay extends their assessment by suggesting that Whiteness is a critical, albeit often overlooked, component of US racism and consequently a major contributor to broader US-based social inequalities and health inequities. It then speculates on several key areas associated with Whiteness that warrant additional scholarly investigation and closes by offering suggestions for how reconsideration of Whiteness might be used to secure broader population health equity.

Whiteness is arguably the least investigated, yet potentially most fundamental, causal social determinant of racialized health inequities. Consequently, there remain many unexamined phenomena associated with the relationship between Whiteness and population health. For instance, how does Whiteness influence health inequities among populations of color and Whites? How might poorly originated or impoverished notions of Whiteness overlook important within-group heterogeneity that should be explored? Finally, how can researchers, practitioners, and activists emphasize that addressing Whiteness is essential to understanding race and racism as well as securing the highest possible health status for broader US and international populations?

Northwestern European colonizers of the emerging United States originated and used voodoo science to argue that race reflects a natural hierarchy of humanity indexed by "superior" physical characteristics (e.g., lighter skin and hair) inherently associated with desirable traits, whereas "inferior" physical characteristics (e.g., darker skin and hair) were inherently associated with undesirable traits.[4] This "natural" hierarchy was used to justify material exploitation of Native Americans through land appropriation, market exploitation of African-descended populations via chattel slavery, and subordination of select European immigrants contingent on national origin, religion, and political orientation.[5]

Racism, broadly defined, entails core guiding principles and subsequent national-level decision-making associated with racial construction and racial hierarchy as well as racial bias (positive supremacy and privilege as well as negative oppression and discrimination) to build a durable socialized system of differential human valuation that was, and remains, a central guiding principle of US national construction and identity.[6,7] These collective social processes reliably advantage racially majoritized Whites at the cost of disadvantaging racially minoritized populations of color as well as select European populations.[8,9]

Accordingly, when compared with minoritized populations of color, White Americans benefit from superior social positioning granting direct privileged access to resources and protection from risks in ways reliably translating into improved social well-being and better health. However, the White racial group is not a social monolith.[9,10] Flawed assumptions of homogeneity informing exclusive or primary focus on White racial identity only obfuscates the ways White Americans are minoritized in other identity domains and social contexts. For example, White immigrants to the United States have better health

AJPH February 2025, Vol. 115, No. 2

profiles than US-born ethnic White Americans.[10] Efird and Griffith rightly highlight rurality as one among many minoritizing constructs that interact with other identity markers across multiple and varied social contexts to compromise health and suggest the value of cultural considerations among ethnic White Americans.

The history of differential US immigration policy also influenced White racial construction. Many Southern and Eastern European immigrants were initially disqualified from, but later integrated into, an increasingly expansive and inclusive White racial category during key historical periods in efforts to expand and consolidate White racial solidarity and power.[9] Non-Protestant faith, liberal political affiliation, and labor support were similarly disqualifying. How might the historical legacies of these variable processes of exclusion and strategic inclusion manifest as contemporary processes influencing social well-being and health? How might their evolution expand to include rural, urban, and suburban distinctions? Moreover, what might be the health implications of these distinguishing processes remaining largely obscured and consequently unexplored under the illusion of a singularly unifying White racial identity? Lastly, how does Whiteness drive poor population health outcomes in the United States compared with high-income peer countries? The COVID-19 pandemic provides one example.

US national COVID-19 mortality rates for Whites converged with those of Black and Native Americans in 2021 through 2022.[3] County-level analyses revealed that percentage vote for Republican presentinal candidate Donald Trump in 2020 was positively associated with increased mortality, and this was particularly the case for rural counties. Speculative explanations for this phenomenon proposed that conservative political narratives disparaging COVID-19 vaccinations and personal mitigation practices, such as distancing, handwashing, and masking, as infringements on liberty may have increased risks. In this case, political ideology and Whiteness drove the largest decline in US life expectancy when compared with high-income national peers.

Social contextual factors from urban settings also influence racialization processes affecting White American health. An investigation using a multiracial/-ethnic sample from Detroit, Michigan, reported poor Whites to have worse health than poor Black and Mexican origin residents and nonpoor residents of all three groups.[11] The authors speculated, but did not measure, that notions of egalitarian meritocracy, racial dominance, supremacy, privilege, and entitlement combined with failed economic success may inform mental, psychological, and physical pathology in ways particularly harmful for poor Detroit Whites.

Given the well-documented historical development of Whiteness, its contemporary social impact, and the brief review offered here of a much larger body of empirical work highlighting compelling findings associated with it, how and why has Whiteness remained relatively ignored in public and population health research? The answer, I believe, is because Whiteness is the normative standard against which all other racial/ethnic identities have been constructed and are compared, including shifts over time in who is considered White. Because Whiteness is the normative standard, its harmful effects are often not considered. Ironically, these normative notions serve to preclude critical examinations of Whiteness to the detriment of select segments of the identity group.

As the central guiding principle in a fundamentally racist society, Whiteness must be addressed to disempower systemic racism and inform the move toward racialized health equity. Additionally, racially majoritized White social advocates are likely better positioned to engage coracial counterparts who may be unaware of or unwilling to support the move toward a more just and equitable society proposing to support and advance racial justice and, by extension, racialized health equity. The difficult work of critical self-examination and answering the question of what might be one's most important or appropriate role in undoing Whiteness remains unrealized.

In conclusion, as an alternative to normative acceptance, prioritizing more explicit acknowledgment of and increased critical examination into the social functioning and heterogeneous nature of Whiteness are essential to US national population health. This is true for racially minoritized and majoritized populations. More complete conceptualizations of White supremacist systems and more precise measurement of White privilege are essential components of this work.[12] Additionally, examining the ways that variable other phenomena associated with Whiteness may work to disadvantage select White subpopulations in the US context as well as the implications these have for other groups, including minoritized populations of color, is facilitated by this movement. AJPH

CORRESPONDENCE

Correspondence should be sent to Jay A. Pearson, Associate Professor, Sanford School of Public Policy, Duke University, 201 Science Dr, SB 211, Box 90245, Durham, NC 27708 (e-mail: jay.pearson@duke.edu). Reprints can be ordered at https://www.ajph.org by clicking the "Reprints" link.

PUBLICATION INFORMATION

Full Citation: Pearson JA. A critical examination of Whiteness as a fundamental causal determinant of US health inequities. *Am J Public Health*. 2025;115(2): 146–148.

Acceptance Date: November 20, 2024.

DOI: https://doi.org/10.2105/AJPH.2024.307952

ORCID iD:
Jay A. Pearson https://orcid.org/0000-0003-4290-0229

CONFLICTS OF INTEREST

The author has no conflicts of interest to declare.

REFERENCES

1. Paradies Y, Ben J, Denson N, et al. Racism as a determinant of health: a systematic review and meta-analysis. *PLoS One*. 2015;10(9):e0138511. https://doi.org/10.1371/journal.pone.0138511
2. Case A, Deaton A. *Deaths of Despair and the Future of Capitalism*. Princeton, NJ: Princeton University Press; 2020. https://doi.org/10.2307/j.ctvpr7rb2
3. Lundberg DJ, Wrigley-Field E, Cho A, et al. COVID-19 mortality by race and ethnicity in US metropolitan and nonmetropolitan areas, March 2020 to February 2022. *JAMA Netw Open*. 2023;6(5): e2311098. https://doi.org/10.1001/jamanetworkopen.2023.11098
4. American Anthropological Association. AAA statement on race. *Am Anthropol*. 1998;100(3):712–713. https://doi.org/10.1525/aa.1998.100.3.712
5. American Sociological Association. *The Importance of Collecting Data and Doing Social Scientific Research on Race*. Washington, DC: American Sociological Association; 2003. Available at: https://www.asanet.org/wp-content/uploads/race_statement.pdf. Accessed November 21, 2024.
6. Bonilla-Silva E. Rethinking racism: toward a structural interpretation. *Am Sociol Rev*. 1997;62(3): 465–480. https://doi.org/10.2307/2657316
7. Anderson E. Durable social hierarchies: how egalitarian movements imagine inequality. July 19, 2016. Available at: https://items.ssrc.org/what-is-inequality/durable-social-hierarchies-how-egalitarian-movements-imagine-inequality. Accessed November 21, 2024.
8. Gee GC, Ford CL. Structural racism and health inequities: old issues, new directions. *Du Bois Rev*. 2011;8(1):115–132. https://doi.org/10.1017/S1742058X11000130
9. Peck G. *Race Traffic: Antislavery and the Origins of White Victimhood, 1619–1819*. Chapel Hill, NC: University of North Carolina Press; 2024.
10. Read JG, West JS, Kamis C. Immigration and health among non-Hispanic Whites: the impact of arrival cohort and region of birth. *Soc Sci Med*. 2020;246:112754. https://doi.org/10.1016/j.socscimed.2019.112754
11. Geronimus AT, Pearson JA, Linnenbringer E, et al. Race–Ethnicity, poverty, urban stressors, and telomere length in a Detroit community-based sample. *J Health Soc Behav*. 2015;56(2):199–224. https://doi.org/10.1177/0022146515582100
12. Leonardo Z. The color of supremacy: beyond the discourse of "White privilege." *Educ Philos Theory*. 2004;36(2):137–152. https://doi.org/10.1111/j.1469-5812.2004.00057.x

Redlining, Root Causes, and a Firearm Injury Scholarship of Consequence

Jonathan Jay, DrPH, JD

ABOUT THE AUTHOR

Jonathan Jay is with the School of Public Health, Boston University, Boston, MA.

See also Whiteness and Redlining, pp. 146–169.

The public health crisis of firearm injuries in the United States has been, and continues to be, severely understudied because of a lack of resources.[1] Scholarship on firearm injuries, therefore, presents unique opportunities to contribute new knowledge and support urgently needed solutions. New scientific knowledge can support solutions, but it does not do so automatically, as Galea and Vaughan argued when they called for a public health of consequence.[2] They encouraged public health scholars to find a north star in consequentialist questions such as, "Does this work matter?" and "How could it matter more?"

In this issue, Hans et al. (p. 161) find that US neighborhoods that were adversely redlined by the Home Owners Loan Corporation (HOLC) in the 1930s experienced greater increases in firearm violence during the COVID-19 pandemic than did those that were not. To reach this finding, the authors exploited an exogenous population threshold that determined whether a city's neighborhoods were eligible for HOLC grading, making exposure to redlining as good as random near that population of 40 000 threshold. This causal identification strategy is innovative and elegant. The study persuasively links HOLC grades and COVID-19 era violence trends. But from a consequentialist perspective we must also ask: What is it good for?

The scholarship linking historical HOLC redlining with present-day firearm violence has grown rapidly in recent years. Analytical approaches have varied, and the prevailing associations do not hold true in every city.[3] But the evidence is now sufficiently robust that Jacoby and South—leading scholars in the field—have suggested that it is time to ask new questions.[4] They have argued that studies on the influence of this 1930s era policy (1) are not highly relevant to contemporary interventions, and (2) could let policymakers off the hook for the many decisions in the intervening decades that have produced today's inequities. In other words, feeding the apparent demand for research on this topic may not be helpful and may even be harmful. These are consequentialist concerns.

Some categories of firearm injury scholarship easily pass the consequentialist test. In my subfield of community firearm violence, for instance, rigorous research on community violence intervention (CVI) programs has clear utility. Using tools such as street outreach, case management, conflict mediation, and intensive mentorship, CVI programs aim to curb violence exposure among the highest-risk individuals. Although there has been important work on CVI from public health scholars,[5,6] a dramatic influx of funding for CVI programming since 2020 has outpaced the production of new scholarship, creating a need and opportunity to advance the scientific understanding of what works, and why, in CVI.

There is also an obvious use for public health scholarship on place-based interventions, such as improvements to the built environment. Recent trials have shown that modest physical upgrades, for example, "cleaning and greening" unkempt vacant lots,[7] can reduce nearby firearm violence. Environmental approaches embody enduring values of public health by providing community-level benefits at a comparatively low cost. More scholarship is needed to understand how these strategies can be scaled up and to expand the toolbox by identifying strategies that will work in settings where vacant properties are not widespread.

But there remains an important role for scholarship to help us uncover and address the root causes of firearm injuries. From a social-ecological perspective, CVI and place-based interventions address key factors at the interpersonal and community levels that drive cycles of firearm violence. However, they do not address the maldistribution of those risk factors, which leads to vast racial and ethnic disparities in firearm injuries. For example, my colleagues and I found that child firearm assault rates for Black children were 100 times those for White children during the COVID-19 pandemic in four major US cities.[8] Even in a country awash in

AJPH February 2025, Vol. 115, No. 2

firearms, even during an unprecedented global health crisis, children from the dominant racial category (i.e., White children) saw no increase in firearm victimization in those cities, unlike children in every minoritized category.[8] These glaring inequities could not arise without forces that systematically array risk factors in racially minoritized communities: structural racism.

Will another redlining study help solve this problem? In my view it could, but it is up to firearm injury scholars to make this work matter. We have not done enough to connect the dots between research on root causes and remedies. One preliminary step is to sharpen our framing: vacant lots are symptoms not of "blight" but of disinvestment,[9] a long-term process that has a solution in the present day (i.e., investment). Going forward, we must continue to grow scientific knowledge on current policies that can address drivers of violence. For instance, we need to test cash transfers for firearm injury survivors and to use natural experiments such as expanding tax credits, raising the minimum wage, and changing local zoning rules to reduce residential racial segregation. Shrinking the criminal legal system's impacts by eliminating cash bail appears not to increase firearm violence,[10] but more work is needed in this area. Studies of historical redlining and firearm injuries are not compelling ends in themselves but could provide important background for work on more proximal, contemporary social determinants.

Addressing root causes could be key to achieving the potential of violence prevention programs. For example, interpersonal interventions such as CVI programs cannot be expected to deliver dramatic results when a community's load of deprivation and trauma is excessively heavy. If intervening in social determinants of violence can ease these burdens—perhaps while place-based interventions simultaneously improve social processes at key locations—CVI workers may have greater opportunities to bend the curve on violence. This multilevel approach to violence prevention is likely the only way to ease such a complex, deeply entrenched problem as community firearm violence. Scholars can support these solutions with conceptual and analytical approaches tailored to complexity, for example, systems science and computer simulation modeling.[11]

Efforts toward a firearm injury scholarship of consequence must also continue to elevate the role of community members affected by firearm injuries, especially survivors. There are clear instrumental reasons for academics to engage and empower communities throughout the research process, because people with relevant lived and frontline experience are likely to have a keen sense of what really matters and a motivation to avoid pointless analytic exercises. (I note this, sheepishly, as a researcher who coauthored a rigorous scientific analysis that essentially found that there is more firearm violence on warmer days[12]—a conclusion so obvious to community violence workers that it has drawn laughs from them in more than one conference room.) Scholarship that addresses community priorities is more likely to have an impact in part because it is viewed as legitimate. Beyond this, academics have obligations to respect the dignity and self-determination of affected communities that cannot be reduced to a calculation of what may be useful in any given instance.

The utility of academic research may not always be immediately evident, but those of us with the privilege to conduct firearm injury scholarship must remain mindful of the urgency of the problem. Another HOLC redlining study might matter, or it might not. The answer depends on whether we put in the work needed to make it matter. AJPH

CORRESPONDENCE

Correspondence should be sent to Jonathan Jay, DrPH, JD, Crosstown 430, 801 Massachusetts Ave, Boston, MA 02118 (e-mail: jonjay@bu.edu). Reprints can be ordered at https://www.ajph.org by clicking the "Reprints" link.

PUBLICATION INFORMATION

Full Citation: Jay J. Redlining, root causes, and a firearm injury scholarship of consequence. *Am J Public Health*. 2025;115(2):149–151.

Acceptance Date: November 8, 2024.

DOI: https://doi.org/10.2105/AJPH.2024.307933

ORCID iD:

Jonathan Jay https://orcid.org/0000-0002-7543-4247

CONFLICTS OF INTEREST

The author has no conflicts to disclose.

REFERENCES

1. Cunningham RM, Ranney ML, Goldstick JE, Kamat SV, Roche JS, Carter PM. federal funding for research on the leading causes of death among children and adolescents. *Health Aff (Millwood)*. 2019;38(10):1653–1661. https://doi.org/10.1377/hlthaff.2019.00476
2. Galea S, Vaughan R. A public health of consequence. *Am J Public Health*. 2016;106(1):10–11. https://doi.org/10.2105/AJPH.2015.302954
3. Mehranbod CA, Gobaud AN, Jacoby SF, Uzzi M, Bushover BR, Morrison CN. Historical redlining and the epidemiology of present-day firearm violence in the United States: a multi-city analysis. *Prev Med*. 2022;165:107207. https://doi.org/10.1016/j.ypmed.2022.107207
4. Jacoby SF, South EC. "Redlining" maps and contemporary firearm violence research: is it time to ask new questions? *Ann Intern Med*. 2024;177(5):678–679. https://doi.org/10.7326/M24-0870
5. Matthay EC, Farkas K, Rudolph KE, et al. Firearm and nonfirearm violence after Operation Peacemaker Fellowship in Richmond, California, 1996–2016. *Am J Public Health*. 2019;109(11):1605–1611. https://doi.org/10.2105/AJPH.2019.305288
6. Buggs SA, Webster DW, Crifasi CK. Using synthetic control methodology to estimate effects of a cure violence intervention in Baltimore, Maryland.

Inj Prev. 2022;28(1):61–67. https://doi.org/10.1136/injuryprev-2020-044056

7. Branas CC, South E, Kondo MC, et al. Citywide cluster randomized trial to restore blighted vacant land and its effects on violence, crime, and fear. *Proc Natl Acad Sci USA.* 2018;115(12):2946–2951. https://doi.org/10.1073/pnas.1718503115
8. Jay J, Martin R, Patel M, Xie K, Shareef F, Simes JT. Analyzing child firearm assault injuries by race and ethnicity during the COVID-19 pandemic in 4 major US cities. *JAMA Netw Open.* 2023;6(3):e233125. https://doi.org/10.1001/jamanetworkopen.2023.3125
9. Gause EL, McLone SG, Cunningham M, Jay J. Community–academic partnership to assess the role of physical disinvestment on firearm violence in Toledo, OH. *J Urban Health.* 2024;101(3):584–594. https://doi.org/10.1007/s11524-024-00870-y
10. Jahn JL, Simes JT, Jay J. Evaluating firearm violence after New Jersey's cash bail reform. *JAMA Netw Open.* 2024;7(5):e2412535. https://doi.org/10.1001/jamanetworkopen.2024.12535
11. Goldstick JE, Jay J. Agent-based modeling: an underutilized tool in community violence research. *Curr Epidemiol Rep.* 2022;9(3):135–141. https://doi.org/10.1007/s40471-022-00292-x
12. Lyons VH, Gause EL, Spangler KR, Wellenius GA, Jay J. Analysis of daily ambient temperature and firearm violence in 100 US cities. *JAMA Netw Open.* 2022;5(12):e2247207. https://doi.org/10.1001/jamanetworkopen.2022.47207

Whiteness: A Fundamental Determinant of the Health of Rural White Americans

Caroline R. Efird, PhD, MPH, and Derek M. Griffith, PhD

See also Whiteness and Redlining, pp. 146–169.

Because residents of rural areas in the United States experience a persistent disadvantage in life expectancy relative to their urban counterparts, it is critical to consider the structural and social determinants that affect the health of rural populations. White Americans constitute 3 out of every 4 (76%) rural residents, and there is growing evidence that rurality is a predictor of poor health status for White Americans in ways that are not present for racially minoritized populations or nonrural White populations.

We offer a framework to describe Whiteness as a fundamental determinant of the health of rural White Americans, which is useful to more precisely characterize and address the heterogeneous yet unique factors that drive their health. While Whiteness is a dynamic system that typically upholds White Americans' social supremacy, we provide examples of intermediate (e.g., rural culture, environment) and intrapersonal (e.g., psychosocial) factors through which Whiteness can harm rural White Americans' health (e.g., chronic disease, mental health).

We conclude with a discussion of implications and recommendations that may help to advance research to promote health and well-being among rural White Americans. (*Am J Public Health*. 2025;115(2): 152–160. https://doi.org/10.2105/AJPH.2024.307904)

AJPH February 2025, Vol. 115, No. 2

According to the 2020 US Census, 20% of the population—more than 60 million people—lives in rural areas.[1] Residents of rural areas in the United States, as compared with their peers who live in nonrural areas, are more likely to experience an excess burden of adverse health outcomes and mortality from heart disease, cancer, chronic lower respiratory disease, suicide, unintentional injury, and stroke, and have a shorter life expectancy.[2,3] Compared with their urban counterparts, rural residents are more likely to face structural and social barriers such as a lack of grocery stores and public transit, persistently high poverty rates, lower educational attainment, and a shortage of high-wage employment opportunities and limited resources to support local public health infrastructure.[4] Furthermore, rural populations are generally older and more likely to live in health care–shortage areas than their nonrural peers.[5–7] To improve US population health, it is critically important to alleviate the burden of health disparities experienced by rural populations.

The 2021–2025 National Institute on Minority Health and Health Disparities strategic plan explicitly names rural populations as a priority because rural health research necessitates "attention to the unique geographic, geopolitical, and cultural context of each community."[8] Rural populations are not a monolith. Rural Americans who are racialized as Black and those who live in counties where the majority of residents are from racially minoritized groups tend to experience the cumulative effects of rural residence and structural racism in ways that are unique,[6,9,10] and it is critical to continue focusing on the health and well-being of racially minoritized populations; however, almost 2 decades of National Vital Statistics Data demonstrate that the rural–nonrural mortality difference is wide and growing, particularly for White Americans.[11] Attempts to improve the health of rural Americans may benefit from investigating racialized health differences within rural populations and more precisely defining subgroups of rural populations.[12–14] In the context of structural racism,[15,16] studying the health of White Americans highlights that structural power and privilege is not universally associated with better health (particularly mental health and behavioral health). Specifically, we highlight how a distinct subgroup of White Americans—those who live in rural areas—can experience a particular set of social and environmental factors that meaningfully impact their health in disparate ways from nonrural White populations.

The goal of the essay is to refine efforts to identify and address the unique factors that influence and characterize the health of rural White Americans by highlighting how racialized framing[17] can enhance our understanding of the health of rural White populations. According to the March 2024 "Revisions to OMB's Statistical Policy Directive No. 15: Standards for Maintaining, Collecting, and Presenting Federal Data on Race and Ethnicity," which created a combined race and ethnicity question, the category "White" only refers to "Individuals with origins in any of the original peoples of Europe, including, for example, English, German, Irish, Italian, Polish, and Scottish."[18(p22 191–22 192)]

To improve the health of rural White Americans, it is essential to name and frame their health in the context of Whiteness to identify areas of future research and points of intervention. Whiteness is a racialized system that endures through policies, processes, and normative beliefs, and Whiteness typically offers social, political, economic, and psychological benefits to White Americans.[19–21] Similar to racism,[22] Whiteness has been defined as a fundamental determinant of the health of racially minoritized and majoritized populations.[20,23,24] Whereas racism delineates and justifies who should be structurally disadvantaged and why, Whiteness indicates and explains who should experience some structural advantage and why. As a structuring force, Whiteness complements racism and contributes to the creation of racial categories and the subsequent experiences of minoritization or majoritization for those who are relegated into different racial groups (see "Fundamental Factors" section). Public health research commonly considers the health effects of oppression (racism) on racially minoritized populations, while it is rare to investigate the health effects of social supremacy (Whiteness) for the racially majoritized population.[20,23,25] This is likely because the structural and normative nature of Whiteness has obscured that White Americans have a race, ethnicity, and culture that can have meaningful implications for their health.

Following a brief description of the poor health of rural White Americans, we use an intersectional approach[26,27] and a fundamental determinants of health framework[22,28–30] to characterize the macrosocial nature of Whiteness and its intersection with rurality to frame the underlying social context that helps to explain the concentration of poor mental health, unhealthy stress coping behaviors, and high mortality among this population. We conclude with a discussion of implications and recommendations that may help to advance research to promote the health and well-being of rural White Americans.

WHY FOCUS ON RURAL WHITE AMERICANS?

White Americans constitute 3 out of every 4 (76%) rural residents, which is similar to the proportion of the US population (75.5%) who identify as non-Hispanic White.[31] While there is a growing amount of data documenting the poor health of rural Americans,[2] the lack of national rural health data that are regularly disaggregated by race and ethnicity make it difficult to depict the rural population in a way that facilitates identifying where and how best to intervene in a way that considers structural racism and Whiteness. Given the size of the rural White population, it is essential to uncover the determinants of White Americans' worsening mortality if we want to improve rural health in the United States.

RURAL WHITE AMERICANS' HEALTH PROFILE

Rural residence is a predictor of poor health status and mortality for White Americans in ways that are different from racially minoritized groups and nonrural White populations. Lack of access to health care in rural areas is a much stronger predictor of all-cause mortality for White Americans than Black Americans.[32] When compared with their Black American, Latinx, and Asian American counterparts, rural White residents have higher drug overdose death rates per 100 000 people (28.8 vs 18.9, 13.7, and 4.5, respectively).[33] Similarly, when compared with their American Indian/ Alaska Native, Black American, Latinx, and Asian/Pacific Islander counterparts, rural White residents have higher chronic lower respiratory disease death rates per 100 000 people (56.8 vs 44.9, 33.0, 20.3, and 13.5, respectively).[34] Relatedly, rural White Americans have a higher prevalence of cigarette smoking, are more likely to report current smoking and binge drinking, and are more likely to be diagnosed with alcohol use disorder than their racially minoritized rural counterparts.[35–37] Rural White Americans also report significantly more days with stress, depression, and problems with emotions than their nonrural White peers, rural Black Americans, and nonrural Black Americans.[38] In addition, rural residence is significantly associated with greater mentally unhealthy days for White Americans while rural residence is associated with fewer mentally unhealthy days for Black Americans.[38] More specifically, rural residence is a predictor of suicide for White American veterans, while rurality is not significantly associated with suicide among Black American or Latinx veterans.[39] Furthermore, rural White men have consistently higher suicide rates than rural and nonrural men who identity as Black, Asian, and Latinx.[40]

WHITENESS AS A FUNDAMENTAL DETERMINANT

Consistent with Schulz et al.,[29] we use fundamental cause and fundamental determinant interchangeably to describe factors that create contexts that shape how inequalities endure despite changes over time in diseases, risk and protective factors, and medical interventions. The health implications of fundamental factors cannot be eliminated by addressing the mechanisms that link the fundamental cause to health; fundamental causes must be addressed directly.[22]

Malat et al.[21] developed a novel theoretical framework to characterize how Whiteness contributes to White Americans' morbidity, mortality, and mental health via societal and social conditions that interact with White Americans' individual characteristics and psychosocial responses,[21] but there is not an organizing conceptual framework that has considered both rurality and Whiteness. Building on the work of Malat et al.,[21] we add rurality to Whiteness and provide examples of intermediate (e.g., rural culture, environment) and intrapersonal (e.g., psychosocial) factors through which Whiteness can contribute to rural White Americans' health (e.g., chronic disease, mental health, mortality) and well-being. Our conceptual framework (Figure 1) is grounded in the work of scholars[28,29,41] who have addressed fundamental determinants of health and seeks to identify pathways that could potentially illuminate points of intervention. Because it is imperative to consider how social and biological factors influence health,[42] our model illustrates how the structural nature of Whiteness interacts with social status, intermediate factors, intrapersonal factors, and health outcomes.

Fundamental Factors

Via ideology and policies predating and throughout US history, Whiteness structurally influences the dynamic process of White racial construction by delineating who holds the power and social status associated with being White.[23,43–47] Land-owning, Protestant colonizers from England and Scandinavian countries were some of the earliest "White Americans," yet the White racial category eventually expanded to include other ethnic groups from Europe, North Africa, and the Middle East,[44,48] and recently it contracted and removed Middle Eastern and North African people and made them their own category.[18] Whiteness presently determines who is "allowed" to be White via its influence on the US Office of Management and Budget (the government entity responsible for setting federal standards of how race and ethnicity should be collected in the United States), White racial construction, and White American ethnic identification.[44,46,49]

Largely invisible in society, particularly to most White people, Whiteness propagates the notion that the United States is an egalitarian meritocracy where all people have access to success and opportunities if they exert enough individual effort.[50–52] While all White Americans benefit from White racial dominance to some extent, the privileges and structural advantages of normative Whiteness are not distributed equally among all White people. For example, the "material share of the benefits of whiteness is low" for low-income and working-class White Americans relative to wealthier White Americans.[19(p187)] This is particularly true for rural White Americans who hold a lower socioeconomic position or who live in communities that have a high rate of poverty. Furthermore, the material share of Whiteness may be even lower for rural White Americans who exist at the intersections of other marginalized identities related to gender or sexual orientation.

Intermediate Factors

Qualitative research[53,54] and survey data[55] suggest that some rural White Americans see their identity as separate from White people who live in urban areas, because they believe there are distinct components of rural White

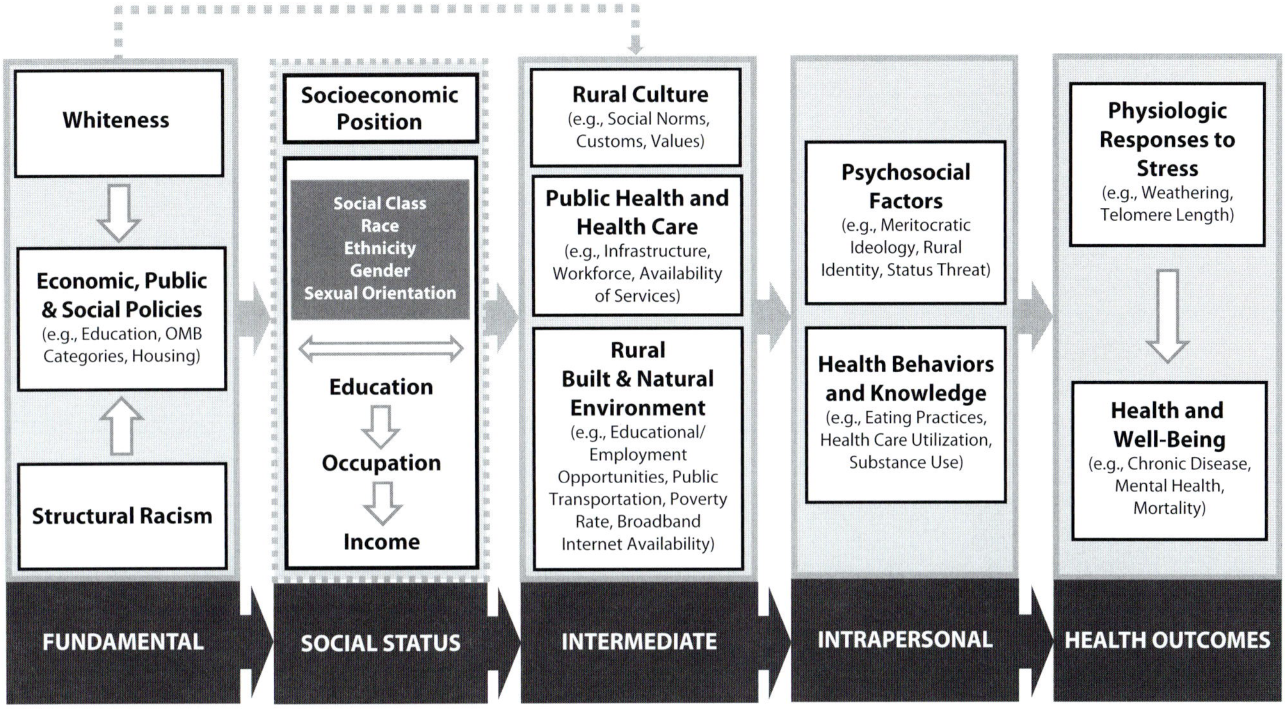

FIGURE 1— Whiteness as a Fundamental Determinant of Rural White Americans' Health

Note. OMB = US Office of Management and Budget. Figure 1 is grounded in Griffith et al.,[28] Schulz et al.,[29] and Williams and Mohammed's[30] conceptualization of racism as a fundamental (or basic) determinant of health.

American culture that are uniquely important. Culture comprises shared social norms, customs, values, and assumptions that "shape a group's beliefs, attitudes, and behavior through their interactions in and with their environments."[12(p197)] We posit that common cultural aspects of rurality—such as local beliefs and values (e.g., individualism, mistrust of outsiders)[50,53,56,57] or attitudes (e.g., normative racial resentment)[53,54,58,59]—may contribute to health disparities among rural White Americans. Notably, these beliefs and attitudes can be adopted by rural White Americans irrespective of higher or lower socioeconomic position.[50,53,60]

Within the context of rurality, Whiteness can promote unhealthy beliefs among some rural White adults—across the socioeconomic gradient—such that they nostalgically remember the era when the social dominance of White Americans was more pronounced.[50,53] For example, rural White Americans in one qualitative study reminisced about how their community was healthier "back in the good ol' days" when they indicated that their community mirrored Mayberry—a fictional, "utopian" town from the popular 1960s television series called *The Andy Griffith Show*.[50] The show rendered the Civil Rights Era experiences of Black Americans invisible throughout its 8 seasons, and there was only 1 episode in which a Black cast member had a speaking role.[61] Similarly, findings from the Community and Environment in Rural America survey highlight that White Americans from distressed rural communities across the nation are nostalgic for the "'heritage' of what used to be."[62(p76)] This nostalgia for the segregated past is a color-blind[19] misperception of what it means to have a healthy community because some rural White Americans' "Mayberry-like failure to acknowledge the past and present effects of structural racism"[50(p7)] mirrors their oversight of the health impact of other social and structural determinants of health, prompting them to believe that individual-level factors are the fundamental causes of many health outcomes. These whitewashed beliefs and attitudes are inaccurate and have the potential to harm rural White Americans' health.

Rural White Americans' meritocratic beliefs and attitudes can be reflected in their interpersonal interactions regarding their own and others' health and health care decisions. Multiple qualitative studies suggest that some rural White patients and providers blame individuals for developing lifestyle diseases and mental illnesses, and criticize medication use unless it serves as treatment of an illness that they perceive to be outside of one's individual control (e.g., genetic conditions, cancer).[50,53,60] Moreover, some rural White patients and health care providers disparage the use of medication-assisted treatment of mental illnesses and substance use disorders.[53,60,63] As such, the meritocratic cultural norms of independence and personal responsibility—which we argue are components of both Whiteness and rural White culture—may inhibit some rural White Americans from seeking out and utilizing health care services because they adhere to local norms and values. As noted, often the economic decline in rural areas shapes the built environment in ways that characterize the physical environment and hinder access to health care, public health services, mental health support, public transit, reliable broadband Internet, full-service grocery stores, and educational and employment opportunities.[4] Increases in rural hospital closures and health workforce shortages also negatively affect rural residents.[64–66] Intermediate barriers that exist in a built environment can increase the likelihood that one engages in unhealthy and risky behaviors because those are the resources the environment affords them to cope with stress.[67] Furthermore, "rates of deep poverty, near poverty, and relative poverty are almost universally higher" in nonmetropolitan US counties than metropolitan counties.[14(p10)] Not all rural White Americans are impoverished, but the clustering of impoverished people in rural areas speaks to the historical nature of the structural disadvantage faced by residents of rural communities (e.g., deindustrialization, resource extraction, lasting effects of plantation economies).[14]

Intrapersonal Factors

We posit that Whiteness contributes to psychosocial factors (e.g., belief in meritocratic ideology, perceived stressors) that can adversely affect the health and well-being of rural White Americans. Because stressors come in a variety of forms (e.g., life events, chronic strains, traumas) it is necessary to identify stressors within their broader social context.[68,69] The narratives of success that are intrinsic to Whiteness can adversely affect White Americans' health if they do not perceive that they are reaping the full benefits of being White.[21,50,51,58,59] Some rural White Americans' perceived threat to their social standing and their frustration with "outsiders"[53,60] is rooted in the ethnocentrism that Whiteness propagates. Ethnocentrism is the "practice and perception of regarding one's own ethnic, racial, or social group as the center of all things."[70] Ethnocentrism is a core component of status threat because it is about maintaining the protection and superiority of the in-group.[71] As such, Whiteness undergirds some rural White Americans' fears that their cultural norms are diminishing and the collective social status of White people in the United States is deteriorating. This experience of status threat likely produces stress and anxiety for rural White Americans because the disruption of meritocratic beliefs and expectations can produce psychological distress for White people.[72]

Because White Americans' beliefs about their position within social hierarchies can affect their health,[73,74] it is plausible that the stress response associated with status threat is contributing to the concentration of poor health among rural White populations.

In addition, qualitative research demonstrates that perceptions of social changes—such as shifting social norms and an influx of "outsiders" moving into their rural community—can be a source of stress for White (but not Black) rural Americans.[60] Relatedly, Straubel's[75] research with older White adults indicates that some White people believe that social changes equate to anti-White discrimination. According to Versey et al.,[72] the stress responses associated with perceptions of discrimination (i.e., "appropriated racial oppression") can produce adverse mental health effects for White Americans.

Furthermore, Cooley et al.[76] found that when White Americans believe that their social status is lower than that of the majority of White Americans, this predicts fewer positive emotions, which results in worse self-reported physical and mental health. Given the "White = wealthy" stereotype in the United States, low-income White Americans may perceive that they are even poorer,[77] and this belief can harm their health.[76] Moreover, perceptions of status incongruency may adversely affect telomere length (an indicator of stress-mediated biological aging) for White Americans, while this is not the case for Black Americans and Mexican immigrants.[51] Geronimus et al.[51] posit that some low-income White Americans have less resources to protect themselves from the potential negative effects of anxiety and environmental stressors than wealthier White Americans, which results in low-income White Americans' relatively shorter telomere length. Regardless of individual-level socioeconomic position, the extent to which rural White Americans believe in meritocratic "American Creed" ideology (e.g., emphasis on rewards for hard work, self-sufficiency) could be detrimental for their individual-level health outcomes because of the stress responses associated with those beliefs[50,51] and how these beliefs and stress responses intersect with their rural environment.

Moreover, rural White Americans' perceived status threat and associated health behaviors could pose a health risk to other marginalized populations. Interestingly, resistance to masking early in the COVID-19 pandemic among some rural White Americans was linked to perceptions of infringement on individual rights.[78] Other studies found that racial prejudice (specifically, anti-Blackness) among White Americans amplified opposition to masking and other health-promoting public health policies that were designed to reduce the spread of severe acute respiratory syndrome coronavirus 2 (SARS-CoV-2).[79,80] Policies that aim to promote equity and "level the playing field" for racially minoritized groups can contribute to feelings of resentment, anger, and threat among White Americans.[72] These perceptions of loss of status potentially adversely affect White Americans' collective morbidity and mortality,[74] and a recent scoping review denotes that feeling threatened by perceived changes in societal conditions can negatively affect White Americans' health at the individual and population level.[73] As such, some rural White Americans' perceived status threat is a pressing public health issue that warrants further investigation because it can negatively affect the health of White Americans and racially minoritized populations.

IMPLICATIONS

To improve health among rural White Americans, we offer a nuanced understanding of what contributes to rural White Americans' collective poor mental health and worsening mortality. Delineating how structural forces like Whiteness interact with aspects of rural culture, individually held beliefs and attitudes, and subsequent stress-related experiences and coping behaviors refines ways to inform policy and programmatic efforts to improve the health of rural White populations.

For example, applying Geronimus's weathering hypothesis,[81] we posit that stress over the life course could adversely affect the health of rural White Americans who experience the challenges of living in a rural area coupled with the perception that White people are losing status. Weathering emphasizes that chronic exposure to social and economic disadvantage contributes to accelerated biological aging and declines in health through psychosocial mechanisms (e.g., high-effort coping) that can lead to general health vulnerability, increased susceptibility to infectious disease, and the early onset of chronic conditions.[51,81] The adverse effects of weathering among racially minoritized groups are well-documented,[81] and it suggests that dominant racial group status does not protect White people from the negative health effects of impoverishment and other forms of perceived or actual marginalization.

Yet, we need empirical evidence to determine if and how the intersections of Whiteness, status threat, and the environmental challenges of living in rural areas affect White Americans' health and well-being over the life course across various levels of the socioeconomic gradient. While we hypothesize that the system of Whiteness is likely to disproportionately negatively affect the health of rural White Americans with lower socioeconomic position (SEP), it is unlikely that rural White Americans with higher SEP are immune to the negative health effects of Whiteness. For example, research on mental health among relatively high-SEP rural White Americans suggests that the ideology of Whiteness can still harm their mental health.[60] Thus, future research is needed to determine how individual-level SEP relates to the influence of Whiteness on White Americans' health and well-being within the context of rurality. While this article focuses on the rural White population in the United States in general, we hypothesize that there could be meaningful cultural and contextual variation among rural White Americans in different geographic regions (e.g., Appalachia, Pacific Northwest, Southeast) that differentially contributes to their health behaviors, psychosocial responses, and health outcomes via the intersections of Whiteness and other identities. Empirical evidence is needed to determine whether Whiteness similarly influences health-related intermediate and intrapersonal factors for rural White Americans who live in particular geographic contexts, given that cultural aspects of what it means to be a rural White person may vary by region and intersectional identities. For example, rural White transgender adolescents in the US South or rural White evangelical Christian older adult men in central Appalachia may experience unique intrapersonal factors that differentially affect their physiological responses to stress and mental health. Thus, we need empirical evidence to expose if and how health beliefs, attitudes, and behaviors vary among rural populations based on identities beyond race (e.g., gender, age, social class, political affiliation, sexual orientation, religion, geographic location, ability status).

Furthermore, we must consider how Whiteness contributes to the effectiveness of health communication and policy. Understanding how Whiteness influences subgroups of rural White Americans' acceptance or aversion to public health policies could enhance our efforts to frame health communication in ways that are culturally appropriate.[12] We posit that policies that emphasize the health of the collective (e.g., wearing a face mask to prevent the spread of SARS-CoV-2) may be contrary to the values of rural White Americans who adhere to the individualism and ethnocentrism espoused by Whiteness. Without considering Whiteness, well-intentioned public health campaigns and policies could exacerbate health inequities.[23] For instance, some White Americans were less concerned about masking and social distancing when they read messages indicating that COVID-19 had a disproportionately negative impact on Black Americans.[79,80] As such, accounting for the ideology of Whiteness could help us avoid framing health communication and policies in ways that inadvertently reinforce racism. More research is needed to determine how Whiteness similarly or dissimilarly influences health beliefs and policy attitudes among rural, nonrural, and other subgroups of White Americans.

In sum, utilizing racialized framing, considering rurality and Whiteness simultaneously, and recognizing Whiteness as a fundamental determinant of health are essential to refining our understanding of, and ability to improve, the health of rural White Americans. AJPH

ABOUT THE AUTHORS

Caroline R. Efird is with the Department of Health Management and Policy, School of Health, Georgetown University, Washington, DC. Derek M. Griffith is with the Department of Family and Community Health, School of Nursing, and Department of Medical Ethics and Health Policy, Perelman School of Medicine, University of Pennsylvania, Philadelphia. Both authors were affiliated with the Racial Justice Institute and Center for Men's Health Equity at Georgetown University during the initial development of this essay.

CORRESPONDENCE

Correspondence should be sent to Caroline R. Efird, Assistant Professor of Health Management and Policy, Georgetown University School of Health, 3700 Reservoir Rd, NW, Washington, DC 20057 (e-mail: caroline.efird@georgetown.edu). Reprints can be ordered at https://www.ajph.org by clicking the "Reprints" link.

PUBLICATION INFORMATION

Full Citation: Efird CR, Griffith DM. Whiteness: a fundamental determinant of the health of rural White Americans. *Am J Public Health*. 2025;115(2): 152–160.

Acceptance Date: October 18, 2024.

DOI: https://doi.org/10.2105/AJPH.2024.307904

ORCID iDs:

Caroline R. Efird https://orcid.org/0000-0001-7258-463X

Derek M. Griffith https://orcid.org/0000-0003-0018-9176

CONTRIBUTORS

C. R. Efird led the conceptualization, writing, and revisions of the article. D. M. Griffith substantially contributed to conceptualization, writing, and editing.

ACKNOWLEDGMENTS

C. R. Efird's contributions to this article were supported in part by a fellowship at the Racial Justice Institute at Georgetown University.

We are grateful to the *AJPH* associate editor Lisa Bowleg, the editorial team, and several anonymous peer reviewers for their thoughtful feedback on this essay.

CONFLICTS OF INTEREST

The authors have no conflicts of interest to report.

HUMAN PARTICIPANT PROTECTION

Institutional review board approval was not necessary for this analytic essay because no human participants were involved in this research.

REFERENCES

1. US Census Bureau. Nation's urban and rural populations shift following 2020 Census. December 29, 2022. Available at: https://www.census.gov/newsroom/press-releases/2022/urban-rural-populations.html. Accessed September 9, 2023.
2. Abrams LR, Myrskylä M, Mehta NK. The growing rural–urban divide in US life expectancy: contribution of cardiovascular disease and other major causes of death. *Int J Epidemiol*. 2022;50(6): 1970–1978. https://doi.org/10.1093/ije/dyab158
3. Centers for Disease Control and Prevention. About rural health. Rural health. May 16, 2024. Available at: https://www.cdc.gov/rural-health/php/about/index.html. Accessed November 8, 2024.
4. Mujuru P, Dinwiddie G, Marshall V, et al. Understanding and addressing health disparities and health care among rural populations. National Institute on Minority Health and Health Disparities. February 7, 2023. Available at: https://www.nimhd.nih.gov/docs/approved-fund-concepts/nacmhd_apprvdConcept_2023feb_ruralHD.pdf. Accessed May 27, 2024.
5. Dobis EA, Krumel TP, Cromartie JC, Conley KL, Sanders A, Ortiz R. *Rural America at a Glance*. Washington, DC: US Department of Agriculture, Economic Research Service; 2021:1–16.
6. Kozhimannil KB, Henning-Smith C. Racism and health in rural America. *J Health Care Poor Underserved*. 2018;29(1):35–43. https://doi.org/10.1353/hpu.2018.0004
7. Ramesh T, Tsai TC. Hospital closures in rural communities of color: a double dose of inequality. *J Rural Health*. 2023;39(1):88–90. https://doi.org/10.1111/jrh.12704
8. National Institute on Minority Health and Health Disparities. Rural health disparities and health care. February 2023. Available at: https://www.nimhd.nih.gov/funding/approved-concepts/2023/rural-health-disparities-and-health-care.html. Accessed September 9, 2023.
9. Ziller E, Milkowski C. A century later: rural public health's enduring challenges and opportunities. *Am J Public Health*. 2020;110(11):1678–1686. https://doi.org/10.2105/AJPH.2020.305868
10. Henning-Smith C, Hernandez AM, Ramirez M, Hardeman R, Kozhimannil K. Dying too soon: county-level disparities in premature death by rurality, race, and ethnicity. University of Minnesota Rural Health Research Center. 2019. Available at: https://rhrc.umn.edu/wp-content/uploads/2019/03/1552267547UMNpolicybriefPrematureDeath.pdf. Accessed November 16, 2020.
11. Monnat SM. Trends in US working-age non-Hispanic White mortality: rural–urban and within-rural differences. *Popul Res Policy Rev*. 2020;39(5): 805–834. https://doi.org/10.1007/s11113-020-09607-6
12. Griffith DM, Efird CR, Baskin ML, Webb Hooper M, Davis RE, Resnicow K. Cultural sensitivity and cultural tailoring: lessons learned and refinements after two decades of incorporating culture in health communication research. *Annu Rev Public Health*. 2024;45(1):195–212. https://doi.org/10.1146/annurev-publhealth-060722-031158
13. Richman L, Pearson J, Beasley C, Stanifer J. Addressing health inequalities in diverse, rural communities: an unmet need. *SSM Popul Health*. 2019;7:100398. https://doi.org/10.1016/j.ssmph.2019.100398
14. Tickamyer AR. Rural poverty: research and policy for U.S. families. In: Glick JE, McHale SM, King V, eds. *Rural Families and Communities in the United States: Facing Challenges and Leveraging Opportunities*. Vol 10. National Symposium on Family Issues. Cham, Switzerland: Springer International Publishing; 2020:3–26. https://doi.org/10.1007/978-3-030-37689-5_1

15. Bailey ZD, Krieger N, Agénor M, Graves J, Linos N, Bassett MT. Structural racism and health inequities in the USA: evidence and interventions. *Lancet.* 2017;389(10077):1453–1463. https://doi.org/10.1016/S0140-6736(17)30569-X
16. Alang S, Hardeman R, Karbeah J, et al. White supremacy and the core functions of public health. *Am J Public Health.* 2021;111(5):815–819. https://doi.org/10.2105/AJPH.2020.306137
17. Bowleg L. The White racial frame of public health discourses about racialized health differences and "disparities": what it reveals about power and how it thwarts health equity. *Front Public Health.* 2023;11:1187307. https://doi.org/10.3389/fpubh.2023.1187307
18. Office of Management and Budget. Revisions to OMB's Statistical Policy Directive No. 15: Standards for Maintaining, Collecting, and Presenting Federal Data on Race and Ethnicity. *Fed Regist.* 2024:22182–22196. Available at: https://www.federalregister.gov/documents/2024/03/29/2024-06469/revisions-to-ombs-statistical-policy-directive-no-15-standards-for-maintaining-collecting-and. Accessed May 25, 2024.
19. Bonilla-Silva E. *Racism Without Racists: Color-Blind Racism and the Persistence of Racial Inequality in America.* 6th ed. Lanham, MD: Rowman & Littlefield; 2022.
20. Efird CR, Wilkins CL, Versey HS. Whiteness hurts society: how Whiteness shapes mental, physical, and social health outcomes. *J Soc Issues.* 2024;80(1):53–79. https://doi.org/10.1111/josi.12598
21. Malat J, Mayorga-Gallo S, Williams DR. The effects of Whiteness on the health of Whites in the USA. *Soc Sci Med.* 2018;199:148–156. https://doi.org/10.1016/j.socscimed.2017.06.034
22. Phelan JC, Link BG. Is racism a fundamental cause of inequalities in health? *Annu Rev Sociol.* 2015;41(1):311–330. https://doi.org/10.1146/annurev-soc-073014-112305
23. Efird CR, Griffith DM. Whiteness: a fundamental determinant of health. In: Ford CL, Griffith DM, eds. *Racism: Science & Tools for the Public Health Professional.* 2nd ed. Washington, DC: American Public Health Association; 2024. https://doi.org/10.2105/9780875533537ch07
24. National Collaborating Centre for Determinants of Health. *Let's Talk: Whiteness and Health Equity.* St Francis Xavier University. 2020. Available at: https://nccdh.ca/images/uploads/comments/Lets-talk-whiteness-and-health-equity_2020_EN.pdf. Accessed November 8, 2024.
25. Pearson JA. Can't buy me Whiteness. *Du Bois Rev.* 2008;5(1):27–48. https://doi.org/10.1017/S1742058X0808003X
26. Crenshaw K. Mapping the margins: intersectionality, identity politics, and violence against women of color. *Stanford Law Rev.* 1993;43(6):1241–1299.
27. Griffith DM. Gender health equity: the case for including men's health. *Soc Sci Med.* 2024;351(suppl 1):116863. https://doi.org/10.1016/j.socscimed.2024.116863
28. Griffith DM, Towfighi A, Manson SM, Littlejohn EL, Skolarus LE. Determinants of inequities in neurologic disease, health, and well-being: the NINDS Social Determinants of Health Framework. *Neurology.* 2023;101(7 suppl1):S75–S81. https://doi.org/10.1212/WNL.0000000000207566
29. Schulz AJ, Williams DR, Israel BK, Bex Lempert L. Racial and spatial relations as fundamental determinants of health in Detroit. *Milbank Q.* 2002;80(4):677–707. https://doi.org/10.1111/1468-0009.00028
30. Williams DR, Mohammed SA. Racism and health I: pathways and scientific evidence. *Am Behav Sci.* 2013;57(8):1152–1173. https://doi.org/10.1177/0002764213487340
31. Johnson K, Lichter D. Growing racial diversity in rural America: results from the 2020 Census. University of New Hampshire, Carsey School of Public Policy. May 22, 2022. Available at: https://carsey.unh.edu/publication/growing-racial-diversity-in-rural-america. Accessed September 9, 2023.
32. James W, Cossman JS. Long-term trends in Black and White mortality in the rural United States: evidence of a race-specific rural mortality penalty. *J Rural Health.* 2017;33(1):21–31. https://doi.org/10.1111/jrh.12181
33. Spencer MR, Garnett MF, Miniño AM. Urban–rural differences in drug overdose death rates, 2020. *NCHS Data Brief.* 2022;(440):1–8. https://doi.org/10.15620/118601
34. Probst JC, Zahnd WE, Hung P, Eberth JM, Crouch EL, Merrell MA. Rural-urban mortality disparities: variations across causes of death and race/ethnicity, 2013–2017. *Am J Public Health.* 2020;110(9):1325–1327. https://doi.org/10.2105/AJPH.2020.305703
35. Arauz RF, Mayer M, Reyes-Guzman C, Ryan BM. Racial disparities in cigarette smoking behaviors and differences stratified by metropolitan area of residence. *Int J Environ Res Public Health.* 2022;19(5):2910. https://doi.org/10.3390/ijerph19052910
36. Dixon MA, Chartier KG. Alcohol use patterns among urban and rural residents: demographic and social influences. *Alcohol Res.* 2016;38(1):69–77.
37. James CV, Moonesinghe R, Wilson-Frederick SM, Hall JE, Penman-Aguilar A, Bouye K. Racial/ethnic health disparities among rural adults—United States, 2012–2015. *MMWR Surveill Summ.* 2017;66(23):1–9. https://doi.org/10.15585/mmwr.ss6623a1
38. Efird CR, Matthews DD, Muessig KE, Barrington CL, Metzl JM, Lightfoot AF. Rural and nonrural racial variation in mentally unhealthy days: findings from the Behavioral Risk Factor Surveillance System in North Carolina, 2015–2019. *SSM Ment Health.* 2023;3:100199. https://doi.org/10.1016/j.ssmmh.2023.100199
39. Peltzman T, Gottlieb DJ, Levis M, Shiner B. The role of race in rural–urban suicide disparities. *J Rural Health.* 2022;38(2):346–354. https://doi.org/10.1111/jrh.12603
40. Centers for Disease Control and Prevention. Disparities in suicide. November 2, 2022. Available at: https://www.cdc.gov/suicide/facts/disparities-in-suicide.html. Accessed February 3, 2023.
41. Williams DR, Collins C. Racial residential segregation: a fundamental cause of racial disparities in health. *Public Health Rep.* 2001;116(5):404–416. https://doi.org/10.1016/S0033-3549(04)50068-7
42. Krieger N. Proximal, distal, and the politics of causation: what's level got to do with it? *Am J Public Health.* 2008;98(2):221–230. https://doi.org/10.2105/AJPH.2007.111278
43. Helms JE. The challenge of making Whiteness visible: reactions to four Whiteness articles. *Couns Psychol.* 2017;45(5):717–726. https://doi.org/10.1177/0011000017718943
44. Painter NI. *The History of White People.* 1st ed. New York, NY: W. W. Norton & Company; 2010.
45. Roediger DR. *The Wages of Whiteness: Race and the Making of the American Working Class.* Revised ed. Brooklyn, NY: Verso; 2007.
46. Torkelson J, Hartmann D. The heart of Whiteness: on the study of Whiteness and White Americans. *Sociol Compass.* 2021;15(11):e12932. https://doi.org/10.1111/soc4.12932
47. Du Bois WEB. *Black Reconstruction in America (The Oxford W. E. B. Du Bois): An Essay Toward a History of the Part Which Black Folk Played in the Attempt to Reconstruct Democracy in America, 1860–1880.* 1st ed. New York, NY: Oxford University Press; 2014:623.
48. Omi M, Winant H. *Racial Formation in the United States From the 1960s to the 1990s.* 3rd ed. New York, NY: Routledge; 2014.
49. Fields K, Fields BJ. *Racecraft: The Soul of Inequality in American Life.* Brooklyn, NY: Verso; 2012:310.
50. Efird CR, Lightfoot AF. Missing Mayberry: how Whiteness shapes perceptions of health among White Americans in a rural Southern community. *Soc Sci Med.* 2020;253:112967. https://doi.org/10.1016/j.socscimed.2020.112967
51. Geronimus AT, Pearson JA, Linnenbringer E, et al. Race-ethnicity, poverty, urban stressors, and telomere length in a Detroit community-based sample. *J Health Soc Behav.* 2015;56(2):199–224. https://doi.org/10.1177/0022146515582100
52. Kwate NOA, Meyer IH. The myth of meritocracy and African American health. *Am J Public Health.* 2010;100(10):1831–1834. https://doi.org/10.2105/AJPH.2009.186445
53. Efird CR. "Different than a regular White": exploring health-related White identity politics in rural Appalachia. *Du Bois Rev.* 2022;19(1):107–128. https://doi.org/10.1017/S1742058X21000333
54. Lensmire TJ. *White Folks: Race and Identity in Rural America.* New York, NY: Routledge; 2017. https://doi.org/10.4324/9781315180359
55. Lunz Trujillo K. Rural identity as a contributing factor to anti-Intellectualism in the US. *Polit Behav.* 2022;44(3):1509–1532. https://doi.org/10.1007/s11109-022-09770-w
56. Cheesmond NE, Davies K, Inder KJ. Exploring the role of rurality and rural identity in mental health help-seeking behavior: a systematic qualitative review. *Rural Mental Health.* 2019;43(1):45–59. https://doi.org/10.1037/rmh0000109
57. Walton E. A culture of Whiteness: how integration failed in cities, suburbs, and small towns. *Sociol Compass.* 2021;15(11):e12930. https://doi.org/10.1111/soc4.12930
58. Daniels J. Whiteness and health and dying in America. *Am J Public Health.* 2019;109(9):1152–1153. https://doi.org/10.2105/AJPH.2019.305225
59. Metzl JM. *Dying of Whiteness.* New York, NY: Hachette Book Group; 2019.
60. Efird CR, Barrington C, Metzl JM, Muessig KE, Matthews DD, Lightfoot AF. "We grew up in the church": a critical discourse analysis of Black and White rural residents' perceptions of mental health. *Soc Sci Med.* 2023;336:116245. https://doi.org/10.1016/j.socscimed.2023.116245
61. McElroy K. Remembering Mayberry in White and Black: The Andy Griffith Show's construction of the South. *Mem Stud.* 2015;8(4):440–453. https://doi.org/10.1177/1750698015581073
62. Ulrich-Schad JD, Duncan CM. People and places left behind: work, culture and politics in the rural United States. *J Peasant Stud.* 2018;45(1):59–79. https://doi.org/10.1080/03066150.2017.1410702

63. Richard EL, Schalkoff CA, Piscalko HM, et al. "You are not clean until you're not on anything": perceptions of medication-assisted treatment in rural Appalachia. *Int J Drug Policy.* 2020;85:102704. https://doi.org/10.1016/j.drugpo.2020.102704
64. Kaufman BG, Thomas SR, Randolph RK, et al. The rising rate of rural hospital closures. *J Rural Health.* 2016;32(1):35–43. https://doi.org/10.1111/jrh.12128
65. Kett PM, Bekemeier B, Patterson DG, Schaffer K. Competencies, training needs, and turnover among rural compared with urban local public health practitioners: 2021 Public Health Workforce Interests and Needs Survey. *Am J Public Health.* 2023;113(6):689–699. https://doi.org/10.2105/AJPH.2023.307273
66. Thomas SR, Holmes GM, Pink GH. To what extent do community characteristics explain differences in closure among financially distressed rural hospitals? *J Health Care Poor Underserved.* 2016;27(4A):194–203. https://doi.org/10.1353/hpu.2016.0176
67. Mezuk B, Abdou CM, Hudson D, et al. "White box" epidemiology and the social neuroscience of health behaviors: the environmental affordances model. *Soc Ment Health.* 2013;3(2):79–95. https://doi.org/10.1177/2156869313480892
68. McLeod JD. The meanings of stress. *Soc Ment Health.* 2012;2(3):172–186. https://doi.org/10.1177/2156869312452877
69. Pearlin LI, Menaghan EG, Liberman MA, Mullen JT. The stress process. *J Health Soc Behav.* 1981;22(4):337–356. https://doi.org/10.2307/2136676
70. American Psychological Association. APA Dictionary of Psychology. 2023. Available at: https://dictionary.apa.org/ethnocentrism. Accessed September 25, 2023.
71. Parker CS. Status threat: moving the right further to the right? *Daedalus.* 2021;150(2):56–75. https://doi.org/10.1162/daed_a_01846
72. Versey H, Cogburn CC, Wilkins CL, Joseph N. Appropriated racial oppression: implications for mental health in Whites and Blacks. *Soc Sci Med.* 2019;230:295–302. https://doi.org/10.1016/j.socscimed.2019.03.014
73. Efird CR, Bennett F, Metzl JM, Siddiqi A. Perceived status threat and health among White Americans: a scoping review. *SSM Popul Health.* 2023;21:101326. https://doi.org/10.1016/j.ssmph.2022.101326
74. Siddiqi A, Sod-Erdene O, Hamilton D, Cottom TM, Darity W. Growing sense of social status threat and concomitant deaths of despair among Whites. *SSM Popul Health.* 2019;9:100449. https://doi.org/10.1016/j.ssmph.2019.100449
75. Straubel MG. *"I Was Raised Not Persecuting at All": How White Southerners Use Privileged Persecution.* Master's thesis. University of North Carolina at Chapel Hill; 2020.
76. Cooley E, Brown-Iannuzzi JL, Lei RF, Philbrook LE, Cipolli W, McKee SE. Investigating the health consequences for White Americans who believe White Americans are wealthy. *Soc Psychol Personal Sci.* 2020;12(3):371–382. https://doi.org/10.1177/1948550620905219
77. Cohen D, Shin F, Liu X, Ondish P, Kraus MW. Defining social class across time and between groups. *Pers Soc Psychol Bull.* 2017;43(11):1530–1545. https://doi.org/10.1177/0146167217721174
78. Shelus VS, Frank SC, Lazard AJ, et al. Motivations and barriers for the use of face coverings during the COVID-19 pandemic: messaging insights from focus groups. *Int J Environ Res Public Health.* 2020;17(24):9298. https://doi.org/10.3390/ijerph17249298
79. Stephens-Dougan L. White Americans' reactions to racial disparities in COVID-19. *Am Polit Sci Rev.* 2022;117(2):1–8. https://doi.org/10.1017/S000305542200051X
80. Miller CA, Wilkins CL, de Paula Couto C, Farias J, Lisnek JA. Anti-Black attitudes predict decreased concern about COVID-19 among Whites in the U.S. and Brazil. *Soc Sci Med.* 2023;320:115712. https://doi.org/10.1016/j.socscimed.2023.115712
81. Geronimus AT, Pearson JA, Linnenbringer E, et al. Weathering in Detroit: place, race, ethnicity, and poverty as conceptually fluctuating social constructs shaping variation in allostatic load. *Milbank Q.* 2020;98(4):1171–1218. https://doi.org/10.1111/1468-0009.12484

Legacy of Racism and Firearm Violence During the COVID-19 Pandemic in the United States

Zainab Hans, PhD, Daniel B. Lee, PhD, Marc A. Zimmerman, PhD, and Douglas J. Wiebe, PhD

See also Whiteness and Redlining, pp. 146–160.

Objectives. To examine whether, through interactions with preexisting socioeconomic status vulnerabilities, the COVID-19 pandemic exacerbated exposure to firearm violence among communities with a legacy of redlining (i.e., grading the creditworthiness of neighborhoods based on their sociodemographic composition).

Methods. We used an exogenous population threshold whereby the Home Owners Loan Corporation graded neighborhoods only in US cities with populations of more than 40 000 and used a difference-in-difference strategy to examine the evolution of fatal firearm incidents between 2017 and October 2022.

Results. After the COVID-19 pandemic began, fatal firearm violence increased significantly in low-graded neighborhoods that the Home Owners Loan Corporation had deemed risky for mortgage lending. The effect held consistently across various model specifications.

Conclusions. Social and environmental constructs can interact in a complex manner to compound disadvantage and exacerbate the consequences of negative shocks for marginalized communities.

Public Health Implications. Home Owners Loan Corporation policies contributed to widening racial disparities in firearm violence, highlighting the need for reinvestment in marginalized communities to keep future shocks from exacerbating vulnerability to adverse outcomes. (*Am J Public Health*. 2025;115(2):161–169. https://doi.org/10.2105/AJPH.2024.307891)

AJPH February 2025, Vol. 115, No. 2

Marginalized communities bear a disproportionate burden of firearm violence—reflecting deep-seated disparities in safety and well-being.[1] Alarmingly, these gaps appear to be widening.[2] Between 2019 and 2020, the overall firearm homicide rate increased by 34.6%, with the largest increases occurring among Black and American Indian/Alaska Native males.[1] The advent of the COVID-19 pandemic and the disruptions it caused in social and economic processes differentially affected people of color,[3,4] likely contributing to increased violence.[5]

Although pandemics are indiscriminate, their consequences can affect certain populations disproportionately by amplifying structural vulnerabilities in socioeconomic status.[4,6]

The differential incidence of COVID-19–related morbidity and mortality among Black and other minority groups demonstrates how social and environmental constructs interact to exacerbate negative shocks among resource deprived communities.[6] Like health risks, exposure to violence is often rooted in longstanding socioeconomic inequities. Given the parallels between the disproportionate burden of COVID-19 and firearm violence on racial minority groups, it is likely that the pandemic increased exposure to firearm violence by reinforcing structural barriers among communities with a history of marginalization.

Redlining—restricting credit access of neighborhoods occupied predominantly by Black and other minoritized individuals—was instrumental in entrenching racial inequities by causing residential segregation and long-term disinvestment.[7] By systematically channeling resources away from these communities, this policy led to concentrated poverty and limited opportunities for upward social mobility.[8,9] The structural vulnerabilities stemming from this economic marginalization have had enduring and devastating impacts on health and safety.[6,10–12]

There is a small nascent literature examining the effects of exogenous disease-related shocks on various forms of violence, including civil unrest and war.[13–16] This literature illustrates the profound impact economic disadvantage has on how resiliently communities can weather public health crises. This body of work highlights the crucial links between economic factors, epidemic outbreaks, and violence and shows that the issue extends beyond the direct impacts of health shocks to how these shocks interact with underlying social and structural inequities.

Although this literature focuses primarily on countries with weak institutional environments and volatile political structures,[13,15,16] the fundamental conclusions may be transferable to marginalized communities irrespective of their country's economic development or political stability. Unsurprisingly, research focusing on the nexus of firearm violence and the COVID-19 pandemic in developed countries has found that racial and economic factors amplify the disparities in firearm violence.[5,12]

However, few studies have explicitly investigated the underlying role of discriminatory policies, such as redlining, in intensifying violence when communities are hit by a negative shock.[12] We exploited an exogenous population threshold to compare neighborhoods assigned low grades by the Home Owners Loan Corporation (HOLC) with similar neighborhoods. We employed a difference-in-difference framework to evaluate whether the COVID-19 pandemic's exacerbation of the socioeconomic vulnerabilities created by HOLC policies led to a disproportionate increase in firearm violence among marginalized communities.

Our research expanded on previous literature on firearm violence and public health crises by examining a specific but important issue: the interaction of an exogenous shock with underlying structural inequities in an economically advanced country. We provide empirical evidence of how racial and economic disparities influenced the distribution of firearm violence during a nationwide public health emergency. In demonstrating the enduring repercussions of historical discriminatory policies, we underscore the urgent need to rectify the structural conditions that foster violence to safeguard these communities against the harmful consequences of future shocks.

METHODS

The HOLC created residential security maps for more than 200 US cities to classify their creditworthiness to stabilize the housing market after the Great Depression. Residential neighborhoods were assigned grades "A" through "D" to symbolize the risk involved in financial lending, with "A" signifying high creditworthiness and "D" a hazardous investment. Of note, the racial composition of a neighborhood was a key determining factor in assigning these grades. Neighborhoods with a growing or high proportion of racial minority residents received lower grades (i.e., C and D), signaling undesirability for mortgage lending. Each grade was represented by a specific color on the maps, with green being the best (A) and red being the worst (D), leading to the colloquial term "redlining."

However, HOLC's focus on larger cities created an exogenous population threshold, whereby cities with fewer than 40 000 residents in the 1930s were not subjected to grading even though many of the neighborhoods in these cities had demographic and socioeconomic characteristics comparable to neighborhoods that were graded. This allowed us to compare similar neighborhoods above and below the threshold and analyze the increase in firearm fatalities in low-graded neighborhoods after the beginning of the COVID-19 pandemic.

Analytical Strategy

To identify appropriate controls for graded neighborhoods, we used a data set created by Hynsjö and Perdoni,[17] who used a machine-learning algorithm to replicate the original HOLC grade assignment for neighborhoods in cities that had fewer than 40 000 residents in the 1930s. Hynsjö and Perdoni used ESRI StreetMap (Redlands, CA) to geocode addresses available in the full count 1930 US census data.[17] The ESRI algorithm assigned each address–coordinate match a score between 100 and 0. Higher scores indicate better matches. To reduce measurement error, Hynsjö and Perdoni excluded matches with a score of 84 or less and used digitized HOLC maps to convert originally graded neighborhoods into a grid of hexagons—each roughly the size of a New York City block. Although Hynsjö and Perdoni chose the size and shape of the hexagons to capture the boundaries of HOLC neighborhoods as precisely and compactly as possible, in some instances a single hexagon occupied more than 1 grade because areas demarked by the HOLC had nonuniform shapes.

To avoid conflating different socioeconomic characteristics, Hynsjö and Perdoni excluded hexagons occupying less than 75% of a single grade and used a random forest algorithm to predict and assign grades to similar sized hexagons in control cities (i.e., cities with < 40 000 residents in the1930s). The random forest approach split the data set recursively using multiple decision trees. In each tree, decision nodes partitioned the data to maximize the predictive power of covariates. The model used a nonlinear multivariate function to classify instances into pure leaves so that all instances belonged to a single grade. Appendix Table A (available as a supplement to the online version of this article at http://www.ajph.org) provides a list of the census variable used in training the machine learning algorithm. More details on the creation of the data set are provided in Hynsjö and Perdoni.[17]

Figure 1 provides an evaluation of the classification model by comparing the predicted and observed grades for cities with populations between 40 000 and 50 000 residents. Overall, the out-of-sample accuracy is greater than 90%.[17]

Figure 2 provides a visual interpretation of the classification model. Panel b shows the digitized versions of the original HOLC maps for Pittsburgh, Pennsylvania, and panel a shows the replication created by the machine-learning algorithm. Given the slight overlap in C and D neighborhoods in the predicted maps, we aggregated these (i.e., low-graded neighborhoods) for our analysis. Aggregation of low- and high-graded neighborhoods is not unusual when studying relatively rare outcomes such as firearm violence,[18] as C and D neighborhoods faced similar constraints and exclusion from financial markets. Although differences between C and D boundaries dissipated over time, differences continued to persist between C and B neighborhoods.[9] Furthermore, the aggregation addresses the problem posed by the very small number of A graded neighborhoods, which makes grade-specific analysis infeasible for that classification.

To minimize confounding by unobservable variables, we limited our analysis to control cities with a 1930 population of between 25 000 and 39 999 and treatment cities with a 1930 population of between 40 000 and 55 000. We estimated a negative binomial model to accommodate the overdispersed nature of our count outcome. Our difference-in-difference model can be specified as

$$\log(Y_{cq}) = \beta_0 + \beta_1 G_c C_q + \beta_2 X_c + \varphi_c + \tau_q + \epsilon_{cq} + \log(\rho_{cq}), \quad (1)$$

where Y_{cq} is the number of firearm fatalities that occurred in low-graded neighborhoods of city c and quarter q; G_c is the treatment indicator signifying if a city was graded by HOLC; $C_q$is the indicator for the period after and takes on the value of 1 for periods after March 2020, signifying the emergence of the COVID-19 pandemic; X_c are city-level covariates; ρ_{cq} is the city-level population included as exposure; and φ_c and τ_q represent city and quarter fixed effects. Bootstrapped SEs account for correlation among observations over time.

We also conducted a series of robustness checks to test the validity of our findings. Because we compared smaller cities with larger ones, if cities were on different trajectories of firearm violence

		Observed Grades			
		A	B	C	D
Predicted Grades	A	866	45	18	3
	B	153	2647	214	36
	C	18	219	4435	233
	D	0	12	117	2139
Class Sensitivity		83.72	90.56	92.70	88.72
Overall Accuracy 90.43%					

FIGURE 1— Random Forest Confusion Matrix: United States

Note. The matrix shows a comparison between the observed and predicted grades for hexagons located in cities with populations under 50 000. The comparison is conducted using a test set comprising of a 25% random subsample of the original dataset that was excluded from the training phase.

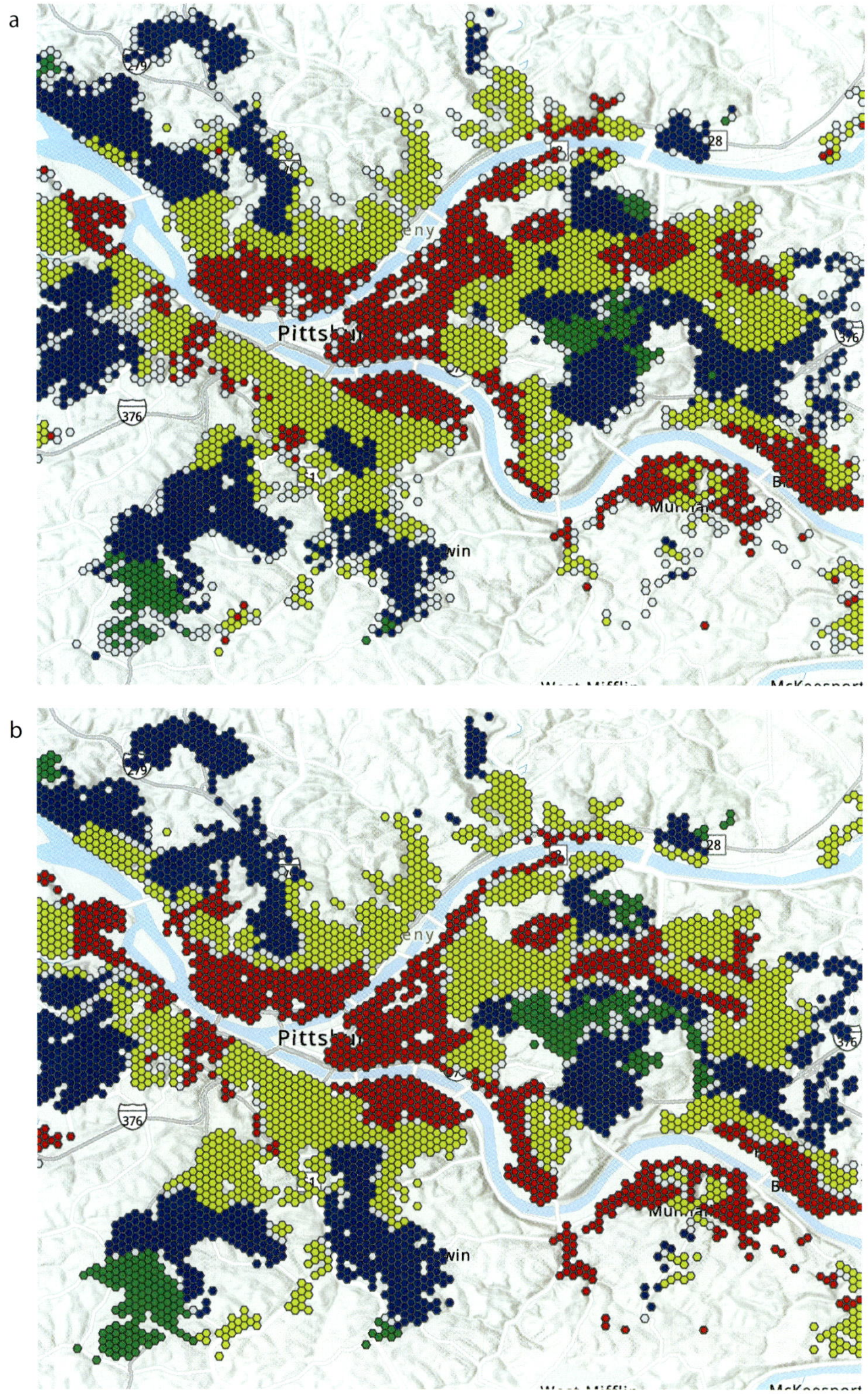

FIGURE 2— Comparison of (a) Predicted and (b) Original Maps: Pittsburgh, PA

Note. Part a shows neighborhood maps predicted by the random forest algorithm, and part b shows digitized versions of the original Home Owners Loan Corporation (HOLC) maps. Green = A, blue = B, yellow = C, and red = D. Gray hexagons had fewer than 20 residents in 1930 and were not included in the random forest algorithm to reduce prediction error.

that were unrelated to the systemic vulnerabilities created by HOLC practices, we might expect to see differences in both high- and low-graded neighborhoods in treatment and control cities. Therefore, we aggregated A- and B-graded neighborhoods and used them as negative controls. We also conducted a falsification test using a placebo population threshold to define a control group comprising cities that had between 40 000 and 55 000 residents in the 1930s and a treatment group of cities with 55 000 to 70 000 residents to evaluate differences in these groups.

We further examined how firearm fatalities evolved in high- versus low-graded neighborhoods in treated and control cities. Lastly, because our primary analysis focused on smaller cities, where the patterns of gun violence may not be as indicative of broader US trends, we conducted additional supplementary analyses using a larger sample. Because it was not possible to create a control group for larger cities, we employed propensity score–weighted difference-in-difference analysis, excluding originally mapped cities with a contemporary population greater than 250 000 to achieve good covariate balance.

Data

We obtained data for firearm fatalities from the Gun Violence Archive (GVA)—a crowdsourced database that provides detailed information on a broad spectrum of firearm violence.[19] We aggregated GVA incidents that occurred between July 2017 and October 2022 to a quarterly level and geocoded them. We then merged quarterly counts of firearm fatalities with the neighborhood hexagons (Appendix Figure A [available as a supplement to the online version of this article at http://www.ajph.org] provides an example). We extended our analysis beyond the initial wave of COVID-19, as different variants continued to cause high levels of mortality until March 2022. Moreover, during the initial peak in the number of infectious cases, many states issued shelter-in-place orders that may have resulted in differential exposure to crime.

Using data from the American Community Survey collected at the city level, we controlled for the percentage of the population that was White, Black, or another racial minority; was unemployed; was living below the poverty level; had less than a high school diploma; and was a man aged between 18 and 49 years. Additionally, we used data from RAND's state Firearm Law Database[20] to construct dichotomous variables to indicate the presence of permit-to-purchase requirements and stand-your-ground laws. Lastly, in estimating the propensity scores, we included the 2020 residential segregation data from the Dissimilarity Index provided by the American Communities Project as well as the percentage of the population that was married and the median income from the American Community Survey.

RESULTS

We began by ensuring that changes in socioeconomic conditions since the 1930s had not rendered control cities an inappropriate comparison group. Appendix Table B (available as a supplement to the online version of this article at http://www.ajph.org) compares key socioeconomic indicators between treated and control cities before the COVID-19 pandemic. There were statistically significant differences in the total population of cities and the percentage of Black residents, which we expected. Treated cities did have higher unemployment rates but were similar to control cities in other sociodemographic characteristics. Table 1 reports the results of our difference-in-difference analysis. Despite aggregating to a quarterly level, zeros constitute more than half (58.7%) of our outcome variable, making the negative binomial model an appropriate choice. Employing an exponential model meant the parallel trends assumption needed to hold in terms of their proportional changes and not necessarily in level.[21] We present the *P* values for the parallel trends test in Table 1 that indicate that this assumption was not violated (Appendix Figure B [available as a supplement to the online version of this article at http://www.ajph.org] provides a visual evaluation of parallel trends). Testing for heterogenous treatment effects, we found no evidence of differential effects among cities. Table 1 presents the results of the negative binomial model without any socioeconomic controls. The results show that, after March 2020, the rate of firearm fatalities increased by 33% in low-graded neighborhoods in treated cities relative to similar neighborhoods in control cities.

Table 1 also includes socioeconomic controls as well as indicator variables for firearm laws. The incidence rate ratio increased somewhat after accounting for covariates, indicating a 35% increase in firearm fatalities in treated cities relative to controls. Poisson specification yielded results that were consistent with the primary model (Appendix Table C, available as a supplement to the online version of this article at http://www.ajph.org). Replicating the analysis using neighborhoods as the primary unit of analysis instead of

TABLE 1— City-Level Analysis of Firearm Fatalities in Low-Graded Neighborhoods: Select US Cities, July 2017–October 2022

	Dependent Variable: Firearm Fatalities	
	Model 1	Model 2
IRR (95% CI)	1.33 (1.11, 1.59)	1.35 (1.09, 1.67)
Pre-trends test, *P*	.12	.18
Heterogenous trends test, *P*	.38	.6
Sociodemographic controls	No	Yes
Observations, no.	1920	1920
Number of clusters	120	120

Note. CI = confidence interval; IRR = incident rate ratio. We based estimates on a difference-in-difference model employing an exponential conditional mean function and used data from the Gun Violence Archive to compare firearm fatalities in low-graded neighborhoods (i.e., neighborhoods assigned C and D grades) in treated cities to neighborhoods that would have received the same grades in cities that the Home Owners Loan Corporation did not redline. Cities with a 1930 population of between 25 000 and 39 999 served as the control cities; cities with a 1930 population between 40 000 and 55 000 served as treated cities. Bootstrapped SEs are clustered at the city level. Model 1 contains no sociodemographic controls. Model 2 includes controls for percentage of population that, per the American Community Survey, was White, Black, or other minority race; unemployed; lived in poverty; faced a language barrier; was a man aged 18–49 years; and had less than a high school diploma. Additional controls included state-level indicators for stand-your-ground laws and permit requirements for firearm purchasing.
Source. We obtained data for these covariates from the RAND Corporation.

cities also showed a differential increase in firearm fatalities in treated cities (Appendix Table D, available as a supplement to the online version of this article at http://www.ajph.org).

Table 2 reports the results of our falsification test using a placebo threshold. Using cities with populations between 40 000 and 55 000 in 1930 as controls and cities with populations between 55 000 and 70 000 as our treated units, we did not observe a statistically significant increase in firearm fatalities in either the low- (C and D) or high- (A and B) graded neighborhoods. Although the parallel trends assumption failed to hold for high-graded neighborhoods, as indicated by the low *P* value, the results of low-graded neighborhoods assure us that the results in Table 1 were not driven merely by differences in population size.

When we compared firearm fatalities among low- and high-graded neighborhoods in treated and control cities (Appendix Table E, available as a supplement to the online version of this article at http://www.ajph.org), we did not find any statistically significant differences in control cities. There was some evidence of a disproportionate increase in low-graded neighborhoods of treated cities; however, the confidence intervals were at the boundary. When evaluating high-graded neighborhoods, we did not detect statistically significant increases in firearm fatalities after March 2020 (Appendix Tables F and G, available as a supplement to the online version of this article at http://www.ajph.org). It should be noted that the class imbalance between grades led to fewer observations even after combining the A and B grades,[17] and the parallel trends assumption was not satisfied for this analysis (Appendix Figure C, available as a supplement to the online version of this article at http://www.ajph.org).

Finally, our propensity score–weighted difference-in-difference analysis yielded results that were similar to our primary findings (Appendix Table H, available as a supplement to the online version of this article at http://www.ajph.org). Although there was an increase in overall firearm fatalities in treated cities, it is not statistically significant. We did observe a

TABLE 2— Difference in Firearm Fatalities Using a Placebo Threshold: Select US Cities, July 2017–October 2022

	Dependent Variable: Firearm Fatalities	
	Model 1, Low-Graded Neighborhoods	Model 2, High-Graded Neighborhoods
IRR (95% CI)	0.79 (0.61, 1.02)	1.08 (0.53, 2.22)
Pre-trends test, *P*	.61	.01
City controls	Yes	Yes
Observations, no.	1328	752
Number of clusters	83	47

Note. CI = confidence interval; IRR = incident rate ratio. We based estimates on a difference-in-difference model employing an exponential conditional mean function. The models compared cities using a placebo threshold. Cities with a 1930 population of between 40 000 and 55 000 served as the control cities, and cities with a 1930 population of between 55 000 and 70 000 served as treated cities. Bootstrapped SEs were clustered at the city level. Low-graded neighborhoods constituted residential areas assigned C and D grades, and high-graded neighborhoods constituted areas assigned A and B grades.
Source. Data for the outcome variable were from the Gun Violence Archive (https://www.gunviolencearchive.org).

significant increase in fatalities occurring in low-graded neighborhoods. However, there was a reduction in fatalities in high-graded neighborhoods. Although some differences remained in covariates even after propensity score weighting (Appendix Table I, available as a supplement to the online version of this article at http://www.ajph.org), the overall results support the main findings, as presented in Table 1.

DISCUSSION

Our study documents the confluence of the COVID-19 pandemic and the structural inequities created by HOLC policies. We found a significant increase in firearm fatalities in neighborhoods that received low grades relative to similar neighborhoods in cities that did not meet the population threshold set by HOLC and therefore were not graded. Specifically, we found that after the onset of COVID-19, firearm fatalities increased by 35% in low-graded neighborhoods. These findings are significant because neighborhoods in treated and control cities were similar in terms of their historic demographic and socioeconomic characteristics.[17] Moreover, there are not many significant differences in important contemporary indicators, such as poverty and median income, among these cities overall. This suggests that the socioeconomic marginalization resulting from HOLC policies set low-graded neighborhoods on different trajectories of violence after March 2020, illustrating how the structural inequities stemming from historical discriminatory policies continue to affect communities to this day. Furthermore, high levels of firearm violence persisted long after the initial shockwaves of the pandemic subsided, indicating that not only are these communities more vulnerable to the adverse effects of exogenous shocks, but they also require longer recovery periods.

Interestingly, our results are consistent with previous findings on the impact of public health crises in Africa[13] despite stark contextual differences and resource availability—underscoring the importance of structural underpinnings and marginalization in driving violence. This is concerning because negative shocks caused by natural disasters or spread of infectious disease can be expected to increase in frequency and intensity owing to environmental changes.[22,23] Therefore, there is an urgent need for reinvestment in marginalized communities to address structural inequities that foster vulnerability to the impacts of future disasters. Given that previous research demonstrates that children who grow up in neighborhoods graded as undesirable for mortgage lending by the HOLC have lower educational attainment, have lower earning potential in adulthood, are more likely to live in high-poverty areas, and are more likely to be incarcerated,[8] investing in education and creating meaningful employment opportunities can offer potential channels through which the systemic barriers that contribute to cycles of poverty and violence can be reduced.

Limitations and Advantages

There are some limitations to our study. We are unable to make broader generalizations because our primary analysis compared cities in a specific band of the 1930 population. Although the results of our propensity score–weighted difference-in-difference model evaluated firearm violence in larger cities and yielded consistent results, differences remain in some socioeconomic metrics. Lastly, we cannot completely rule out the possibility that prediction errors in the classification algorithm or reporting errors in GVA data can exaggerate or attenuate our estimates.

Despite these shortcomings, our approach offers several advantages. First, the number of cities included in our analysis was not trivial, and by comparing cities located all over the country, we avoided spatial spillovers and endogeneity concerns implicit in border discontinuity designs. Second, we used an exogenous shock to isolate the effects of a historic policy. Finally, many of the cities that had small populations in the 1930s have grown significantly over the past decades and therefore may provide a more accurate picture of violence plaguing cities in the United States today. We also tried to avoid bias by excluding GVA data for the initial year, as coverage has been noted to improve over time.[24] This combined with our robustness checks supports the causal interpretation of our findings.

Conclusions

Overall, the stark increase in firearm fatalities in neighborhoods beset by racial discrimination speaks to the enduring effects of inequitable policies and how they continue to influence public health and safety. Our findings add to the growing body of evidence that calls for a reevaluation of resources and investment in marginalized communities to foster resilience and promote equity. This is critical because although redlining left a tangible legacy of structural racism, it is only one aspect of the larger institutional framework that created and reinforced racial inequities through exclusionary practices. Evidence indicates that the Federal Housing Administration's lending practices were far more restrictive than the HOLC maps indicate.[25] Future research should investigate the impact of discriminatory policies followed by other institutions to quantify the full scale of negative impacts on socioeconomic factors that compromise public health and safety.

Public Health Implications

Marginalization creates conditions in which violence proliferates. Through influencing redistribution of resources and consequently the socioeconomic status of communities, racial segregation has played a role in how resilient communities are in the face of negative shocks. The COVID-19 pandemic highlights how historic and systemic inequities are further compounded through interactions with negative shocks. Our findings emphasize the necessity of deliberate and sustained interventions aimed at redressing these long-standing disparities. AJPH

ABOUT THE AUTHORS

All authors are with the Institute of Firearm Injury Prevention, University of Michigan, Ann Arbor. Marc A. Zimmerman and Douglas J. Wiebe are also with the School of Public Health, University of Michigan, Ann Arbor.

CORRESPONDENCE

Correspondence should be sent to Zainab Hans, Institute for Firearm Injury Prevention, 1109 Geddes Ave, Ann Arbor, MI 48109 (e-mail: zanhans@umich.edu). Reprints can be ordered at https://www.ajph.org by clicking the "Reprints" link.

PUBLICATION INFORMATION

Full Citation: Hans Z, Lee DB, Zimmerman MA, Wiebe DJ. Legacy of racism and firearm violence during the COVID-19 pandemic in the United States. *Am J Public Health*. 2025;115(2):161–169.

Acceptance Date: September 29, 2024.

DOI: https://doi.org/10.2105/AJPH.2024.307891

ORCID iDs:

Zainab Hans https://orcid.org/0000-0002-3328-0155

Douglas J. Wiebe https://orcid.org/0000-0002-6434-8693

CONTRIBUTORS

Z. Hans conceptualized and designed the study, conducted statistical analyses, and drafted and finalized the article. D. B. Lee and M. A. Zimmerman contributed to writing. D. J. Wiebe contributed to the study design and supervised the analyses. All authors critically reviewed the article.

ACKNOWLEDGMENTS

Research reported in this publication was supported by the Eunice Kennedy Shriver National Institute of Child Health and Human Development, National Institutes of Health (NIH; award T32HD10854).

Note. The content of this article is solely the responsibility of the authors and does not necessarily represent the official views of the NIH.

CONFLICTS OF INTEREST

The authors have no financial or nonfinancial conflicts of interest to disclose.

HUMAN PARTICIPANT PROTECTION

This study used publicly available data and did not include human participants and was therefore exempted by the University of Michigan's institutional review board.

REFERENCES

1. Centers for Disease Control and Prevention. Vital signs: changes in firearm homicide and suicide rates—United States, 2019–2020. *MMWR Morb Mortal Wkly Rep*. 2022;71(19):656–663. https://doi.org/10.15585/mmwr.mm7119e1
2. Pino EC, Gebo E, Dugan E, Jay J. Trends in violent penetrating injuries during the first year of the COVID-19 pandemic. *JAMA Netw Open*. 2022;5(2):e2145708. https://doi.org/10.1001/jamanetworkopen.2021.45708
3. Schleimer JP, McCort CD, Shev AB, et al. Firearm purchasing and firearm violence during the coronavirus pandemic in the United States: a cross-sectional study. *Inj Epidemiol*. 2021;8(1):43. https://doi.org/10.1186/s40621-021-00339-5
4. Benfer EA, Vlahov D, Long MY, et al. Eviction, health inequity, and the spread of COVID-19: housing policy as a primary pandemic mitigation strategy. *J Urban Health*. 2021;98(1):1–12. https://doi.org/10.1007/s11524-020-00502-1
5. Jay J, Martin R, Patel M, Xie K, Shareef F, Simes JT. Analyzing child firearm assault injuries by race and ethnicity during the COVID-19 pandemic in 4 major US cities. *JAMA Netw Open*. 2023;6(3):e233125. https://doi.org/10.1001/jamanetworkopen.2023.3125
6. Ogedegbe G, Ravenell J, Adhikari S, et al. Assessment of racial/ethnic disparities in hospitalization and mortality in patients with COVID-19 in New York City. *JAMA Netw Open*. 2020;3(12):e2026881. https://doi.org/10.1001/jamanetworkopen.2020.26881
7. Rothstein R. *The Color of Law: A Forgotten History of How Our Government Segregated America*. New York, NY: Liveright; 2017.
8. Aaronson D, Hartley D, Mazumder B, Stinson M. The long-run effects of the 1930s redlining maps on children. *J Econ Lit*. 2023;61(3):846–862. https://doi.org/10.1257/jel.20221702
9. Aaronson D, Faber J, Hartley D, Mazumder B, Sharkey P. The long-run effects of the 1930s HOLC "redlining" maps on place-based measures of economic opportunity and socioeconomic success. *Reg Sci Urban Econ*. 2021;86:103622. https://doi.org/10.1016/j.regsciurbeco.2020.103622
10. Poulson M, Neufeld MY, Dechert T, Allee L, Kenzik KM. Historic redlining, structural racism, and firearm violence: a structural equation modeling approach. *Lancet Reg Health Am*. 2021;3:100052. https://doi.org/10.1016/j.lana.2021.100052.
11. Dalve K, Gause E, Mills B, Floyd AS, Rivara FP, Rowhani-Rahbar A. Neighborhood disadvantage and firearm injury: does shooting location matter? *Inj Epidemiol*. 2021;8(1):1–9. https://doi.org/10.1186/s40621-021-00304-2
12. Schleimer JP, Buggs SA, McCort CD, et al. Neighborhood racial and economic segregation and disparities in violence during the COVID-19 pandemic. *Am J Public Health*. 2022;112(1):144–153. https://doi.org/10.2105/AJPH.2021.306540
13. Gonzalez-Torres A, Esposito E. Epidemics and conflict: evidence from the Ebola outbreak in Western Africa. October 23, 2022. Available at: https://doi.org/10.2139/ssrn.3544606. Accessed October 15, 2024.
14. Iacoella F, Justino P, Martorano B. *Do Pandemics Lead to Rebellion? Policy Responses to COVID-19, Inequality, and Protests in the USA*. Helsinki, Finland: United Nations University World Institute for Development Economics Research; March 2021. WIDER working paper no. 2021/57. Available at: https://www.wider.unu.edu/sites/default/files/Publications/Working-paper/PDF/wp2021-57-pandemics-rebellion-policy-responses-COVID-19-inequality-protests-USA.pdf. Accessed October 15, 2024.
15. Cervellati M, Esposito E, Sunde U. Epidemic shocks and civil violence: evidence from malaria outbreaks in Africa. *Rev Econ Stat*. 2022;104(4):780–796. https://doi.org/10.1162/rest_a_01050
16. Cervellati M, Esposito E, Sunde U. Long-term exposure to malaria and development: disaggregate evidence for contemporaneous Africa. *J Demogr Economics*. 2017;83(1):129–148. https://doi.org/10.1017/dem.2016.27
17. Hynsjö DM, Perdoni L. The effects of federal "redlining" maps: a novel estimation strategy. Presented at: Labor/Public Economics Workshop. Yale University Department of Economics; October 21, 2022.
18. Uzzi M, Aune KT, Marineau L, et al. An intersectional analysis of historical and contemporary structural racism on non-fatal shootings in Baltimore, Maryland. *Inj Prev*. 2023;29(1):85–90. https://doi.org/10.1136/ip-2022-044700
19. Gun Violence Archive. General methodology. 2019. Available at: https://www.gunviolencearchive.org/methodology. Accessed November 26, 2023.
20. Cherney S, Morral AR, Schell TL, Smucker S, Hoch E. Development of the RAND State Firearm Law Database and supporting materials. 2018.

Available at: https://www.rand.org/pubs/tools/TLA243-2-v2.html. Accessed October 15, 2024. https://doi.org/10.7249/TL283

21. Wooldridge JM. Simple approaches to nonlinear difference-in-differences with panel data. *Econom J.* 2023;26(3):C31–C66. https://doi.org/10.1093/ectj/utad016
22. Tollefson J. Why deforestation and extinctions make pandemics more likely. *Nature.* 2020;584(7820):175–177. https://doi.org/10.1038/d41586-020-02341-1
23. Kumar A, Nagar S. Climate change and existential threats. In: Singh S, Singh P, Rangabhashiyam S, Srivastava KK, eds. *Global Climate Change.* Amsterdam, Netherlands: Elsevier; 2021:1–31. https://doi.org/10.1016/C2019-0-05200-4
24. Gobaud AN, Mehranbod CA, Kaufman E, et al. Assessing the gun violence archive as an epidemiologic data source for community firearm violence in 4 US cities. *JAMA Netw Open.* 2023;6(6):e2316545. https://doi.org/10.1001/jamanetworkopen.2023.16545
25. Fishback P, Rose J, Snowden KA, Storrs T. *New Evidence on Redlining by Federal Housing Programs in the 1930s.* Chicago, IL: Federal Reserve Bank of Chicago. January 3, 2022. Working paper no. 2022-01. https://doi.org/10.21033/wp-2022-01

Laws Limiting Access to SNAP Benefits for People With Felony Drug Convictions: A Policy-Mapping Study

Hridika Shah, MSPH, Alexander D. McCourt, JD, PhD, MPH, and Sachini Bandara, PhD, MS

See also Dong, p. 113.

Objectives. To map US state Supplemental Nutrition Assistance Program (SNAP) bans for individuals with felony drug convictions between 2004 and 2021.

Methods. Using standard legal-mapping methodology, we categorized states as maintaining the lifetime ban imposed by federal law, modifying the lifetime ban, or fully opting out of the lifetime ban in each year. Among states with modified bans in 2021, we coded types of modifications.

Results. As of 2021, 26 states and the District of Columbia fully opted out of the lifetime ban, 23 states modified bans, and 1 state maintained a lifetime ban. Among states with modified bans in 2021, 13 states required compliance with parole and probation, 12 states required drug treatment, 7 states required drug testing, and 9 states limited eligibility to certain populations.

Conclusions. Most states effectively de-implemented the federal lifetime ban on SNAP for people with felony drug convictions by fully opting out or modifying bans over time. However, some states still had stringent modified ban provisions.

Public Health Implications. These findings underscore the need to study the effects of this patchwork of drug conviction–related ban policies on substance use and nutrition-related outcomes. (*Am J Public Health*. 2025;115(2):170–177. https://doi.org/10.2105/AJPH.2024.307873)

AJPH February 2025, Vol. 115, No. 2

People reentering communities following incarceration face an increased risk of morbidity and mortality during this critical transition period, particularly because of substance use and overdose.[1] In addition to the increased risk of adverse physical and mental health outcomes, individuals who were previously incarcerated are more likely to experience housing instability, food insecurity, and unemployment.[2–5]

Food is essential for everyone's health and well-being, yet people with previous criminal legal system involvement face structural barriers to food access. People who have been previously incarcerated are nearly 2 times as likely to experience food insecurity as are individuals without a history of incarceration.[4] This compounds the challenges this population faces in meeting basic needs, which several qualitative studies find are associated with negative effects on health and well-being, successful reentry, upward mobility, and recidivism.[6–8] Food insecurity may also worsen physical and mental health challenges among individuals with previous criminal legal system involvement, widening existing health inequities.[9,10] Given these structural obstacles, access to the Supplemental Nutrition Assistance Program (SNAP), which provides nutrition assistance to low-income households in the United States and is associated with reduced poverty and improved food security,[11] is vital to facilitating successful reentry following release from incarceration.

Despite the relationship between reentry and food insecurity, federal SNAP policy is highly restrictive. In 1996, as part of bipartisan efforts to substantially restructure and restrict public welfare programs, the Personal Responsibility and Work Opportunity Reconciliation Act imposed a lifetime disqualification for SNAP and cash assistance benefits among individuals with a felony drug conviction.[12] In the first 5 years of enactment, nearly

90 000 individuals with felony drug convictions were denied SNAP benefits.[13] The potential implications of this policy have persisted, with approximately 244 000 individuals sent to prison annually for drug-related crimes in the United States.[14] A pilot study in California, Texas, and Connecticut found that 91% of individuals convicted of drug felonies were food insecure on release.[15]

Although the federal lifetime ban has been in place since 1996, provisions of the Personal Responsibility and Work Opportunity Reconciliation Act allow states discretion to modify or completely opt out of the lifetime SNAP ban.[12] Many states have enacted legislative reform addressing this ban, electing to either fully opt out of the ban or modify eligibility criteria for individuals with a felony drug conviction. This has resulted in a shifting patchwork of SNAP eligibility policies over the past few decades.[16] Previous studies have documented state decisions regarding SNAP bans through 2015 and suggest a shift away from maintaining the lifetime ban to completely opting out or modifying the lifetime ban.[17–19] However, the progression of state policies past 2015 and a characterization of the specific modification provisions that have been enacted are not well documented in the research literature. In the gray literature, the Center for Law and Social Policy has published important work documenting the overall status of SNAP bans but does not systematically document the details of state by state modifications over time.[20]

We aimed to fill this gap by mapping trends in state SNAP provisions between 2004 and 2021 for individuals with drug felony convictions and providing a detailed characterization of modified bans by state.

METHODS

We identified and mapped SNAP policies related to assistance and benefit eligibility for individuals with felony drug convictions for all 50 states and the District of Columbia every year between 2004 and 2021. Our study team of 3 included 1 public health lawyer with experience in legal epidemiology and mapping (A. D. M.) and a subject matter expert in US health policy (S. B.). We collected data between June 2022 and January 2023.

First, we gathered policy data from the US Department of Agriculture's State Options Reports from 2004 through 2019, which are reports that provide state-level descriptions of SNAP options that states may adopt, including opting out of lifetime bans for people with felony drug convictions.[21]

Second, because the state option reports were not available consistently during the study period, we searched the Thomas Reuters Westlaw legal research database, used in previous public health legal-mapping studies,[22] to validate policy data gathered from the state options reports and to fill missing data points during the study period. We conducted state-specific searches in the Statutes & Court Rules database on Westlaw using standardized search terms related to SNAP and the federal ban enactment date, including "SNAP, food stamps, or August 22, 1996." This search strategy was based on existing peer-reviewed and gray literature and reports and descriptions of the policy from the US Department of Agriculture. We pilot tested and refined the search strategy. For example, we included the date in the search terms because the federal ban applied only to individuals with a felony conviction on or after the date.

Third, for state years that still had missing policy information, we used state-level legal data sources, such as state legislature Web sites using the same search terms. Using these search terms in the Westlaw and state-level sources, we abstracted subsections of state code relevant to SNAP policy that documented policies regarding benefit eligibility for individuals with a felony drug conviction, which were most often located in sections of the code related to social and human services. We used the credits and history of each relevant code section to determine when the statute was first enacted and whether there were any subsequent amendments. We included all of these abstracted sections for detailed review using the coding instrument we describe later. We excluded sections of the code not relevant to SNAP eligibility from this detailed review.

Using the abstracted text, for each state and each year, we coded the ban status and effective date. We coded ban status as (1) no ban, (2) a modified ban, or (3) a lifetime ban. We identified states as having no ban if the policy text included an "opt-out" from the federal ban with no additional provisions stipulating alternative eligibility requirements for individuals with felony drug convictions. If states opted out of the federal ban but had additional requirements for eligibility, we classified them as a modified ban state. We determined that states had a lifetime ban if they had no policies related to benefit eligibility for individuals with felony drug convictions or had a ban identical to the federal ban.

In states with modified bans in 2021, we developed additional measures in the coding instrument to categorize the types of modifications states enacted. Modification categories included whether the state had enacted a (1) compliance with parole or probation requirement, (2) drug treatment requirement, (3) drug-testing requirement, or (4) provision limiting the population for whom the permanent disqualification applied. We identified states as in category 2 or 3 if they required satisfactory completion of a drug treatment program or drug testing to be eligible for SNAP. We identified states as having a temporary disqualification if the state applied a ban from SNAP benefits for all individuals with a felony drug conviction for a time less than a lifetime. We classified temporary disqualifications contingent on drug testing or for people with certain types of felony convictions in other relevant categories.

Eligibility rules were modified for specific subgroups by restricting ineligibility or imposing additional requirements on individuals with certain types of felony drug convictions, multiple convictions, or noncompliance with parole or probation conditions. We included some states in multiple categories, as there were multiple types of modifications. The research team resolved disagreements in policy categorization with review and discussion.

Finally, we examined abstracted policy text and the legal-mapping results to identify policy themes during the entire study period. Through an iterative hybrid inductive and deductive coding process, we developed a list of policy themes and then coded all abstracted policies according to whether they fit into the following themes:

1. Enacting less restrictive SNAP ban provisions. The state either fully opted out of the ban or maintained a modified ban but over time enacted less restrictive modifications related to drug testing, treatment, and limited populations;
2. Enacting stricter ban provisions. The state enacted stricter modification provisions over time;
3. Enacting modifications that contradict 2 best practices. The state enforced mandatory treatment without any exemptions in the statute text and punitive measures for positive drug testing[23]; and
4. Enacting other provisions. The state's code specified additional SNAP eligibility requirements for people with felony drug convictions but was unclear about what recipients must do to confirm eligibility and who was responsible for making decisions regarding drug treatment and benefit receipt.

RESULTS

Between 2004 and 2021, we found a shift away from lifetime bans to the enactment of no bans and modified bans (Figure 1). In 2004, 17 states had a lifetime ban, 18 states had modified bans, and 15 states and the District of Columbia had no ban. By 2010 this shifted to 11 states with a lifetime ban, 20 states with a modified ban, and 19 states and the District of Columbia with no ban. In 2014, 10 states had lifetime bans, 22 states had modified bans, and 18 states and the District of Columbia had no ban. By the end of 2021, only 1 state, South Carolina, maintained a lifetime ban, 23 states had modified bans, and 26 states and the District of Columbia had no ban. One distinct case was Oregon. Although classified as a no ban state for the entirety of the study period, Oregon's code includes a provision granting parole or postprison supervisors the authority to recommend benefit suspension, specifically for individuals with manufacture- or delivery-related drug convictions.

Types of Modified Bans

For the 23 states with a modified ban in 2021, there was significant variation in the types of modifications that states enacted (Table A [available as a supplement to the online version of this article at http://www.ajph.org] provides a detailed summary of the provisions for each state with a modified ban in 2021). In 2021, the most common modification type required compliance with parole and probation to receive benefits (n = 13 states) followed by modifications that required the satisfactory completion of a drug treatment program (n = 12 states; Table 1). In some cases, the statute specified that drug treatment was mandated only "if necessary," which was often stated to be determined by a "licensed medical provider" or "mental health authority." Connecticut and Montana did not require drug treatment for all individuals.

Seven states mandated drug testing as a component of SNAP benefit eligibility for individuals with a felony drug conviction, and 4 states designated punitive measures for positive drug tests, specified as a reduction in benefits or a temporary disqualification from SNAP. However, the number of positive drug tests permitted and the disqualification period varied considerably from state to state. Kansas had the shortest period, with a 30-day disqualification, whereas Pennsylvania had the longest, with a 10-year disqualification for the second positive drug test. Minnesota had the most stringent provisions, with a 30% cut in benefits for the first positive

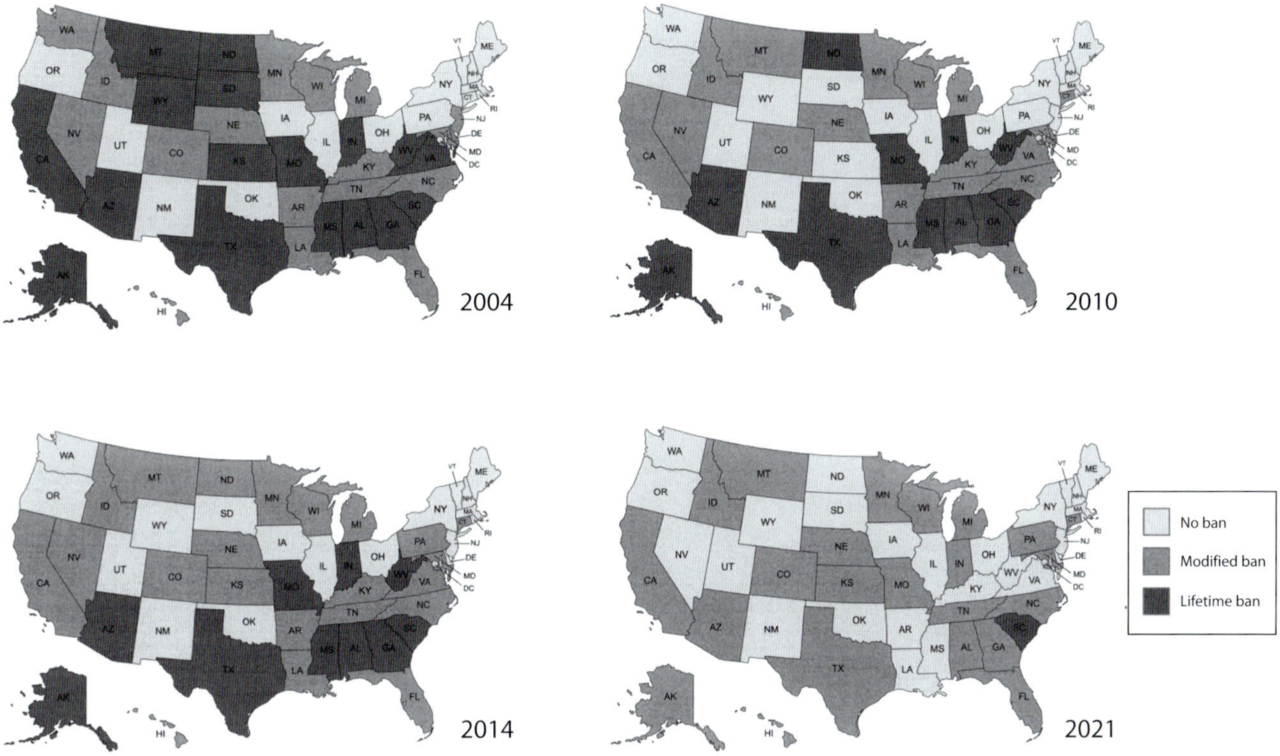

FIGURE 1— US State Supplemental Nutrition Assistance Program (SNAP) Bans for People With Felony Drug Conviction in 2004, 2010, 2014, and 2021

drug test and a permanent disqualification for any subsequent positive test.

Several modification provisions limited ineligibility to certain subpopulations among people with felony drug convictions. Four states restricted limited ineligibility to certain higher-level felony drug convictions (i.e., sale, distribution, trafficking, or manufacture of controlled substances). For example, in Nebraska only individuals with a conviction related to sale or distribution of controlled substances were subject to the lifetime ban on benefits. Similarly, 3 states limited ineligibility to individuals with multiple (more than either 2 or 3) felony drug convictions. Notably, the Texas SNAP provisions stipulated that any subsequent felony conviction (not limited to drug-related convictions) resulted in lifetime ineligibility, which was distinct

TABLE 1— Modification Provisions Among 22 US States With Modified SNAP Bans for People With Felony Drug Convictions in 2021

Modifications	Description	States
Parole/Probation (n = 13 states)	Requires compliance with parole or probation requirements to obtain SNAP	AL, AK, AZ, CA, CT, GA, ID, IN, MI, MO, MT, NE, TX
Treatment (n = 12 states)	May require satisfactory completion of a drug treatment program to obtain SNAP	AL, AK, AZ, CT, HI, KS, MO, MT, NE, NC, PA, TN
Drug testing (n = 7 states)	Requires drug testing to obtain SNAP	AZ, CT, KS, MN, MO, PA, WI
Limited populations: multiple convictions (n = 4 states)	Limits ineligibility to or imposes additional eligibility requirements for individuals with multiple felony drug convictions	KS, MO, NE, TX[a]
Limited populations: high-level vs low-level drug conviction (n = 4 states)	Limits ineligibility to or imposes additional eligibility requirements for individuals with higher-level felony drug conviction (i.e., sale, distribution, trafficking, or manufacture of controlled substances)	FL, MD, NE, TN

Note. SNAP = Supplemental Nutrition Assistance Program.
[a]Any subsequent felony conviction (not just drug related) results in ineligibility.

from the ineligibility criteria of multiple felony drug convictions present in other states. One state, North Carolina, had a 6-month temporary disqualification period that applied to all people with a felony drug conviction.

In 2021, 12 states enacted a combination of these modifications. For example, Missouri required compliance with parole and probation, drug testing, and drug treatment, if necessary. In addition, individuals with 2 subsequent drug felony convictions were permanently ineligible for benefits in the state.

Trends in Bans Over Time

In examining abstracted state policies between 2004 and 2021 and types of modification provisions, several themes emerged (Table 2). Overall, 23 states enacted less restrictive SNAP ban policies over the study period, moving from a lifetime ban to a modified ban, from a modified ban to no ban, or from a lifetime ban to no ban. Some states maintained a modified ban but enacted less restrictive provisions affecting drug testing, treatment, and limited populations, or they transitioned from a modified ban to fully opted out.

Whereas 23 states shifted to less restrictive policies over time, 3 states enacted stricter modifications in the study period. For example, in 2013, Kansas added to their modified ban that required drug treatment of SNAP eligibility an additional provision blocking SNAP benefits for individuals with more than 1 drug felony conviction. Similarly, in 2011, Pennsylvania shifted from no ban to a modified ban requiring drug testing and treatment. In 2018, Pennsylvania added an additional provision prohibiting eligibility for individuals convicted of drug distribution.

In the modified bans, 11 states had provisions conflicting with best practices. Several states had mandatory treatment requirements. For example, since 1997, Hawaii has exempted only "persons who are complying with treatment or who have not refused or failed to comply with treatment" from the ban on SNAP benefits. In other states, such as Minnesota and Pennsylvania, there are punitive measures (either a reduction in benefits or a disqualification period) for positive drug test results among SNAP benefit recipients.

Finally, 3 states with modified bans had other provisions and eligibility requirements. In these cases, states had unclear requirements about who decided on the type of substance use disorder treatment completion that

TABLE 2— Themes in Policy Changes to SNAP Bans for People With Felony Drug Convictions: United States, 2004–2021

Theme Name	Theme Description	Example
Enacting less restrictive SNAP ban provisions (n = 23 states)	States have either maintained a modified ban and enacted less restrictive modifications or fully opted out of the ban	California: Between 2005 and 2015, CA had a modified ban in place that limited ineligibility to individuals with a conviction related to sale, manufacture, or trafficking. The modified ban also required drug treatment of individuals who were not ineligible under this restriction. In 2015, these restrictions eased up, with any individual eligible for benefits, provided they comply with terms of parole/probation. Cal. Welf. & Inst. Code § 18901.3 (2021) Other examples: AL (2016), AK (2016), AZ (2017), AR (2017), DE (2011), GA (2016), IN (2020), KY (2021), LA (2017), MD (2017), MS (2019), MO (2015), MT (2005), NV (2021), NJ (2009), ND (2017), SD (2009), TX (2015), VA (2020), WA (2005), WV (2019), WY (2005)
Enacting stricter ban provisions (n = 3 states)	States enact more strict modifications over time (2004–2021)	Kansas: Between 2006 and 2013, there was a modified ban in place that provided assistance to any individual who completed a drug treatment program. In 2013, Kansas modified the provisions of benefits to exclude individuals with more than 1 felony conviction. Kan. Stat. Ann. § 39-709(13) (2021) Other examples: MI (2015–2020), PA (2011, 2018)
Enacting modifications that contradict clinical guidelines (n = 11 states)	States have provisions regarding mandatory treatment and punitive measures for drug testing that directly contradict clinical guidelines	Hawaii: Since 1997, Hawaii has exempted "persons who are complying with treatment or who have not refused or failed to comply with treatment" from the ban on SNAP benefits. Haw. Rev. Stat. § 346-53.3 (2021) Other examples: DE (2003–2011), CA (2005–2015), KS (since 2013), KY (1998–2020), MN (since 2001), NC (since 1997), NE (since 2003), NJ (1997–2009), PA (since 2011), WI (since 1997)
Other provisions (n = 3 states)	Code specifies additional requirements for recipients but is unclear	Colorado: Since 1997, Colorado implemented a modified ban whereby individuals are ineligible for benefits "unless such person is determined by the county department to have taken action toward rehabilitation such as, but not limited to, participation in a drug treatment program." Colo. Rev. Stat. Code § 26-2-706 (2021) Other examples: KS (since 2006), NC (since 1997)

Note. SNAP = Supplemental Nutrition Assistance Program.

satisfied eligibility requirements. For example, in Colorado between 2005 and 2015, individuals with a felony drug conviction were ineligible for SNAP unless they had "taken action toward rehabilitation such as, but not limited to, participation in a drug treatment program" (Colo. Rev. Stat. § 26–2-706 [2021]). What types of actions "toward rehabilitation" would satisfy this eligibility requirement other than the 1 listed and who approved the action were not specified in the statute. In Kansas, there was a provision stating that "food assistance shall not be provided unless a drug test is successfully passed, and a drug treatment plan is approved by the secretary" (Kan. Stat. Ann. § 39–709(13) [2021]).

DISCUSSION

Our study examined the status of state SNAP provisions between 2004 and 2021 for individuals with drug felony convictions and detailed characterizations of modified bans in 2021 by state. There was a general trend toward less stringent SNAP policy over the study period, as some states eliminated the lifetime ban for individuals with felony drug convictions. Despite the maintenance of a stringent federal ban through the entire study period, all but 1 state contributed to effectively de-implementing this federal policy by opting out or modifying the lifetime ban.

The current patchwork of policies underscores the need to understand the effect of various SNAP ban policies for individuals with a felony drug conviction. One study found that among men convicted of drug trafficking in Florida, a lifetime ban on SNAP benefits was associated with a 58% increase in recidivism.[24] In another study, which examined SNAP bans nationwide, state actions that fully opted out of the lifetime ban were associated with a 2.2% reduction in recidivism, but having a modified ban had no effect on recidivism.[25] Future work should examine the relationship between SNAP bans—particularly the effects of various modification provisions—and other key outcomes such as food insecurity and drug use–related outcomes. Understanding the effects of eligibility restrictions on recovery and well-being can help identify mechanisms to create a more trauma-informed SNAP policy for people with criminal legal involvement.[26]

Our legal research and mapping demonstrate that most states chose to de-implement the federal lifetime ban and replace it with a state-level modified ban. Understanding the implications of these modifications on people with felony drug convictions is of public health importance. We found that 12 states had modifications requiring drug treatment to maintain SNAP eligibility in 2021. A 2016 review found limited evidence on the effectiveness of compulsory drug treatment, which indicates that such an approach may not improve drug-related outcomes for people with felony drug convictions.[27] Finally, some individuals convicted of a drug felony might not have a substance use disorder or be in need of drug treatment services.

A common modification was the enactment of punitive consequences for positive drug tests. Although the literature on drug testing as part of SNAP eligibility is scarce, previous evidence on drug testing and welfare benefits more broadly demonstrates that the requirement is both costly and ineffective.[28] Reports from advocacy groups stated that substance use was lower among Temporary Assistance for Needy Families recipients than among the general population.[29] Moreover, administering drug tests was more costly than the savings from denying welfare benefits for positive test results.[30] We might expect to see similar effects of drug-testing requirements for people with felony drug convictions; however, more research is needed to understand this relationship. In addition, creating more stringent eligibility for SNAP may exacerbate food insecurity, which previous studies have shown to be linked with challenges in treatment and recovery.[31,32]

Further research is needed to understand the implementation of such policies. For example, in states that require drug treatment, it is unknown whether certain types of drug treatment are preferred to others and how participation in drug treatment is enforced. Studies focused on the criminal legal system have found that courts are less likely to refer people to the highest standard of drug treatment than are other bodies that make referrals.[23,33] Whether there are similar trends among agencies that implement and enforce SNAP requirements for mandated treatment is unknown, and other questions remain about how various modification provisions are administered more broadly.

Eliminating lifetime bans and enacting modified SNAP bans may have implications for intergenerational outcomes as well. Parental incarceration significantly increases the risk of food insecurity among children, and childhood food insecurity has significant and persistent effects on cognitive development, behavioral outcomes, and social and economic mobility.[34–36] More than half of individuals who are incarcerated and have minor children have a drug-related conviction.[37] Most SNAP recipients are women and children,[38] suggesting that restricting

SNAP access for individuals with felony drug conviction may exacerbate the intergenerational effects of the overdose crisis and widen existing health disparities.

Limitations

This study should be considered in the context of several limitations. First, we based policy mapping on text in each state's statutory code found via state options reports, the Westlaw database, and state legislature Web sites. Although we attempted to be comprehensive by consulting multiple sources, we did not examine regulatory codes and agency-level guidance documents related to the state statutes we identified, and any relevant details therein may not be captured in this study. These types of materials may be particularly relevant for states with modified bans in which the statutes are unclear on how the modifications should be implemented.

Next, we identified state policies by year, which means that policies were coded as first present in the first full year they were in effect. As a result, our legal data do not describe details of midyear changes. Future research seeking to assess the effects of these policy changes may need to modify this coding to reflect exact implementation dates. Finally, the categories for modification provisions that we developed may have not captured all possible modifications states enacted.

Public Health Implications

To our knowledge, this study is the first to map changes to SNAP ban policies over a 17-year period and provide a detailed mapping of modifications to lifetime SNAP bans. We found that between 2004 and 2021, all but 1 state effectively de-implemented the stringent federal lifetime ban on SNAP for people with felony drug convictions. Nearly half of all states have fully opted out of the federal lifetime ban, and a little more than half of states have modified bans in place. We found, however, that these modifications may still place stringent requirements and limit access to SNAP for people with felony drug convictions.

Both movement to fully opt out of the lifetime ban and state action to enact stringent modification provisions could have significant implications for food insecurity, drug-related outcomes, recidivism, and intergenerational outcomes, but this is not yet well explored in the literature. However, data on high levels of food insecurity among individuals who were previously incarcerated and the broader body of research demonstrating SNAP's association with reduced food insecurity and improved health among a general population suggest that policies expanding access to SNAP for individuals leaving the criminal legal system may be particularly beneficial because of the vulnerable nature of reentry.[4,39] AJPH

ABOUT THE AUTHORS

All authors are with the Department of Health Policy and Management, Johns Hopkins Bloomberg School of Public Health, Baltimore, MD. Sachini Bandara is also with the Department of Mental Health, Johns Hopkins Bloomberg School of Public Health.

CORRESPONDENCE

Correspondence should be sent to Hridika Shah, 615 N. Wolfe St, Baltimore, MD 21205 (e-mail: hshah25@jh.edu). Reprints can be ordered at https://www.ajph.org by clicking the "Reprints" link.

PUBLICATION INFORMATION

Full Citation: Shah H, McCourt AD, Bandara S. Laws limiting access to SNAP benefits for people with felony drug convictions: a policy-mapping study. *Am J Public Health*. 2025;115(2):170–177.

Acceptance Date: September 18, 2024.

DOI: https://doi.org/10.2105/AJPH.2024.307873

ORCID iDs:
Hridika Shah https://orcid.org/0000-0002-1727-1929

Alexander D. McCourt https://orcid.org/0000-0002-3524-3454

CONTRIBUTORS

The authors contributed equally to this study.

ACKNOWLEDGMENTS

Funding for this research was provided through Bloomberg Philanthropies.

Findings from this study were previously presented at the 2023 APHA Annual Meeting and Expo. Atlanta, GA; November 13.

CONFLICTS OF INTEREST

The authors have no conflicts of interest to disclose.

HUMAN PARTICIPANT PROTECTION

No institutional review board approval was required because no human participants were involved in this study. We conducted a policy-mapping study and used data from legal databases and state legislature Web sites.

REFERENCES

1. Binswanger IA, Nowels C, Corsi KF, et al. Return to drug use and overdose after release from prison: a qualitative study of risk and protective factors. *Addict Sci Clin Pract.* 2012;7(1):3. https://doi.org/10.1186/1940-0640-7-3
2. Link NW, Ward JT, Stansfield R. Consequences of mental and physical health for reentry and recidivism: toward a health-based model of desistance. *Criminology*. 2019;57(3):544–573. https://doi.org/10.1111/1745-9125.12213
3. Herbert CW, Morenoff JD, Harding DJ. Homelessness and housing insecurity among former prisoners. *RSF*. 2015;1(2):44–79. https://doi.org/10.7758/RSF.2015.1.2.04
4. Testa A, Jackson DB. Food insecurity among formerly incarcerated adults. *Crim Justice Behav.* 2019;46(10):1493–1511. https://doi.org/10.1177/0093854819856920
5. Visher CA, Debus-Sherrill SA, Yahner J. Employment after prison: a longitudinal study of former prisoners. *Justice Q.* 2011;28(5):698–718. https://doi.org/10.1080/07418825.2010.535553
6. Western B, Braga AA, Davis J, Sirois C. Stress and hardship after prison. *Am J Sociol.* 2015;120(5):1512–1547. https://doi.org/10.1086/681301
7. Harding DJ, Wyse JJB, Dobson C, Morenoff JD. Making ends meet after prison. *J Policy Anal Manage.* 2014;33(2):440–470. https://doi.org/10.1002/pam.21741
8. Morenoff JD, Harding DJ. Incarceration, prisoner reentry, and communities. *Annu Rev Sociol.* 2014;40:411–429. https://doi.org/10.1146/annurev-soc-071811-145511

9. Porter LC. Incarceration and post-release health behavior. *J Health Soc Behav*. 2014;55(2):234–249. https://doi.org/10.1177/0022146514531438
10. Testa AM. Access to healthy food retailers among formerly incarcerated individuals. *Public Health Nutr*. 2019;22(4):672–680. https://doi.org/10.1017/S1368980018002720
11. Bartfeld J, Gundersen C, Smeeding TM, Ziliak JP, eds. *SNAP Matters: How Food Stamps Affect Health and Well-Being*. Stanford, CA: Stanford University Press; 2015.
12. Personal Responsibility and Work Opportunity Reconciliation Act, Pub L No. 104-193, § 862a (1996).
13. Gustafson K. Criminal law: the criminalization of poverty. *J Crim Law Criminol*. 2009;99(3):643–716.
14. National Center for Drug Abuse Statistics. Drug related crime statistics. 2023. Available at: https://drugabusestatistics.org/drug-related-crime-statistics. Accessed March 15, 2023.
15. Wang EA, Zhu GA, Evans L, Carroll-Scott A, Desai R, Fiellin LE. A Pilot study examining food insecurity and HIV risk behaviors among individuals recently released from prison. *AIDS Educ Prev*. 2013;25(2):112–123. https://doi.org/10.1521/aeap.2013.25.2.112
16. Polkey C. Most states have ended SNAP ban for convicted drug felons. July 30, 2019. Available at: https://www.ncsl.org/news/details/most-states-have-ended-snap-ban-for-convicted-drug-felons. Accessed March 15, 2023.
17. Cramer R, Hexem S, Thompson K, LaPollo AB, Chesson HW, Leichliter JS. State policies in the United States impacting drug-related convictions and their consequences in 2015. *Drug Sci Policy Law*. 2019;5:10.1177/2050324519863491. https://doi.org/10.1177/2050324519863491
18. Luallen J, Edgerton J, Rabideau D. A quasi-experimental evaluation of the impact of public assistance on prisoner recidivism. *J Quant Criminol*. 2018;34(3):741–773. https://doi.org/10.1007/s10940-017-9353-x
19. Sheely A. State supervision, punishment and poverty: the case of drug bans on welfare receipt. *Punish Soc*. 2021;23(3):413–435. https://doi.org/10.1177/1462474520959433
20. Center for Law and Social Policy. No more double punishments: lifting the ban on SNAP and TANF for people with prior felony drug convictions. April 2022. Available at: https://www.clasp.org/publications/report/brief/no-more-double-punishments. Accessed July 15, 2024.
21. US Department of Agriculture, Food and Nutrition Service. State options report. June 27, 2019. Available at: https://www.fns.usda.gov/snap/waivers/state-options-report. Accessed April 13, 2023.
22. White SA, McCourt A, Bandara S, Goodman DJ, Patel E, McGinty EE. Implementation of state laws giving pregnant people priority access to drug treatment programs in the context of coexisting punitive laws. *Womens Health Issues*. 2023;33(2):117–125. https://doi.org/10.1016/j.whi.2022.09.001
23. Mancher M, Leshner AI, eds. *Medications for Opioid Use Disorder Save Lives*. Washington, DC: National Academies Press; 2019. Available at: http://www.ncbi.nlm.nih.gov/books/NBK538936. Accessed February 18, 2023.
24. Tuttle C. Snapping back: food stamp bans and criminal recidivism. *Am Econ J: Econ Policy*. 2019;11(2):301–327. https://doi.org/10.1257/pol.20170490
25. Yang CS. Does public assistance reduce recidivism? *Am Econ Rev*. 2017;107(5):551–555. https://doi.org/10.1257/aer.p20171001
26. Bowen EA, Murshid NS. Trauma-informed social policy: a conceptual framework for policy analysis and advocacy. *Am J Public Health*. 2016;106(2):223–229. https://doi.org/10.2105/AJPH.2015.302970
27. Werb D, Kamarulzaman A, Meacham MC, et al. The effectiveness of compulsory drug treatment: a systematic review. *Int J Drug Policy*. 2016;28:1–9. https://doi.org/10.1016/j.drugpo.2015.12.005
28. Palacio V. Drug testing SNAP applicants is ineffective and perpetuates stereotypes. July 2017. Available at: https://www.clasp.org/sites/default/files/publications/2017/08/Drug-testing-SNAP-Applicants-is-Ineffective-Perpetuates-Stereotypes.pdf. Accessed May 12, 2023.
29. Covert B, Israel J. States spend millions to drug test the poor, turn up few positive results. April 20, 2017. Available at: https://archive.thinkprogress.org/states-spend-millions-to-drug-test-the-poor-turn-up-few-positive-results-81f826a4afb7. Accessed May 13, 2023.
30. Center for Law and Social Policy. Random drug testing of TANF recipients is costly, ineffective and hurts families. October 2013. Available at: https://www.clasp.org/sites/default/files/public/resources-and-publications/files/520.pdf. Accessed May 12, 2023.
31. Marks SJ, Pham H, McCray N, et al. Associations between patient-reported experiences with opioid use disorder treatment and unmet treatment needs and discontinuation among Virginia Medicaid members. *Subst Abuse*. 2023;44(3):196–208. https://doi.org/10.1177/08897077231186218
32. Summers NA, Colasanti JA, Feaster DJ, et al. Predictors for poor linkage to care among hospitalized persons living with HIV and co-occurring substance use disorder. *AIDS Res Hum Retroviruses*. 2020;36(5):406–414. https://doi.org/10.1089/aid.2019.0153
33. Krawczyk N, Picher CE, Feder KA, Saloner B. Only one in twenty justice-referred adults in specialty treatment for opioid use receive methadone or buprenorphine. *Health Aff (Millwood)*. 2017;36(12):2046–2053. https://doi.org/10.1377/hlthaff.2017.0890
34. Jackson DB, Vaughn MG. Parental history of disruptive life events and household food insecurity. *J Nutr Educ Behav*. 2017;49(7):554–560.e1. https://doi.org/10.1016/j.jneb.2017.04.010
35. Gallegos D, Eivers A, Sondergeld P, Pattinson C. Food insecurity and child development: a state-of-the-art review. *Int J Environ Res Public Health*. 2021;18(17):8990. https://doi.org/10.3390/ijerph18178990
36. Jackson DB, Newsome J, Vaughn MG, Johnson KR. Considering the role of food insecurity in low self-control and early delinquency. *J Crim Justice*. 2018;56:127–139. https://doi.org/10.1016/j.jcrimjus.2017.07.002
37. Glaze LE, Maruschak LM. Parents in prison and their minor children. August 2008. Available at: https://www.ojp.gov/ncjrs/virtual-library/abstracts/parents-prison-and-their-minor-children. Accessed November 20, 2023.
38. Cronquist K. *Characteristics of Supplemental Nutrition Assistance Program Households: Fiscal Year 2019*. March 29, 2021. Available at: https://fns-prod.azureedge.us/sites/default/files/resource-files/Characteristics2019.pdf. Accessed November 20, 2023.
39. Keith-Jennings B, Llobrera J, Dean S. Links of the Supplemental Nutrition Assistance Program with food insecurity, poverty, and health: evidence and potential. *Am J Public Health*. 2019;109(12):1636–1640. https://doi.org/10.2105/AJPH.2019.305325

US State Recreational and Medical Cannabis Delivery Laws, 2024

Todd Ebling, PhD, Sunday Azagba, PhD, Mark Hall, JD, and Jessica King Jensen, PhD

Objectives. To provide a legal epidemiology review of state-level policies that regulate the direct delivery of recreational and medical cannabis in the United States.

Methods. We conducted a comprehensive review to identify all relevant policies as of July 1, 2024. Specifically, we developed a coding scheme to capture laws governing (1) direct delivery of recreational cannabis, (2) licensing for direct delivery of recreational cannabis, (3) direct delivery of medical cannabis to qualifying patients, and (4) medical cannabis delivery solely from caregivers to qualified patients.

Results. Fourteen states authorized the direct delivery of recreational cannabis to adults. Twenty-six states and the District of Columbia permitted the direct delivery of medical cannabis to qualifying patients. Twelve states allowed the delivery of medical cannabis to patients exclusively through caregivers. There were numerous variations in the licensing and authorization of recreational and medical cannabis delivery.

Conclusions. States varied in how the delivery of cannabis was regulated.

Public Health Implications. A comprehensive review of state-level policies on cannabis delivery highlights the diverse approaches and their implications for recreational and medical cannabis access.
(*Am J Public Health*. 2025;115(2):178–190. https://doi.org/10.2105/AJPH.2024.307874)

AJPH February 2025, Vol. 115, No. 2

The cannabis policy landscape has seen substantial changes in recent years. Despite cannabis still being federally restricted, a significant number of states have passed laws legalizing its medical and recreational use among adults.[1] It is estimated that 74% of people in the United States reside in a state where cannabis is legal for recreational use, medical use, or both, as of 2024.[1] Scholars have noted that the existing situation, where state cannabis laws conflict with federal regulation, poses challenges to rational drug control and cooperative federalism.[2,3] However, in May 2024, the US Justice Department proposed regulations to ease federal restrictions on cannabis,[4] which could potentially resolve the conflict and allow more permissive state legislation.

The rapid evolution of cannabis legalization in the United States has introduced some ambiguity regarding the public health impact of its regulatory status.[5] Evidence suggests that cannabis use is associated with health risks, including respiratory symptoms, potential development of schizophrenia, and immediate effects such as impaired cognition and driving.[6–10] Prolonged cannabis use can lead to cannabis use disorder, a psychiatric condition characterized by the inability to stop consuming cannabis even when it causes physical or psychological harm to an individual's life.[6] Cannabis use disorder affects nearly 1 in 3 cannabis users in the United States, with a higher risk among individuals who start using cannabis early and those who use it more frequently.[6,11–13] By one estimate, cannabis use disorder accounted for approximately 690 000 disability-adjusted life years globally in 2019.[14] There are also cannabis use risks to youths and young adults, such as neurodevelopmental decline, poor school performance, and adverse mental health outcomes.[15–17]

Notwithstanding the potential risks associated with using cannabis, there are also reported medical benefits. A national report and systematic reviews support the use of cannabinoids (i.e., chemicals found in cannabis) and tetrahydrocannabinol (THC) for treating chronic pain and spasticity in adults.[12,18,19] In addition, oral cannabinoids have been used to treat chemotherapy-induced nausea and vomiting, as well as patient-reported multiple sclerosis spasticity symptoms. Other studies suggest that cannabinoids may not be highly effective in managing chronic noncancer pain, but they could potentially serve as a modest therapeutic option.[20,21] As of 2024, 38 states and the District of Columbia allow the medical use of cannabis products to treat certain conditions such as cancer, Crohn's disease, epilepsy, multiple sclerosis, anxiety disorders, and terminal illnesses.[1]

A crucial factor to consider in regulating products that pose health risks yet offer certain health or social benefits is the method of sale. In contrast to brick-and-mortar outlet sales, where consumers purchase products from vendors in person, "direct-delivery" sales involve placing an order with a vendor remotely through phone, online, or apps such as Leafly and receiving the product directly at the user's location. A significant regulatory challenge for direct-delivery sales is the ability of consumers to place orders remotely.[22] The direct delivery of recreational cannabis products, similar to tobacco products, can inadvertently enhance access for youths and young adults if regulations do not adequately cover various policy dimensions, such as age verification requirements and delivery-specific licensing and enforcement.[23–26] Indeed, a recent study found that most online dispensaries lack adequate age verification measures.[27] Furthermore, consumer habits may have been modified by the regular direct delivery of some substances, such as cannabis, during the COVID-19 pandemic, thereby influencing policy considerations.[23] There has been a growing concern about the home delivery of substances that are prone to misuse, with a call to investigate further the potential health implications and preventive measures associated with this emerging trend.[23]

At the same time, direct delivery of medical cannabis allows qualifying patients to order medical cannabis to be delivered from medical dispensaries or through means similar to those for recreational use. Almost all states that permit medical cannabis use have mandated a statewide registry for patients with qualifying conditions. Direct delivery of medical cannabis can enhance patient access by providing patients with additional choices about when and how they can order and receive their medication, particularly those who are homebound because of certain illnesses.[28] Some states have recognized this and passed legislation allowing direct delivery from medical dispensaries to patients to improve patient access. The extent to which direct delivery of cannabis to consumers may affect patterns of cannabis access and use within states is unclear, given that our understanding of its regulation remains limited.

In the rapidly changing landscape of cannabis policy in the United States, where legalization and access are expanding, we investigated the underexplored legal epidemiology area of state-level direct-delivery laws for both recreational and medical cannabis. Through a systematic legal analysis, we identified and coded relevant statutes and regulations, focusing on elements that potentially have significant implications for public health. This research contributes to a deeper understanding of specific policy dimensions surrounding cannabis direct-delivery legalization, which is particularly important given the ongoing changes in cannabis policy across the United States. The findings from our study could guide further research into the health impacts of these laws and their enforcement.

METHODS

We conducted a comprehensive search of state laws related to the direct delivery of recreational and medical cannabis using the Westlaw legal database. In 2023, we compiled an archive of pertinent statutory and regulatory enactments. We subsequently updated the archive to include all laws in effect as of July 1, 2024.

Legal Variable Coding

The study team reviewed each section within every enactment to identify explicit laws related to cannabis delivery or laws with implicit language on delivery (e.g., "transportation of marijuana"). Laws that did not focus on intrastate direct-delivery sales of recreational and medical cannabis to consumers or qualifying patients were deemed irrelevant to the study and removed from the archive. We also excluded laws addressing only cross-state (interstate) delivery sales or delivery further up the supply chain (e.g., to distributors).

After compiling and reviewing the relevant laws, we developed a coding scheme to capture several salient characteristics: (1) laws permitting direct delivery of recreational cannabis to consumers; (2) licensing laws for direct delivery of recreational cannabis; (3) laws permitting direct delivery of medical cannabis to qualified individuals, including licensing and authorization laws; and (4) laws permitting caregivers to deliver medical cannabis to registered qualified patients in states without laws permitting other forms of direct delivery. Although we use the term "cannabis" in general, we align with the terminology used by individual states in their laws when discussing policy components. For instance, the findings in our tables refer to "marijuana" as used in Massachusetts, or the alternate spelling "marihuana" as used in Michigan statutes. Because of the differences between state-mandated qualifying patient registries for medical consumers and the absence of registry requirements for recreational consumers, our measures focus on slightly different legal domains for recreational versus medical direct delivery.

Measures

Recreational cannabis direct-delivery laws. We identified laws that permit the direct delivery of recreational cannabis to consumers and coded the following aspects: (1) age verification requirements, (2) school and university restrictions, and (3) preemption of local laws prohibiting delivery. Age verification requirements specify procedures for authorized recreational cannabis delivery agents to ensure delivery to legal adults. School and university restrictions prohibit the delivery of recreational cannabis on school or university premises to reduce access to recreational cannabis on institutional grounds. Preemption of local laws restricts municipal governments from prohibiting the direct delivery of recreational cannabis within their jurisdictions.

Recreational cannabis direct-delivery licensing laws. Our research team coded specific provisions related to the licensing of direct delivery of recreational cannabis. These provisions included (1) delivery licensing, (2) penalties for license violations, and (3) local authority. Delivery licensing refers to the types of licenses or permits required to initiate the direct delivery of recreational cannabis, allowing states to monitor delivery activities and ensure compliance. Penalties for license violations consist of fines or sanctions imposed on licensees or delivery agents to deter illicit behavior. Local authority provisions relate to whether states allow or prohibit local laws governing delivery, including whether local licenses are explicitly permitted, whether local approval is required for state licensing, or whether local zoning (i.e., time, place, and manner regulations) applies to licensees. Documenting whether local regulation is permitted is crucial for understanding the scope of state laws, their impact, and the potential for local involvement in cannabis delivery activities.

Medical cannabis direct-delivery laws. We identified laws that permitted the delivery by or from medical cannabis establishments, capturing provisions addressing (1) delivery licensing or authorization, (2) delivery access specification, and (3) local authority. Delivery licensing or authorization relates to the types of licenses or authorizations necessary for delivery. The delivery access specification captures the specified individuals who have obtained authorization to receive direct delivery of medical cannabis. Local authority refers to whether states allow or prohibit local laws governing delivery.

Medical cannabis delivery from caregivers to qualified patients. Lastly, we identified laws that allow caregivers to deliver medical cannabis to qualified patients in states where there are no laws permitting the direct delivery of recreational cannabis to consumers or medical cannabis to qualifying individuals. While caregivers can deliver medical cannabis to assist patients in the states identified, patients in these states do not have the legal option of direct delivery. In these states, we also coded explicit prohibitions on statewide direct delivery.

RESULTS

States varied widely in how the delivery of cannabis was regulated.

Recreational Cannabis Direct-Delivery Laws

Table 1 lists the 14 states that allowed direct recreational cannabis delivery to adult consumers. These states were California, Colorado, Connecticut, Maine, Massachusetts, Michigan, Minnesota, Missouri, Nevada, New Jersey, New Mexico, New York, Oregon, and Rhode Island. States varied in how they regulated age verification. For instance, New Jersey required a signature upon delivery, while Connecticut permitted the use of an online age verification interface. Massachusetts mandated that delivery personnel undergo age verification training and permitted preverification through approved electronic means. Nine of these states, including California, had laws prohibiting the direct delivery of recreational cannabis to schools or universities. Eleven states had laws that explicitly preempted local prohibitions on recreational cannabis direct delivery. Some states, like Connecticut, specifically preempted local prohibitions on cannabis delivery. Others, such as New Mexico, adopted a broader approach by banning local control over cannabis transportation within local jurisdictions, which could include delivery.

TABLE 1— Recreational Cannabis Direct-Delivery Laws: United States, as of July 1, 2024

State[a]	Laws Permitting Recreational Cannabis Direct Delivery	Age Verification Requirements	School and University Delivery Restrictions	Preemption of Local Delivery Prohibitions
CA	Cal. Bus. & Prof. Code § 26001	Cal. Bus. & Prof. Code § 26140; Cal. Code Regs. tit. 4, §§ 15404, 15415	Cal. Code Regs. tit. 4, § 15416	Cal. Bus. & Prof. Code § 26090
CO	Colo. Rev. Stat. § 44-10-601	Colo. Rev. Stat. § 44-10-601; 1 Colo. Code Regs. § 212-3:3-615	Colo. Rev. Stat. §§ 44-10-501, 601; 1 Colo. Code Regs. § 212-3:3-615	NA
CT	Conn. Gen. Stat. § 21a-420	Conn. Gen. Stat. § 21a-420z	NA	Conn. Gen. Stat. § 21a-422 g
ME	Me. Stat. tit. 28-B, § 102	Me. Stat. tit. 28-B, § 504	Me. Stat. tit. 28-B, § 504; 18-691 Me. Code R. Ch. 1, § 1.4	Me. Stat. tit. 28-B, § 504
MA	Mass. Gen. Laws Ch. 94G, §§ 1, 9	Mass. Gen. Laws Ch. 94G, § 4; 935 Mass. Code Regs. 500.105, 500.145	935 Mass. Code Regs. 500.145	Mass. Gen. Laws Ch. 94G, § 3
MI	Mich. Admin. Code r. 420.207	Mich. Admin. Code r. 420.207	Mich. Admin. Code r. 420.207	Mich. Comp. Laws § 333.27956
MN	Minn. Stat. § 342.10	Minn. Stat. §§ 342.27, 342.42	NA	Minn. Stat. § 342.13
MO	Mo. Const. Art. 14 § 2	Mo. Code Regs. Ann. tit. 19, § 100-1.140	NA	Mo. Const. Art. 14 § 2
NV	Nev. Admin. Code § 453D.572	Nev. Admin. Code §§ 453D.572, 453D.558	Nev. Admin. Code § 453D.578	NA
NJ	N.J. Stat. Ann. § 24:6I-33	N.J. Stat. Ann. § 24:6I-44; N.J. Admin. Code § 17:30-15.2	N.J. Admin. Code § 17:30-14.8	N.J. Stat. Ann. § 24:6I-44; N.J. Admin. Code § 17:30-5.1
NM	N.M. Stat. Ann. § 26-2C-2	N.M. Code R. §§ 16.8.2.40, 41	NA	N.M. Stat. Ann. § 26-2C-12
NY	McKinney's Cons. Laws of N.Y. Ann., Cannabis Law § 61	McKinney's Cons. Laws of N.Y. Ann., Cannabis Law § 85; N.Y. Comp. Codes R. & Regs. tit. 9, § 123.20	N.Y. Comp. Codes R. & Regs. tit. 9, § 123.20	McKinney's Cons. Laws of N.Y. Ann., Cannabis Law § 131
OR	Or. Rev. Stat. § 475C.009	Or. Rev. Stat. § 475C.109; Or. Admin. R. 845-025-2880	Or. Admin. R. 845-025-2880	NA
RI	21 R.I. Gen. Laws § 21–28.11-24	21 R.I. Gen. Laws § 21–28.11-5	NA	21 R.I. Gen. Laws § 21–28.11-16

Note. NA = not applicable.
[a]Arizona, per Ariz. Rev. Stat. § 36-2854, will adopt rules allowing and regulating recreational delivery by marijuana establishments by January 1, 2025.

Recreational Direct-Delivery Licensing Laws

Table 2 indicates that states permitting direct delivery of recreational cannabis to consumers had varying regulations concerning authorization and licensees, penalties for license violations, and local authority. For example, Colorado required a "delivery permit" for recreational cannabis delivery, whereas Oregon mandated a "marijuana handler permit" for the same purpose. Other states had unique licensing requirements based on their specific systems. In Massachusetts, there were 2 types of licenses related to cannabis delivery: a "Marijuana Courier" licensee, who could transport marijuana from a retailer to a consumer but could not sell it, and a "Marijuana Delivery Operator" licensee, who had broader privileges, including the ability to purchase wholesale cannabis, store it in a warehouse, and sell and deliver it directly to consumers. Connecticut required a license for any "delivery service" that transported cannabis from licensed microcultivators, retailers, and hybrid retailers to end consumers. Penalties for license infractions varied by state, with fines ranging from $500 for minor infractions in New Jersey to $100 000 for violations that affected public safety in states like Colorado and Maine. These penalties often involved additional sanctions such as license suspensions, revocations, or further restrictions. Provisions involving local authority also differed by state. Some states, like California, allowed local licensing, while others, such as Connecticut, required proof of local zoning approval for state licensure.

Medical Cannabis Direct-Delivery Laws

Table 3 presents the states with laws permitting direct delivery of medical

TABLE 2— Recreational Cannabis Direct-Delivery Licensing Laws: United States, as of July 1, 2024

State	Delivery Licensing	Penalties for License Violations	Local Authority
CA	Cal. Bus. & Prof. Code §§ 26001, 26090; Cal. Code Regs. tit. 4, §§ 15000, 15415, 15415.1 Licensed retailers and microbusinesses by delivery employees only, may contract with technology platform service to take orders	Cal. Bus. & Prof. Code §§ 26031, 26031.5; Cal. Code Regs. tit. 4, § 17802 License suspension and revocation, up to $5000 per violation (each day is a separate violation)	Cal. Bus. & Prof. Code § 26200; Cal. Code Regs. tit. 4, § 15018 Local licensing, local zoning
CO	Colo. Rev. Stat. §§ 44-10-601, 605; 1 Colo. Code Regs. §§ 212-3:3-105, 615, 1105 Licensed retail marijuana store, accelerator store, and licensed retail marijuana transporter (retail marijuana delivery permit required)	1 Colo. Code Regs. § 212-3:8-235 License suspension, revocation, or additional restrictions, up to $10 000 (infraction), $50 000 (violation), $100 000 (violation affecting public safety)	Colo. Rev. Stat. §§ 44-10-203, 601, 605; 1 Colo. Code Regs. §§ 212-3:3-135, 615 Local licensing, local approval is required for retail marijuana delivery permit
CT	Conn. Gen. Stat. §§ 21a-420, 420c Licensed delivery service, microcultivators, retailers, and hybrid retailers	Conn. Gen. Stat. § 21a-421p License or registration suspension or revocation, fines up to $25 000 per violation, compromise offer or renewal refusal, license probation or conditions	Conn. Gen. Stat. § 21a-422f Local zoning
ME	Me. Stat. tit. 28-B, §§ 501, 504; 18-691 Me. Code R. Ch. 1 § 2.2 Limited delivery service including by Tier 1 (not more than 500 square feet of mature plant canopy) and Tier 2 (not more than 2 000 square feet) cultivation facility	Me. Stat. tit. 28-B, § 802; 18-691 Me. Code R. Ch. 1 § 10.3 License suspension or revocation, not more than $10 000 per minor violation, not more than $50 000 per major violation, and not more than $100 000 per major violation affecting public safety	Me. Stat. tit. 28-B, §§ 206, 402, 403; 18-691 Me. Code R. Ch. 1 § 2.7 Local conditions cause for denial, local authorization of establishments required
MA	Mass. Gen. Laws Ch. 94G, § 19; 935 Mass. Code Regs. 500.002, 500.145 Delivery licensees, marijuana establishments with delivery endorsement, marijuana retailers (done by a delivery operator or marijuana courier), may contract with third-party technology platforms	935 Mass. Code Regs. 500.360 Administrative fine of up to $50 000 for each violation (each day is a separate violation)	935 Mass. Code Regs. 500.103 Local compliance for approval
MI	Mich. Admin. Code r. 420.207 Marihuana sales locations licensed under MRTMA (recreational), may only deliver to customers upon approval by the agency of the licensee's delivery procedures	Mich. Comp. Laws § 333.27958; Mich. Admin. Code r. 420.806 License suspension, revocation, or restriction, up to $10 000 (each day is a separate violation)	Mich. Comp. Laws § 333.27956 Local zoning
MN	Minn. Stat. §§ 342.41, 342.42 Licensed cannabis delivery service may purchase from licensed businesses and deliver to customers	Minn. Stat. § 342.19 Up to $10 000, an amount that deprives the business of any economic advantage gained by the violation, or both	Minn. Stat. § 342.13 Local zoning
MO	Mo. Const. Art. 14 § 2; Mo. Code Regs. Ann. tit. 19, §§ 100-1.010, 1.180, 1.190 Licensed comprehensive marijuana dispensary facilities or microbusiness dispensary facilities	Mo. Const. Art. 14 § 2; Mo. Code Regs. Ann. tit. 19, § 100-1.030 Authorized administrative fines (up to an amount equal to the average daily gross receipts of the previous calendar month of the facility per day) and suspension, revocation, or restriction of a license	Mo. Const. Art. 14 § 2 Local zoning is permitted but must not conflict with state laws
NV	Nev. Rev. Stat. §§ 678A.065, 678A.250; Nev. Admin. Code § 453D.572 Licensed adult-use retail marijuana store via marijuana establishment agent with registration card; store must get preapproval for delivery procedures	Nev. Admin. Code § 453D.905 License suspension and revocation, scalar fines $750–$35 000 (categories I–V)	Nev. Rev. Stat. §§ 678B.300, 678B.320; Nev. Admin. Code § 453D.282 Local business license, local zoning for approval
NJ	N.J. Stat. Ann. §§ 24:6I-43, 44; N.J. Admin. Code § 17:30-1.2 Licensed delivery service, certified cannabis handler, approved contractor	N.J. Stat. Ann. § 24:6I-29 License suspension or revocation, not less than $500 nor more than $10 000	N.J. Stat. Ann. § 24:6I-44, 45; N.J. Admin. Code § 17:30-5.1 Local delivery licensing is optional, local may prohibit delivery licensing but may not prohibit delivery

Continued

TABLE 2— Continued

State	Delivery Licensing	Penalties for License Violations	Local Authority
NM	N.M. Stat. Ann. §§ 26-2C-2, 6, 9; N.M. Code R. § 16.8.2.40 Licensed vertically integrated cannabis establishment, cannabis retailer, and integrated cannabis microbusiness via cannabis couriers (with delivery agreement)	N.M. Stat. Ann. § 26-2C-8 Not exceed $10 000 per violation, license suspension, or revocation	N.M. Stat. Ann. § 26-2C-12; N.M. Code R. §§ 16.8.2.36, 42 Local business license is required, local zoning but must not conflict with state laws
NY	McKinney's Cons. Laws of N.Y. Ann., Cannabis Law § 74; N.Y. Comp. Codes R. & Regs. tit. 9, § 123.20 Licensed retailers and microbusinesses but independent contractors must disclose deliveries. The delivery license allows the delivery of cannabis and cannabis products independent of other licenses, but licensees are prohibited from selling	N.Y. Comp. Codes R. & Regs. tit. 9, §§ 133.7, 114.17 License suspension or revocation. Up to $1 000 for the first violation, $5 000 for a second violation within 3 years, $10 000 for a third violation, and each subsequent violation within 3 years	McKinney's Cons. Laws of N.Y. Ann., Cannabis Law §§ 76, 131; N.Y. Comp. Codes R. & Regs. tit. 9, § 119.3 Municipal opinions on licensure, local zoning
OR	Or. Rev. Stat. §§ 475C.117, 269 Licensed retailer via agent with marijuana handler permit	Or. Rev. Stat. § 475C.405; Or. Admin. R. 845-025-8590 License suspension or revocation, scalar fines varied (categories I–V)	Or. Rev. Stat. §§ 475C.113, 117, 449, 950 City or county ordinance may permit or prohibit delivery; local zoning
RI	21 R.I. Gen. Laws § 21–28.11-3 Licensed retailer	21 R.I. Gen. Laws § 21–28.11-9 License suspension or revocation, fines established by the department of business regulation, cease and desist or compliance order, or penalty combination	21 R.I. Gen. Laws § 21–28.11-16 Local zoning recognized

Note. MRTMA = Michigan Regulation and Taxation of Marihuana Act.

cannabis. All 14 states that allowed direct delivery of recreational cannabis also permitted medical cannabis delivery to qualified patients. In addition to these, 13 more jurisdictions—Arizona, Arkansas, Delaware, the District of Columbia, Florida, Kentucky, Louisiana, Maryland, Montana, New Hampshire, Utah, Vermont, and Virginia—allowed medical cannabis direct delivery. The type of authorizations that permitted medical cannabis direct delivery and the recipients of this service varied by state. For instance, most states allowed medical cannabis delivery from registered medical dispensaries, compassion centers, or treatment centers to registered qualifying patients and caregivers. States like Colorado, Massachusetts, Montana, New Jersey, New Mexico, and Utah permitted direct delivery through couriers. The District of Columbia, New Hampshire, and New Mexico even allowed nonresident cardholders to receive medical cannabis direct delivery. Local licensing provisions also differed by state. Some states, such as Colorado, allowed local licensing, and others, like Utah, required compliance with local zoning for state approval.

Caregiver-to-Patient Cannabis Delivery

Table 4 shows states that only permitted medical cannabis delivery from caregivers to qualified patients. Twelve states with recreational or medical cannabis legalization did not permit direct delivery of cannabis. Among the states that had legalized recreational cannabis use, Alaska, Illinois, Ohio, and Washington did not allow direct delivery. Similarly, among the states that had legalized medical cannabis use, Alabama, Hawaii, Mississippi, North Dakota, Oklahoma, Pennsylvania, South Dakota, and West Virginia did not permit direct delivery. However, they all allowed caregivers to deliver medical cannabis to registered qualified patients.

DISCUSSION

As the landscape of cannabis legalization continues to evolve, a critical yet underexplored aspect is the laws governing its direct delivery. This study is the first, to our knowledge, to document and categorize the direct-delivery laws for both recreational and medical cannabis at the state level. Our findings reveal a significant heterogeneity in the legal status of cannabis direct delivery across states. Among the 25 jurisdictions that had legalized recreational cannabis, 14

TABLE 3— Medical Cannabis Direct-Delivery Laws From Medical Cannabis Establishments: United States, as of July 1, 2024

State	Laws Permitting Medical Cannabis Delivery From Medical Cannabis Establishments	Delivery Licensing or Authorization	Delivery Access Specification	Local Authority
AZ	Ariz. Rev. Stat. § 36-2801	Ariz. Rev. Stat. §§ 36-2801, 2804 Registered nonprofit medical marijuana dispensary	Ariz. Rev. Stat. § 36-2806 Registered qualifying patients or through designated caregivers	Ariz. Rev. Stat. § 36-2806.01 Local zoning
AR	Ar. Const. Amend. 98 § 2	Ar. Const. Amend. 98 § 8 Licensed dispensary	Ar. Const. Amend. 98 § 8 Registered qualifying patients and designated caregivers	Ar. Const. Amend. 98 § 8 Local zoning
CA	Cal. Bus. & Prof. Code § 26321	Cal. Bus. & Prof. Code §§ 26050, 26321 Licensed medicinal cannabis business (M-License)	Cal. Bus. & Prof. Code § 26321 Registered qualified patients and primary caregivers	Cal. Bus. & Prof. Code §§ 26322, 26325 Medical cannabis patients' right to access is "a matter of statewide concern and not a municipal affair"
CO	Colo. Rev. Stat. § 44-10-103	Colo. Rev. Stat. §§ 44-10-313, 301, 401 Licensed medical marijuana business or medical marijuana transporter licensee with medical marijuana delivery permit	Colo. Rev. Stat. § 44-10-501; Colo. Const. Art. 18 § 14 Delivery only to registered patients, parents, or guardians	Colo. Rev. Stat. § 44-10-301 Local licensing
CT	Conn. Admin. Code § 21a-408-1	Conn. Admin. Code § 21a-408-1 Licensed dispensary facility	Conn. Admin. Code § 21a-408-35 Registered qualifying patients and primary caregivers	Conn. Admin. Code § 21a-408-15 Local zoning and approval
DE	16 Del. Admin. Code § 4470-7.0	16 Del. Admin. Code § 4470-7.0 Registered compassion centers with approval of delivery plan	16 Del. Admin. Code § 4470-7.0 Registered patients and designated caregivers	16 Del. Admin. Code § 4470-7.0 Local zoning
DC	D.C. Mun. Regs. tit. 22-C, § 5703	D.C. Mun. Regs. tit. 22-C, § 5703 Dispensary	D.C. Mun. Regs. tit. 22-C, § 5703 Registered qualifying patients or caregivers, nonresident qualifying patients	No local provisions were identified
FL	Fla. Stat. § 381.986, Fla. Admin. Code Ann. r. 64ER22-7	Fla. Stat. § 381.986 Licensed medical marijuana treatment center	Fla. Stat. § 381.986 Registered qualifying patients	Fla. Stat. § 381.986 Local amendments to state building and fire prevention codes apply to compliance
KY	Ky. Rev. Stat. Ann. § 218B.110	Ky. Rev. Stat. Ann. § 218B.110 Licensed dispensaries may operate a delivery service	Ky. Rev. Stat. Ann. § 218B.110 Registered cardholders' addresses	Ky. Rev. Stat. Ann. § 218B.130 Local zoning
LA	La. Admin. Code tit. 46, Pt. LIII § 2441	La. Stat. Ann § 40:1046; La. Admin. Code tit. 46, Pt. LIII § 2451 Licensed marijuana pharmacy	La. Stat. Ann § 40:1046; La. Admin. Code tit. 46, Pt. LIII § 2451 Required to offer home delivery to patients in each zip code within the region at least once per month; patients need a doctor's signed certification as identification	La. Admin. Code tit. 46, Pt. LIII § 2441 Local zoning
ME	Me. Stat. tit. 22, § 2428	Me. Stat. tit. 22, § 2428; 18-691 Me. Code R. Ch. 2 § 7 Registered dispensary	Me. Stat. tit. 22, § 2428; 18-691 Me. Code R. Ch. 2 § 7 Registered qualifying patients and caregivers	Me. Stat. tit. 22, § 2429-D Municipal approval via conditional use or site plan approval
MD	Md. Code Regs. 10.62.30.04	Md. Code Regs. 10.62.30.04 Registered dispensary	Md. Code Regs. 10.62.30.01 Registered qualifying patients and caregivers with written certification of delivery request	Md. Code Regs. 10.62.27.02 Local zoning and planning conformity required

Continued

TABLE 3— Continued

State	Laws Permitting Medical Cannabis Delivery From Medical Cannabis Establishments	Delivery Licensing or Authorization	Delivery Access Specification	Local Authority
MA	935 Mass. Code Regs. 501.145	935 Mass. Code Regs. 501.145 Licensed marijuana treatment center by marijuana courier	Mass. Gen. Laws Ch. 94I, § 5935; 935 Mass. Code Regs. 501.050, 501.145 Registered qualifying patients and personal caregivers	935 Mass. Code Regs. 501.101 Local compliance, local licensing authority requirements in application
MI	Mich. Comp. Laws § 333.26423	Mich. Comp. Laws § 333.27504; Mich. Admin. Code r. 420.101 Provisioning center licensed under MMFLA (medical)	Mich. Comp. Laws § 333.27504 Registered qualifying patients and primary caregivers	Mich. Comp. Laws § 333.27205 Local authorization is required with local zoning compliance
MN	Minn. Stat. § 342.51	Minn. Stat. §§ 342.42, 342.51 Cannabis business with a medical cannabis retail endorsement and also must hold a cannabis delivery service license (also subject to recreational operations)	Minn. Stat. § 342.51 Registered person	Minn. Stat. § 342.13 Local zoning
MO	Mo. Const. Art. 14 § 1	Mo. Const. Art. 14 § 1 Licensed medical marijuana dispensary facility	Mo. Const. Art. 14 § 1 Registered qualifying patients and primary caregivers	Mo. Const. Art. 14 § 1 Local zoning is permitted but must not conflict with state laws
MT	Mont. Code Ann. § 16-12-222	Mont. Code Ann. § 16-12-222 Licensed marijuana transporter	Mont. Code Ann. §§ 16-12-222, 513 Registered cardholders and 2 authorized individuals to deliver from a licensed dispensary	Mont. Code Ann. § 16-12-207 Local zoning
NV	Nev. Rev. Stat. § 678C.450	Nev. Rev. Stat. §§ 678C.440, 678C.450 Licensed medical cannabis dispensary (may contract with third-party or intermediary business)	Nev. Rev. Stat. §§ 678C.420, 678C.450 An electronic verification system is required for registered cardholders or with a letter of approval	No local provisions were identified
NH	N.H. Rev. Stat. §§ 126-X:1, 2	N.H. Rev. Stat. §§ 126-X:1, 2; N.H. Code Admin. R. Ann. He-C 401.02 Registered not-for-profit alternative treatment center	N.H. Rev. Stat. § 126-X:8 Registered qualifying patients, designated caregivers, visiting qualifying patients	N.H. Rev. Stat. § 126-X:7; N.H. Code Admin. R. Ann. He-C 402.09 Local zoning and compliance
NJ	N.J. Stat. Ann. § 24:6I-1	N.J. Stat. Ann. § 24:6I-1, 20; N.J. Admin. Code § 17:30-7.1 Licensed alternative treatment center via medical cannabis handler with delivery certification, and unlicensed expanded alternative treatment center with certification including "plan for prioritizing and meeting the needs of" patients	N.J. Stat. Ann. § 24:6I-3 Registered qualifying patients, designated caregivers, or institutional caregivers	N.J. Stat. Ann. §§ 24:6I-7.2, 20 Local zoning approval is required; a municipality may not restrict or prohibit delivery
NM	N.M. Stat. Ann. § 26-2B-3	N.M. Stat. Ann. § 26-2C-2; N.M. Code R. § 16.8.2.41 Licensed cannabis courier	N.M. Stat. Ann. §§ 26-2B-3, 7, 7.1 Registered qualified patients and primary caregivers, reciprocal participants (out of state with proof to participate in medical cannabis program of another state)	N.M. Stat. Ann. § 26-2C-12; N.M. Code R. § 16.8.2.41 Local prohibitions on cannabis transportation are preempted, but the permitted time of delivery must comply with local laws

Continued

TABLE 3— Continued

State	Laws Permitting Medical Cannabis Delivery From Medical Cannabis Establishments	Delivery Licensing or Authorization	Delivery Access Specification	Local Authority
NY	McKinney's Cons. Laws of N.Y. Ann., Cannabis Law § 31	McKinney's Cons. Laws of N.Y. Ann., Cannabis Law § 31; N.Y. Comp. Codes R. & Regs. tit. 9, § 113.14 Registered organization (for-profit business or not-for-profit corporation)	McKinney's Cons. Laws of N.Y. Ann., Cannabis Law § 34 Registered qualifying patients and designated caregivers	McKinney's Cons. Laws of N.Y. Ann., Cannabis Law § 131; N.Y. Comp. Codes R. & Regs. tit. 9, § 113.7 Local zoning and local compliance
OR	Or. Rev. Stat. § 475C.205	Or. Rev. Stat. § 475C.205 Licensed retailer	Or. Rev. Stat. § 475C.205 Registered identification cardholders and designated primary caregivers	Or. Rev. Stat. §§ 475C.113, 117, 449, 950 City or county ordinance may permit or prohibit delivery, local zoning
RI	21 R.I. Gen. Laws § 21–28.6-12	21 R.I. Gen. Laws § 21–28.6-12; 230-80-05 R.I. Code R. § 1.6 Licensed compassion center	21 R.I. Gen. Laws § 21-28.6-12; 230-80-05 R.I. Code R. § 1.6 Patient cardholders, qualified patients' primary caregivers, authorized purchasers	230-80-05 R.I. Code R. § 1.6 Local zoning
UT	Utah Code Ann. § 4-41a-102	Utah Code Ann. §§ 4-41a-1201, 1202, 1203 Medical cannabis pharmacy with approved home delivery designation via licensed medical cannabis courier	Utah Code Ann. §§ 4-41a-1202, 1205 Medical cannabis cardholder (at home through state electronic verification system or at a facility)	Utah Code Ann. § 4-41a-1105 Local zoning
VT	Vt. Stat. Ann. tit. 7, § 971	Vt. Stat. Ann. tit. 7, § 971 Licensed dispensary	Vt. Stat. Ann. tit. 7, § 971 Registered patients and caregivers	Vt. Stat. Ann. tit. 7, § 863; Vt. Admin. Code 26-1-2.14 Local control license, a municipality may not regulate an establishment that has the effect of prohibiting the operation of the establishment
VA	Va. Code Ann. § 4.1-600	Va. Code Ann. § 4.1-1603 Permitted pharmaceutical processor or cannabis dispensing facility	Va. Code Ann. § 4.1-1603 Resident patients or temporary resident patients, patients' registered agents, patients' parents or legal guardians	3 Va. Admin. Code §§ 10-30-130, 140 Local compliance

Note. MMFLA = Michigan Medical Marihuana Facilities Licensing Act.

TABLE 4— **Medical Cannabis Delivery Laws From Caregivers to Qualified Patients: United States, as of July 1, 2024**

State	Laws Permitting Medical Cannabis Delivery From Caregivers to Qualified Patients in States With No Recreational or Medical Direct-Delivery Laws	Delivery Prohibitions
AL	Ala. Code § 20-2A-3	Ala. Code § 20-2A-3 Licensed dispensaries are only "authorized to dispense and sell medical cannabis at dispensing sites."
AK	Alaska Stat. § 17.37.040	Alaska Admin. Code tit. 3, § 306.990 Delivering "does not include transferring or transporting to a consumer off licensed premises."
HI	Haw. Rev. Stat. § 329D-1	Haw. Rev. Stat. § 329D-6 Dispensary "prohibited from off-premises delivery of cannabis or manufactured cannabis products."
IL	Ill. Admin. Code tit. 77, § 946.10	410 Ill. Comp. Stat. 705/15-70, 8 Ill. Admin. Code tit. 8, § 1300.40 Dispensing organizations may not "transport cannabis to residences or other locations where purchasers may be for delivery." A cannabis business establishment may not "Sell, deliver, transport or distribute cannabis to any person or entity other than a cannabis business organization licensed by the Department."
MS	Miss. Code Ann. § 41-137-3	35 Miss. Admin. Code Pt. XI, R. 24 A dispensary must not "Sell or distribute cannabis products using . . . a delivery service."
ND	N.D. Cent. Code § 19-24.1-01	N.D. Cent. Code § 19-03.1-23 Marijuana delivery is prohibited as a controlled substance.
OH	Ohio Admin. Code 3796:6-3-22	Ohio Admin. Code 3796:6-3-22 "No medical marijuana shall be sold, dispensed, or distributed to a patient or caregiver via a delivery service or any other manner outside of a dispensary, except that a caregiver may deliver medical marijuana to the caregiver's registered patient."
OK	Okla. Stat. tit. 63, § 427.11	Okla. Admin. Code § 442:10-5-16 "No commercial licensee shall allow for or provide the delivery of medical marijuana or medical marijuana products to licensed patients or caregivers."
PA	28 Pa. Code § 1141a.21	28 Pa. Code § 1161a.27 A dispensary may not "deliver, or contract to a third party the delivery of, medical marijuana products to a patient or caregiver at the patient's or caregiver's home or any other location."
SD	S.D. Codified Laws § 34-20G-1	S.D. Admin. Code 44:90:08:04 "No cannabis or cannabis product sale may take place at any location other than at a certified medical cannabis dispensary. All sales must take place at a certified medical cannabis dispensary in clear view of security cameras."
WA	Wash. Rev. Code 69.51A.010	Wash. Admin. Code § 314-55-079 "Internet sales and delivery of product to customers is prohibited."
WV	W. Va. Code § 16A-2-1	W. Va. Admin. Code § 64-112-4 "A dispensary may only dispense medical cannabis to a patient or caregiver who presents a valid identification card to an employee at the facility who is authorized to dispense medical cannabis at the facility."

had permitted direct delivery to adult consumers. Of the 39 jurisdictions that had legalized medical cannabis, direct delivery to qualifying patients was permitted in 26 states and the District of Columbia. All states that allowed recreational cannabis direct delivery also allowed medical cannabis direct delivery. Twelve states allowed medical cannabis delivery to patients solely through caregiver delivery.

Furthermore, our results highlight wide variations in the regulation of cannabis direct-delivery laws. Regarding recreational cannabis delivery, there were variations in age verification requirements, restrictions on schools and universities, and the preemption of local prohibition of direct delivery. These laws also differed in delivery licensing, penalties for license violations, and whether local licensing was permitted or local zoning was recognized. State laws varied similarly for medical cannabis direct delivery, including which entities were authorized or licensed to make direct medical-use deliveries and whether local regulation was permitted. There were also differences in who is authorized to access and receive deliveries. In states that had legalized recreational or medical cannabis but did not permit direct delivery, only designated caregivers were allowed to deliver cannabis to registered qualifying patients to assist them in their medical use.

Public Health Significance

The rapidly evolving landscape of cannabis use warrants the need to catalog policies with potential public health ramifications for access, particularly those concerning direct delivery. Previous research has highlighted public health issues, such as underage access, associated with the direct delivery of substances like alcohol and tobacco.[22,25,29,30] It is plausible that cannabis direct delivery could present similar challenges. Our study provides a detailed catalog of existing cannabis policies and reveals significant variations in their legal status, content, and scope across states.

As recreational cannabis use becomes increasingly legal across the United States, it may be advisable to regulate its direct delivery to reduce underage access. States should consider mandating stringent age verification requirements to limit unauthorized access. Examples include preverification, identification checks before delivery, signatures upon delivery, and training requirements for delivery personnel. Age verification is particularly important in online delivery environments where youths may conceal their transactions.[27] Jurisdictions that have not explicitly prohibited delivery to schools and universities may also consider doing so, as this will also limit underage access on school and university grounds.

Although state preemption of local recreational cannabis regulation may streamline oversight, it also poses public health risks. Local authorities should retain the power to prohibit or regulate recreational cannabis direct delivery more stringently than minimum state standards. Potential conflicts may arise between state and local regulations because of variations in regulatory frameworks. However, establishing a minimum state standard with additional local safeguards permitted by states may benefit public health by allowing for tailored approaches that address specific community needs.[31,32] Moreover, state regulatory agencies' issuance of delivery-specific licenses is crucial for effective monitoring. Evidence suggests that retail licensing laws can reduce substance availability and density.[26,33,34] Implementing such laws for recreational cannabis direct delivery and enforcing penalties for violations may help curtail underage access.

In contrast, states with legalized medical cannabis require patients with qualifying conditions to register in statewide medical cannabis registries. This facilitates compliance and enforcement for direct delivery to only legitimate patients, a process not feasible for recreational direct-delivery regulation. Accordingly, states with legalized medical cannabis typically permit direct delivery to qualifying patients eventually. For example, New Jersey initially legalized medical cannabis in 2010 allowing only caregiver assistance,[35] albeit later regulations allowed dispensaries to deliver medical marijuana to patients directly. California has also enabled medical cannabis direct delivery in the Medical Cannabis Patients' Right of Access Act. States should consider adopting similar policies as this may enhance patient choice and health care access. As the cannabis policy landscape evolves, ongoing monitoring of delivery laws will benefit researchers and public health practitioners.

Limitations

While this study provides a detailed overview of the current state of cannabis delivery laws, a few study limitations should be noted. First, we focused on state provisions addressing local licensing, zoning, or approval but did not document specific municipal regulations that might impact direct delivery. Second, our study did not code the specifics of cannabis product types or delivery amount limits. Third, our research is based on state laws in effect as of July 1, 2024. As such, it provides a snapshot of existing delivery laws rather than a historical record of all amendments related to cannabis regulations. Fourth, the study did not consider the enforcement mechanisms present in the laws. Despite these limitations, our study offers valuable insights into an emerging policy issue with significant public health implications. As new laws evolve, future research could benefit from a more detailed analysis of these aspects.

Conclusions

Our study offers, to our knowledge, the first catalog and analysis of state-level cannabis delivery laws. The environment for recreational cannabis direct delivery appears to be more challenging in terms of preventing underage access compared with medical cannabis direct delivery, primarily because of the absence of an adult consumer registry similar to that for qualifying patients. Implementing certain provisions, such as mandatory age verification procedures or delivery-specific licensing, could potentially mitigate underage access to recreational cannabis. However, numerous states do not permit direct delivery of medical cannabis, which could limit the medical access of registered qualifying patients who have mobility restrictions. Striking a balanced policy approach is crucial to ensure protection for underage consumers from the potential hazards of recreational cannabis access while also ensuring optimal access to medical cannabis for registered qualifying patients. AJPH

ABOUT THE AUTHORS

Todd Ebling and Sunday Azagba are with the Ross and Carol Nese College of Nursing, Pennsylvania State University, University Park, PA. Mark Hall is with the Department of Social Science and Health Policy, Wake Forest School of Medicine, Winston-Salem, NC. Jessica King Jensen is with the Rutgers Institute for Nicotine and Tobacco Studies, Rutgers Biomedical and Health Sciences, New Brunswick, NJ.

CORRESPONDENCE

Correspondence should be sent to Todd Ebling, College of Nursing, University Park, PA 16802 (e-mail: txe5134@psu.edu). Reprints can be ordered at https://www.ajph.org by clicking the "Reprints" link.

PUBLICATION INFORMATION

Full Citation: Ebling T, Azagba S, Hall M, Jensen JK. US state recreational and medical cannabis delivery laws, 2024. *Am J Public Health.* 2025;115(2):178–190.

Acceptance Date: September 18, 2024.

DOI: https://doi.org/10.2105/AJPH.2024.307874

ORCID iD:

Todd Ebling https://orcid.org/0000-0002-7199-4108

CONTRIBUTORS

T. Ebling designed and conceptualized the study. T. Ebling and S. Azagba collected and coded laws and conducted legal analysis. M. Hall oversaw legal analysis and legal interpretation. T. Ebling, S. Azagba, M. Hall, and J. K. Jensen contributed to article drafting and interpretation of findings. All authors thoroughly reviewed and revised the article and approved this version.

CONFLICTS OF INTEREST

The authors have no conflicts of interest to disclose.

HUMAN PARTICIPANT PROTECTION

Data were obtained from secondary sources, so no protocol approval was necessary.

REFERENCES

1. Chapekis A, Shah S. Most Americans now live in a legal marijuana state—and most have at least one dispensary in their county. Pew Research Center. February 29, 2024. Available at: https://www.pewresearch.org/short-reads/2024/02/29/most-americans-now-live-in-a-legal-marijuana-state-and-most-have-at-least-one-dispensary-in-their-county. Accessed June 28, 2024.
2. Haffajee RL, MacCoun RJ, Mello MM. Behind schedule—reconciling federal and state marijuana policy. *N Engl J Med.* 2018;379(6):501–504. https://doi.org/10.1056/NEJMp1804408
3. Grabarsky T. Conflicting federal and state medical marijuana policies: a threat to cooperative federalism. *West VA Law Rev.* 2013;116(1):1–32.
4. US Department of Justice, Office of Public Affairs. Justice Department submits proposed regulation to reschedule marijuana. May 16, 2024. Available at: https://www.justice.gov/opa/pr/justice-department-submits-proposed-regulation-reschedule-marijuana. Accessed June 28, 2024.
5. Hall W, Stjepanović D, Caulkins J, et al. Public health implications of legalising the production and sale of cannabis for medicinal and recreational use. *Lancet.* 2019;394(10208):1580–1590. https://doi.org/10.1016/S0140-6736(19)31789-1
6. Connor JP, Stjepanović D, Le Foll B, Hoch E, Budney AJ, Hall WD. Cannabis use and cannabis use disorder. *Nat Rev Dis Primers.* 2021;7(1):16. https://doi.org/10.1038/s41572-021-00247-4
7. Volkow ND, Baler RD, Compton WM, Weiss SRB. Adverse health effects of marijuana use. *N Engl J Med.* 2014;370(23):2219–2227. https://doi.org/10.1056/NEJMra1402309
8. Volkow ND, Swanson JM, Evins AE, et al. Effects of cannabis use on human behavior, including cognition, motivation, and psychosis: a review. *JAMA Psychiatry.* 2016;73(3):292–297. https://doi.org/10.1001/jamapsychiatry.2015.3278
9. Tetrault JM, Crothers K, Moore BA, Mehra R, Concato J, Fiellin DA. Effects of marijuana smoking on pulmonary function and respiratory complications: a systematic review. *Arch Intern Med.* 2007;167(3):221–228. https://doi.org/10.1001/archinte.167.3.221
10. Campeny E, López-Pelayo H, Nutt D, et al. The blind men and the elephant: systematic review of systematic reviews of cannabis use related health harms. *Eur Neuropsychopharmacol.* 2020;33:1–35. https://doi.org/10.1016/j.euroneuro.2020.02.003
11. Hasin DS. US epidemiology of cannabis use and associated problems. *Neuropsychopharmacology.* 2018;43(1):195–212. https://doi.org/10.1038/npp.2017.198
12. National Academies of Sciences, Engineering, and Medicine; Health and Medicine Division; Board on Population Health and Public Health Practice; Committee on the Health Effects of Marijuana: An Evidence Review and Research Agenda. *The Health Effects of Cannabis and Cannabinoids: The Current State of Evidence and Recommendations for Research.* Washington, DC: National Academies Press; 2017.
13. Leung J, Chan GCK, Hides L, Hall WD. What is the prevalence and risk of cannabis use disorders among people who use cannabis? A systematic review and meta-analysis. *Addict Behav.* 2020;109:106479. https://doi.org/10.1016/j.addbeh.2020.106479
14. Shao H, Du H, Gan Q, et al. Trends of the global burden of disease attributable to cannabis use disorder in 204 countries and territories, 1990–2019: results from the Disease Burden Study 2019. *Int J Ment Health Addict.* 2023;22(4):2485–2507. https://doi.org/10.1007/s11469-022-00999-4
15. Lorenzetti V, Hoch E, Hall W. Adolescent cannabis use, cognition, brain health and educational outcomes: a review of the evidence. *Eur Neuropsychopharmacol.* 2020;36:169–180. https://doi.org/10.1016/j.euroneuro.2020.03.012
16. Hammond CJ, Chaney A, Hendrickson B, Sharma P. Cannabis use among US adolescents in the era of marijuana legalization: a review of changing use patterns, comorbidity, and health correlates. *Int Rev Psychiatry.* 2020;32(3):221–234. https://doi.org/10.1080/09540261.2020.1713056
17. Substance Abuse and Mental Health Services Administration. *Preventing Marijuana Use Among Youth.* National Mental Health and Substance Use Policy Laboratory; 2021:1–73. Available at: https://store.samhsa.gov/sites/default/files/pep21-06-01-001.pdf. Accessed March 1, 2024.
18. Whiting PF, Wolff RF, Deshpande S, et al. Cannabinoids for medical use: a systematic review and meta-analysis. *JAMA.* 2015;313(24):2456–2473. https://doi.org/10.1001/jama.2015.6358
19. Koppel BS, Brust JCM, Fife T, et al. Systematic review: efficacy and safety of medical marijuana in selected neurologic disorders. *Neurology.* 2014;82(17):1556–1563. https://doi.org/10.1212/WNL.0000000000000363
20. Lynch ME, Ware MA. Cannabinoids for the treatment of chronic non-cancer pain: an updated systematic review of randomized controlled trials. *J Neuroimmune Pharmacol.* 2015;10(2):293–301. https://doi.org/10.1007/s11481-015-9600-6
21. Stockings E, Campbell G, Hall WD, et al. Cannabis and cannabinoids for the treatment of people with chronic noncancer pain conditions: a systematic review and meta-analysis of controlled and observational studies. *Pain.* 2018;159(10):1932–1954. https://doi.org/10.1097/j.pain.0000000000001293
22. Cohen JE, Sarabia V, Ashley MJ. Tobacco commerce on the internet: a threat to comprehensive tobacco control. *Tob Control.* 2001;10(4):364–367. https://doi.org/10.1136/tc.10.4.364
23. Matthay EC, Schmidt LA. Home delivery of legal intoxicants in the age of COVID-19. *Addiction.* 2021;116(4):691–693. https://doi.org/10.1111/add.15289
24. Matthay EC, Gupta A, Mousli L, Schmidt LA. Using online crowdsourced data to measure the availability of cannabis home delivery: a pilot study. *J Stud Alcohol Drugs.* 2023;84(2):330–334. https://doi.org/10.15288/jsad.22-00171
25. Azagba S, Ebling T, Adekeye OT, Hall M, Jensen JK. Loopholes for underage access in e-cigarette delivery sales laws, United States, 2022. *Am J Public Health.* 2023;113(5):568–576. https://doi.org/10.2105/AJPH.2023.307228
26. Patel M, Donovan EM, Perks SN, et al. E-cigarette tobacco retail licensing laws: variance across US states as of January 1, 2020. *Am J Public Health.* 2020;110(9):1380–1385. https://doi.org/10.2105/AJPH.2020.305771
27. Terala A, Sangiuolo K, Milanaik RL. Access to marijuana by minors via online dispensaries. *JAMA Pediatr.* 2023;177(12):1356. https://doi.org/10.1001/jamapediatrics.2023.3656

28. Marijuana Policy Project. Safe access to cannabis in times of COVID-19. Available at: https://www.mpp.org/issues/medical-marijuana/safe-access-to-cannabis-in-times-of-covid-19. Accessed October 9, 2023.
29. Fletcher LA, Nugent SM, Ahern SM, Willenbring ML. The use of alcohol home delivery services by male problem drinkers: a preliminary report. *J Subst Abuse*. 1996;8(2):251–261. https://doi.org/10.1016/S0899-3289(96)90293-X
30. Fletcher LA, Toomey TL, Wagenaar AC, Short B, Willenbring ML. Alcohol home delivery services: a source of alcohol for underage drinkers. *J Stud Alcohol*. 2000;61(1):81–84. https://doi.org/10.15288/jsa.2000.61.81
31. Pomeranz JL, Zellers L, Bare M, Sullivan PA, Pertschuk M. State preemption: threat to democracy, essential regulation, and public health. *Am J Public Health*. 2019;109(2):251–252. https://doi.org/10.2105/AJPH.2018.304861
32. Pomeranz JL, Pertschuk M. State preemption: a significant and quiet threat to public health in the United States. *Am J Public Health*. 2017;107(6):900–902. https://doi.org/10.2105/AJPH.2017.303756
33. Azagba S, Shan L, Latham K. E-cigarette retail licensing policy and e-cigarette use among adolescents. *J Adolesc Health*. 2020;66(1):123–125. https://doi.org/10.1016/j.jadohealth.2019.06.010
34. Campbell CA, Hahn RA, Elder R, et al. The effectiveness of limiting alcohol outlet density as a means of reducing excessive alcohol consumption and alcohol-related harms. *Am J Prev Med*. 2009;37(6):556–569. https://doi.org/10.1016/j.amepre.2009.09.028
35. State of New Jersey. Pub L 2009, c.307 (S119 3R). 2010. Available at: https://pub.njleg.gov/bills/2008/PL09/307_.HTM. Accessed October 9, 2023.

Bills to Restrict Access to and Harm From Indoor Tanning Facilities in US State Legislatures, 1992–2023

David B. Buller, PhD, Julia Berteletti, MSW, Carolyn Heckman, PhD, Kevin R. J. Schroth, JD, Alan C. Geller, RN, MPH, Jerod L. Stapleton, PhD, Irene Adjei, BS, Anna Mitarotondo, BA, Samantha R. Guild, JD, Jeffrey E. Gershenwald, MD, Robert Dellavalle, MD, and Sherry Pagoto, PhD

Objectives. To describe progression, content, and stringency of state legislation regulating indoor tanning and association with state government political party leadership.

Methods. Trained research assistants used legal mapping methods to code legislative bills on indoor tanning introduced in US states, the District of Columbia, and Puerto Rico. We calculated composite scores on the stringency of age restrictions and of warnings, operator requirements, and enforcement. We evaluated associations of the political party of the legislative sponsor and legislature majority.

Results. Between 1992 and 2023, 184 bills were introduced in 49 of 50 states and DC (56 laws were enacted, and 126 bills failed). An under-18 ban was enacted in 22 states and DC. Party affiliation of the bill sponsor and legislature majority combined to affect bill passage and age restrictions.

Conclusions. In many states, it took several years and proposed bills before a law on indoor tanning was enacted. Enacted bills were more stringent than failed bills.

Public Health Implications. Increasing support for stringent regulations on indoor tanning is evident and may motivate other states or the federal government to prohibit minors from using indoor tanning facilities. (*Am J Public Health*. 2025;115(2):191–200. https://doi.org/10.2105/AJPH.2024.307894)

AJPH February 2025, Vol. 115, No. 2

Skin cancer is a highly prevalent, potentially deadly, and expensive disease.[1,2] Indoor tanning is a well-established cause of melanoma and keratinocyte carcinomas.[3–6] In the most recent estimates, nearly 6% of adolescents and 5% of adults indoor tan in the United States.[7,8] Stringent state indoor tanning laws that include age bans for minors instead of just parental consent are associated with less indoor tanning,[9,10] as most individuals begin indoor tanning as adolescents or young adults. These laws may prevent many melanomas and keratinocyte cancers over the lifetime of the 60 million US youths.[11]

Indoor tanning is regulated by both state legislation and US Food and Drug Administration (FDA) regulations. Laws restricting indoor tanning have been enacted in several states. An FDA regulation to ban indoor tanning by minors was originally proposed in 2015 but later was paused during the first Trump administration and has still not been finalized.[12] Research on the process of how policy efforts translate into actual state indoor tanning laws is limited,[13,14] mainly focused on describing existing laws and consequences of outlawing indoor tanning facilities in certain states or US regions.[15,16] Indoor tanning regulations may have contributed to the recent decrease in indoor tanning prevalence among adolescents.[8,17,18]

Using legal mapping methods[19] that involved collecting and coding content of all available state indoor tanning legislation in 50 US states, the District of Columbia (DC), and Puerto Rico, we sought to address 3 primary research objectives: (1) to describe the progression of state indoor tanning legislation (i.e., enacted or failed); (2) to detail the content and stringency of bills with special attention to whether bills banned indoor tanning by minors (i.e., individuals aged younger than 18 years, hereafter "under-18 ban"); and (3) to explore the potential impact of political party affiliation of state government leadership when bills were proposed. This analysis expanded on one by Gosis et al. in 2012[20] and was more historically comprehensive than a comparison of international laws by Diehl et al. in 2022.[21]

METHODS

We collected all available legislative bills related to indoor tanning in the 50 US states, DC, and Puerto Rico from 1992 through 2023. This included bills that were enacted into law and bills that were proposed but never passed, either not brought to a vote or voted down. Enacted laws were usually passed by vote of legislature and approved by the governor, although the type of executive action (e.g., signed, vetoed but overridden by legislature) was not recorded. The documents were identified and collected through the National Conference of State Legislatures online database, AIM at Melanoma Foundation Web site, and extensive online searching, using the bill name, legislative year, and state, and keywords "tanning," "indoor tanning," and "radiation," on each state's legislative statute Web site and the Google search engine. We also used Westlaw for clarifying some bills. For each state, we recorded titles, history, and dates of the bills. We also consulted an advisory board of individuals involved in education on risks of indoor tanning, advocating for indoor tanning legislation, or researching indoor tanning behavior, including 2 physicians, to locate bills.

Coding Protocol

We developed a coding protocol, modified in part from one used by Gosis et al.[20] Coding categories included age bans, parental involvement (accompaniment or consent), warnings, operator requirements, and enforcement policy components (Appendix A, available as a supplement to the online version of this article at https://ajph.org). Age ban included the age at which indoor tanning is legally prohibited, regardless of parental involvement provisions (0 = no regulation; 2 = under 14 years; 4 = under 15 years; 6 = under 16 years; 8 = under 17 years; and 10 = under 18 years [including 1 bill with under-21 restriction classified as 10]). Parental involvement included requirements for parents to provide consent (in-person or not; consent renewal required or not) or to accompany minors to the indoor tanning facility (or both), with applicable ages recorded. For warnings (12 items), operator requirements (27 items), and enforcement (8 items; Appendix A), coders scored each item as not addressed (0); addressed, but not explicitly (1); or addressed explicitly (2). For each category, we converted initial codes into 6 stringency levels—no regulation, very weak, weak, moderate, strong, or very strong (Table 1). We combined scores on warning, operator requirements, and enforcement into a score for policy provisions applied to minors and to adults and analyzed them separately. We recorded exceptions for medical use of indoor tanning and definition of indoor tanning facilities.

Two trained research assistants coded the text of the legislative bills using the adapted coding protocol. Each bill was coded by a single research assistant. To establish interrater reliability, n = 25 bills were coded by both research assistants (average interrater reliability across all categories: $\kappa = 0.93$). Coders agreed on any discrepancies in discussion with 2 of the authors; for some bills, advisors reviewed a policy to ensure coding accuracy.

We created an overall age restriction stringency score (possible range = 0–10) by combining age ban and parental involvement codes. First, a score was assigned for the oldest age at which any age restriction was applied: 0 = no restriction; 2 = under age 14 years; 4 = under age 15 years; 6 = under age 16 years; 8 = under age 17 years; 10 = under age 18 years. Parent involvement provisions appeared to be intended to weaken age restrictions, so the initial age restriction score was discounted for each year that parental involvement applied. Requirements that did not involve parents being present at indoor tanning facilities (consent, not in-person) were considered weaker (minus 1 for each year it applied) than those that did (in-person consent or accompaniment; minus 0.5 for each year that they applied). For example, if a bill stated that no child aged 14 years or younger could use an indoor tanning facility, and children aged 15 to 16 years could indoor tan with parental accompaniment, an initial score of "8" was assigned (under-age-17 restriction unless accompanied by a parent), and the score was reduced by 0.5 × 2 years = 1 (ages 15 and 16 years) to which accompaniment provision applied, for a final score of 8–1 = 7. If a bill did not specify an age at which a child was banned without exception but contained parent involvement provisions, initial age-restriction score was discounted to age 13, because the lowest age ban restricted those aged 13 years or younger. Thus, a bill that only stated that individuals aged younger than 16 years needed parental consent but not in person would have a final score of 6 [under-16 restriction]–3 [1 × 3 years; ages 13, 14, and 15] = 3.

TABLE 1— Combined Stringency Scores for Enacted and Failed Bills on Indoor Tanning: United States, 1992–2023

	No Under-18 Ban	Under-18 Ban	All Bills
	Enacted bills		
Total no.	28	28	56
Age restriction score			
0 (no regulation), no. (%)	2 (7.1)	0 (0.0)	2 (3.6)
1–3.5 (very weak regulation), no. (%)	0 (0.0)	0 (0.0)	0 (0.0)
4–5.5 (weak regulation), no. (%)	5 (17.9)	0 (0.0)	5 (8.9)
6–7.5 (moderate regulation), no. (%)	12 (42.9)	0 (0.0)	12 (21.4)
8–9.5 (strong regulation), no. (%)	9 (32.1)	0 (0.0)	9 (16.1)
10 (very strong regulation), no. (%)	0 (0.0)	28 (100)	28 (50.0)
Mean (SD)	6.7 (2.4)	10.0 (0)	8.3 (2.4)
Median (IQR)	7.5 (2.5)	10.0 (0)	9.75 (2.5)
Warnings, operator requirements, and enforcement (for minors)			
0 (no regulation), no. (%)	0 (0.0)	13 (46.4)	13 (23.2)
1–6 (very weak regulation), no. (%)	10 (35.7)	15 (53.6)	25 (44.6)
7–12 (weak regulation), no. (%)	5 (17.9)	0 (0.0)	5 (8.9)
13–18 (moderate regulation), no. (%)	12 (42.9)	0 (0.0)	12 (21.4)
19–24 (strong regulation), no. (%)	1 (3.6)	0 (0.0)	1 (1.8)
25–30 (very strong regulation), no. (%)	0 (0.0)	0 (0.0)	0 (0.0)
Mean (SD)	10.6 (5.8)	1.1 (1.1)	5.9 (6.3)
Median (IQR)	12.0 (8.0)	2.0 (2.0)	2.0 (10.0)
Warnings, operator requirements, and enforcement (for adults)			
0 (no regulation), no. (%)	0 (0.0)	1 (3.6)	1 (1.8)
1–6 (very weak regulation), no. (%)	7 (25.0)	16 (57.1)	30 (53.6)
7–12 (weak regulation), no. (%)	8 (28.6)	7 (25.0)	15 (26.8)
13–18 (moderate regulation), no. (%)	12 (42.9)	1 (3.6)	13 (23.2)
19–24 (strong regulation), no. (%)	1 (3.6)	3 (10.7)	4 (7.1)
25–30 (very strong regulation), no. (%)	0 (0.0)	0 (0.0)	0 (0.0)
Mean (SD)	11.4 (5.4)	8.6 (6.1)	10.0 (5.9)
Median (IQR)	12.0 (9.0)	6.0 (6.0)	8.0 (8.0)
	Failed bills		
Total no.	56	72	128
Age restriction score			
0 (no regulation), no. (%)	2 (3.6)	0 (0.0)	2 (1.6)
1–3.5 (very weak regulation), no. (%)	1 (1.8)	0 (0.0)	1 (0.8)
4–5.5 (weak regulation), no. (%)	9 (16.1)	0 (0.0)	9 (7.0)
6–7.5 (moderate regulation), no. (%)	23 (41.1)	0 (0.0)	23 (18.0)
8–9.5 (strong regulation), no. (%)	21 (37.5)	0 (0.0)	21 (16.4)
10 (very strong regulation), no. (%)	0 (0.0)	72 (100)	72 (56.3)
Mean (SD)	6.8 (2.1)	10.0 (0)	8.6 (2.1)
Median (IQR)	7.0 (2.0)	10.0 (0)	10.0 (2.5)
Warnings, operator requirements, and enforcement (for minors)			
0 (no regulation), no. (%)	2 (3.6)	32 (44.4)	34 (26.6)
1–6 (very weak regulation), no. (%)	42 (75.0)	40 (55.5)	82 (61.1)
7–12 (weak regulation), no. (%)	6 (10.7)	0 (0.0)	6 (4.7)

Continued

TABLE 1— Continued

	No Under-18 Ban	Under-18 Ban	All Bills
13–18 (moderate regulation), no. (%)	5 (8.9)	0 (0.0)	5 (3.9)
19–24 (strong regulation), no. (%)	1 (1.8)	0 (0.0)	1 (0.8)
25–30 (very strong regulation), no. (%)	0 (0.0)	0 (0.0)	0 (0.0)
Mean (SD)	5.6 (4.9)	1.1 (1.1)	3.1 (4.0)
Median (IQR)	4.0 (4.0)	2.0 (2.0)	2.0 (4.0)
Warnings, operator requirements, and enforcement (for adults)			
0 (no regulation), no. (%)	12 (21.4)	7 (9.7)	19 (14.8)
1–6 (very weak regulation), no. (%)	32 (57.1)	38 (52.8)	70 (54.7)
7–12 (weak regulation), no. (%)	5 (8.9)	15 (20.8)	20 (15.6)
13–18 (moderate regulation), no. (%)	5 (8.9)	10 (13.9)	14 (10.9)
19–24 (strong regulation), no. (%)	3 (5.4)	2 (2.8)	5 (3.9)
25–30 (very strong regulation), no. (%)	0 (0.0)	0 (0.0)	0 (0.0)
Mean (SD)	5.5 (5.5)	7.2 (4.9)	6.5 (5.2)
Median (IQR)	4.0 (4.0)	6.0 (6.0)	6.0 (4.0)

Note. IQR = interquartile range.

State Characteristics

We collected political affiliation of the governor, legislator sponsoring the bill, and majority party in the legislature for the year in which each bill was proposed from state legislative Web sites. We considered including state annual skin cancer incidence rates and average UV (ultraviolet radiation) index of the state's largest city. However, there were substantial missing data because of lack of reporting, so these data were not analyzed.

Statistical Analysis

We analyzed research objective 1, to describe progression of the legislation, by using a graphic to display indoor tanning bills over time. For research objective 2, to describe bill content, we summarized scores on each policy component and combined age-restriction stringency scores with descriptive statistics (counts, percentages, means, and standard deviations) and displayed content of currently enacted indoor tanning laws in a graphic. Also, for bills with age restrictions, we compared the stringency codes for warnings, operator requirements, and enforcement between bills enacted and bills that failed, using the *t* test. For objective 3, to examine political party predictors of bill enactment, we initially estimated regression models, but statistical suppression was evident because of collinearity of predictors, altering the size and signs of regression weights. So, we compared bill enactment and age restrictions for political party of the bill sponsor and in the majority of the legislature, using the χ^2 test for bill enactment and analysis of variance for age restriction score. We evaluated all tests with a 2-tailed .05 *P* value.

RESULTS

We obtained a total of 184 state indoor tanning bills (range = 0–32 bills per year) from 49 of 50 states and DC between 1992 and 2023. The number of bills proposed ranged from 1 bill in 6 states and DC to 7 bills or more in 6 states. Neither Alaska nor Puerto Rico have had a bill regulating indoor tanning proposed. To date, 56 bills were passed and enacted (hereafter, "enacted bills") in 46 states and DC (range = 0–12 per year), and 126 bills failed to pass in 41 states (range = 0–25 per year; 19 were never voted on, and 107 did not pass when voted on). Three states have thus far had indoor tanning bills proposed but never enacted (Montana = 4 bills; New Mexico = 3; and South Dakota = 3). Notably, 33 states enacted bills containing language broadly defining indoor tanning facilities; the most common definition was any location, place, area, structure, or business that provides customers access to any tanning device.

Timeline of Indoor Tanning Laws and Bills

Figure 1 shows a graphic timeline of indoor tanning bills proposed and enacted in state legislatures by year.

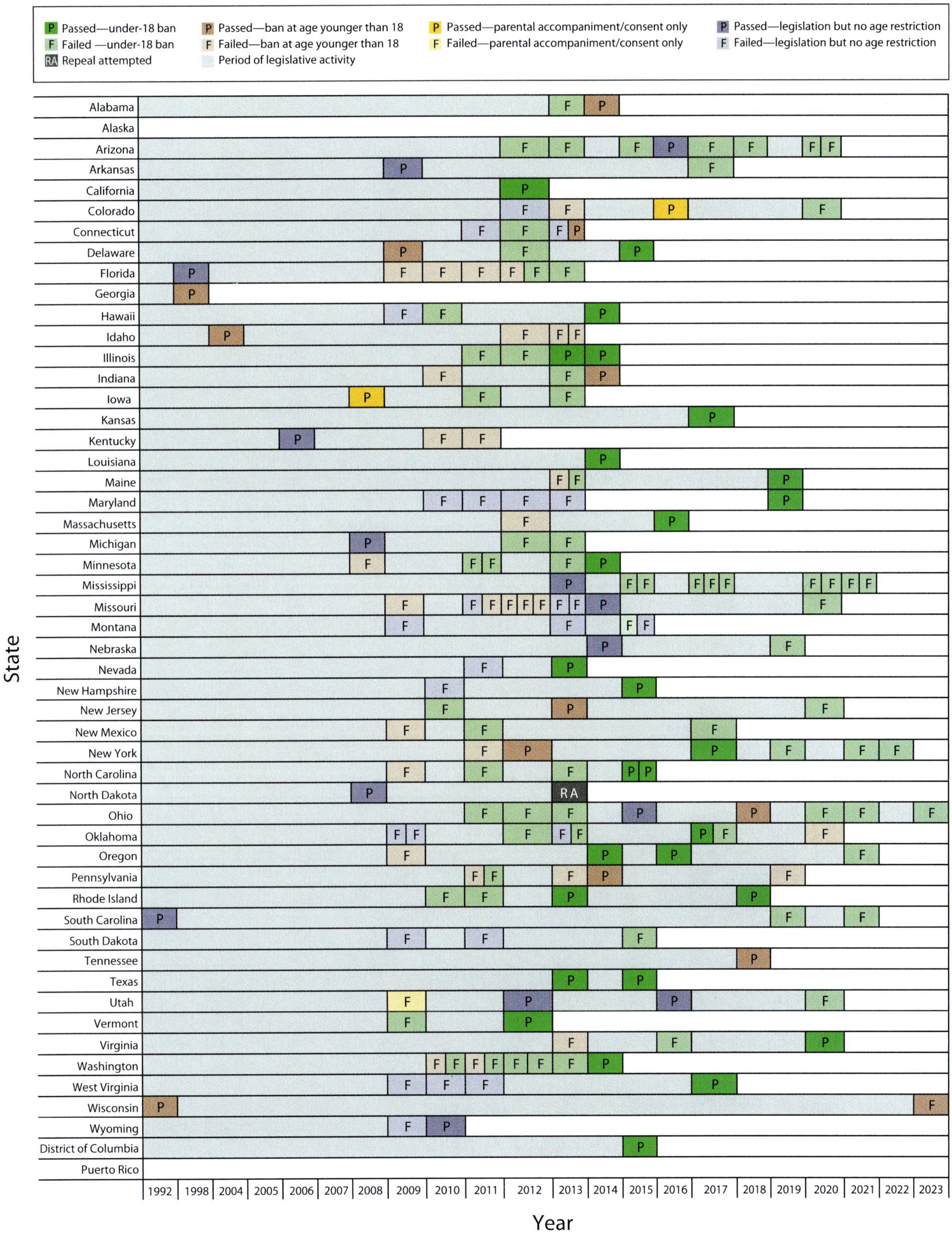

FIGURE 1— **Bills on Indoor Tanning in US State Legislatures: 1992–2023**

To illustrate, the first data row is for the state of Alabama. In Alabama, a bill to ban minors aged younger than 18 years failed in 2013. In 2014, a bill to ban minors at an age younger than 18 years was enacted. The first indoor tanning bill was enacted in Wisconsin in 1992, banning minors aged younger than 16 years, but very few bills were proposed before 2009. Before 2012, bills most commonly contained parental accompaniment or consent requirements or bans on use of indoor tanning facilities by minors aged younger than 14 or 16 years. The first law banning all minors aged younger than 18 years was enacted in 2012 in California, followed soon after in Vermont, although bills with under-18 bans failed in 16 states between 2009 and 2011. The most recent bill was enacted in 2020 in Virginia (7 bills failed in 2020, 1 in 2022, and 2 in 2023).

Figure 1 shows that it took several legislative years for many states to enact an indoor tanning law after a bill was first proposed and failed. In 29 states, 2 to 10 years passed between first proposal and first enactment of an indoor tanning bill (e.g., Arizona had a 4-year span from the first failed bill in 2012 to an enacted bill in 2016). In 18 states, a bill on indoor tanning was enacted the first time one was proposed. A similar pattern occurred for bills including under-18 bans. Nineteen states enacting bills with under-18 bans did so after failed attempts over 3 to 10 years. Nevertheless, 4 states enacted a bill with an under-18 ban in the first year it was introduced. In most states where more than 1 indoor tanning bill was proposed, the dominant pattern was that subsequent bills became more restrictive. However, in 8 states, a less-stringent bill was enacted after a more-stringent bill failed. Four states formally considered only bills that contained under-18 bans. Once states enacted bills with under-18 bans, no more legislative action on indoor tanning occurred in most of these states. However, bills were proposed in 5 states seeking to change the under-18 ban (reducing it to 16 years or increasing it to 21 years), to remove medical or parental exceptions, or to place other regulations on facilities. In one state, a bill to repeal an existing indoor tanning law was proposed. None of the attempts to weaken these laws succeeded.

Bill Content and Stringency

Age restrictions. Figure 2 shows the policy provisions enacted in each state as

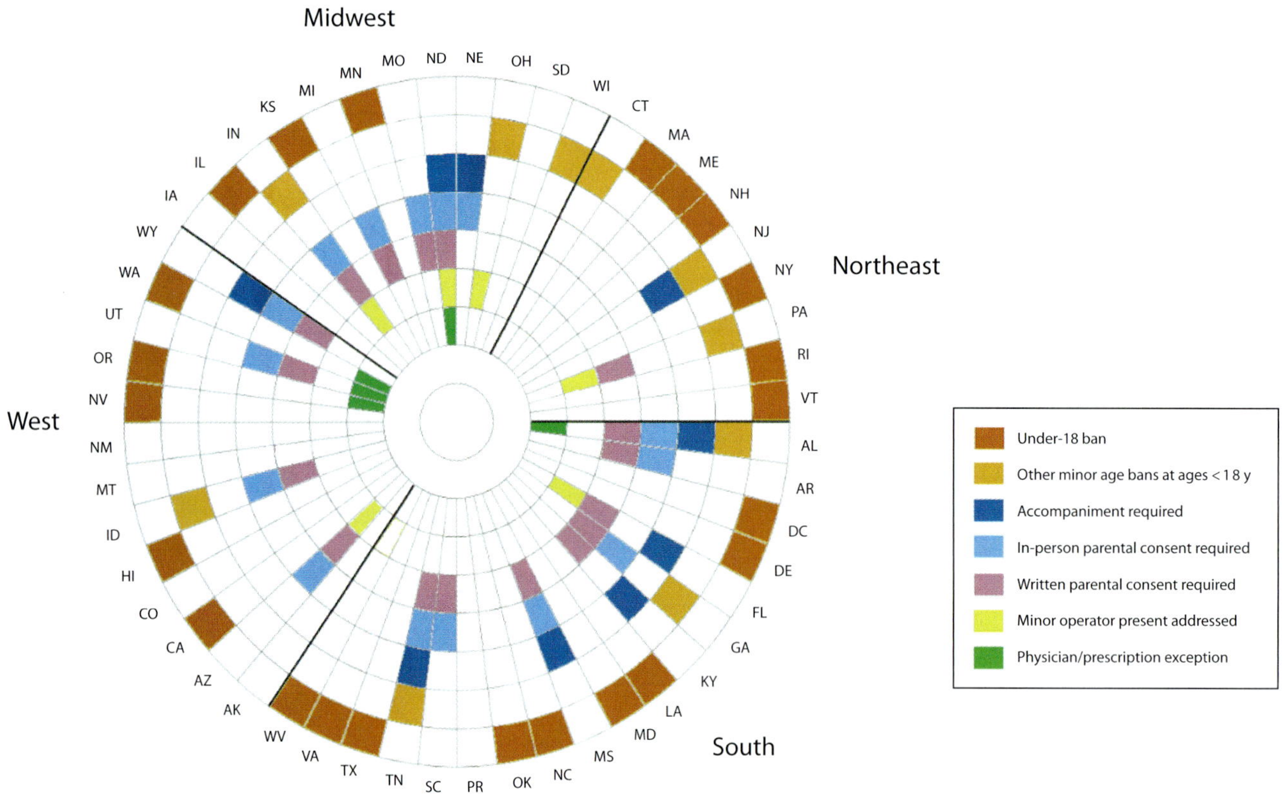

FIGURE 2— **Restrictions on Use of Indoor Tanning Facilities in Current US State Laws by US Census Regions as of January 2024**

of January 2024. The outer orange ring shows that 22 states (44.0%) and DC have enacted laws prohibiting all minors aged younger than 18 years from using indoor tanning facilities (66.7% in the Northeast, 50.0% in the South, 38.5% in the West, 25.0% in the Midwest). Of these, 20 have no exceptions (blue and magenta rings), and 2 state laws have medical exceptions (Oregon and Washington; inner green ring). In addition, 75 of 126 failed bills (59.5%) contained under-18 bans. Under-18 bans were more common in recently enacted bills than in earlier bills (Figure 1). Another 10 states have enacted bills with age restrictions ranging from age 14 years to 17.5 years (2 under age 14 years, 1 under age 15 years, 2 under age 16 years, 4 under age 17 years, and 1 under age 17.5 years; Figure 2, inner orange ring). Nine of these states allow indoor tanning by older minors (typically 16- and 17-year-olds) with parental involvement (Figure 2, blue and magenta rings). Of the remaining, 18 states and Puerto Rico have no age restrictions, and 12 allow children to use indoor tanning facilities with parental involvement.

Stringency of policy components. Stringency scores for policy components, combined age-restriction score, and combined warnings, operator requirements, and enforcement for minors and adults, are displayed in Appendix B (available as a supplement to the online version of this article at https://ajph.org) and Table 1. Approximately one third of indoor tanning bills without an under-18 age ban, regardless of whether they passed, had moderate to strong age-restriction component scores (enacted = 9/28 [32.1%]; failed = 21/56 [37.5%]), but two thirds of enacted (19/28; 67.9%) and failed bills (35/56; 62.5%) had weak or no restrictions (Appendix B). Warning, operator requirement, and enforcement components showed generally weak or nonexistent provisions in most bills (Appendix B). Enacted bills without under-18 age bans appeared to have stronger warning, operator requirement, and enforcement provisions than failed bills. Five states had a medical exemption that allowed minors to use indoor tan facilities with a physician's prescription (Figure 2, innermost ring).

Stringency of bills with age bans. Table 1 shows that enacted laws without under-18 bans, on average, had very weak age bans, moderate parental involvement provisions, weak warning requirements, moderate operator requirements, and weak enforcement stipulations. Failed bills without complete minor bans had weak age bans and parental involvement provisions and very weak provisions on warnings, operator requirements, and enforcement. For bills with age restrictions, stringency of provisions on warnings ($t = 3.45$; $P = .001$), operator requirements ($t = -3.71$; $P < .001$), and enforcement ($t = -2.51$; $P = .013$) was statistically significantly lower in failed than enacted bills. Similarly, for bills related only to adult use (no age restrictions), stringency of provisions on warnings ($t = -8.87$; $P < .001$) and operator requirements ($t = -4.61$; $P < .001$) was also statistically significantly lower for failed than enacted bills, but not enforcement provisions ($t = -1.60$; $P = .111$).

Political Affiliation, Age Restriction, and Enactment

Analyses showed that the combination of the political party of the bill sponsor relative to the party in control of the legislature was associated with both age restriction score (sponsor × legislature; $F = 2.14$; $P = .036$) and bill enactment ($\chi^2 = 63.39$; $P < .001$). Figure 3a shows that age restriction in any bill was highest when bills were proposed in Republican-majority legislatures or when sponsored by a Democrat or bipartisan legislators in a Democrat-majority legislature. Indoor tanning bills sponsored by a Republican compared with Democrat or bipartisan sponsors were more likely to be enacted in Republican-majority legislatures, while those sponsored by Democrat and bipartisan sponsors were more likely to be enacted in Democrat-majority legislatures. Democrat- and bipartisan-sponsored bills were unlikely to be enacted in legislatures with divided control (Figure 3b).

DISCUSSION

There has been considerable activity in the United States regarding state laws regulating indoor tanning in the past 15 years.[20] Laws on indoor tanning were proposed in all legislatures except Alaska and Puerto Rico and enacted in 46 states and DC. Twenty-two states and DC have enacted laws banning individuals aged younger than 18 years from using indoor tanning facilities since 2012.

The political agenda around preventing health risks posed by indoor tanning appeared to garner support across the political spectrum, especially in Republican-majority state legislatures and when sponsored by Democrat or bipartisan legislators in Democrat-majority legislatures where bills proposed by controlling party may be more likely to be considered. Indoor tanning restrictions emerged on legislative agendas at the same time

AJPH February 2025, Vol. 115, No. 2

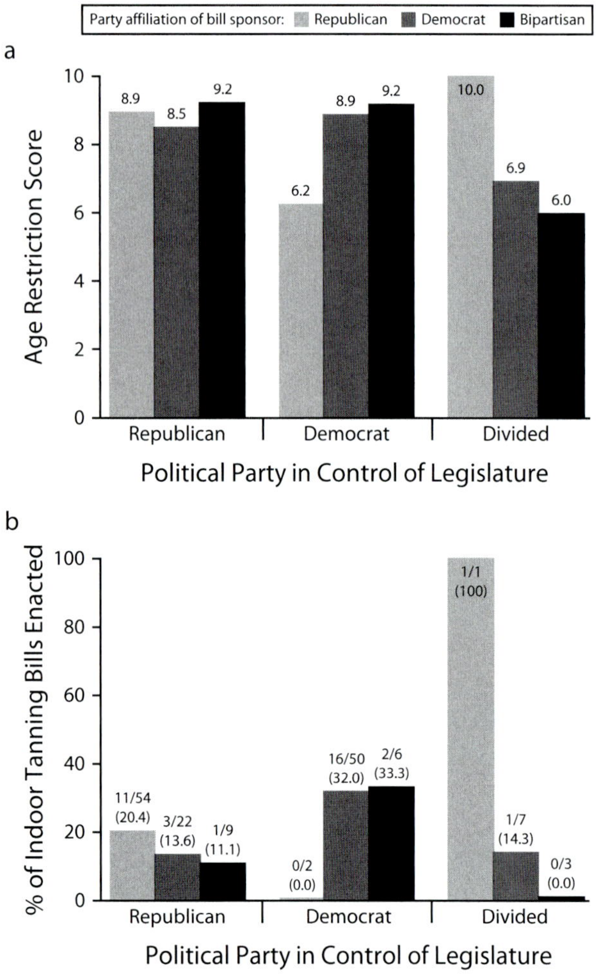

FIGURE 3— **Political Party of Bill Sponsor and Party in Majority and (a) Age Restriction Score (Range = 0–10) and (b) Percentage of Indoor Tanning Bills Enacted: United States, 1992–2023**

that (1) strong evidence was published that indoor tanning increases risk for melanoma and keratinocyte skin cancers[3–6]; (2) the federal government took actions on indoor tanning by levying a 10% excise tax on tanning facility use in the Affordable Care Act in 2012,[22] publishing a call from the US Surgeon General for adopting restrictions on indoor tanning in 2014,[1] and proposing FDA rulemaking with an under-18 ban in 2015[12]; (3) the World Health Organization recommended prohibiting commercial indoor tanning facilities and enacting legally binding age limits in 2017[23]; and (4) 3 international governments outlawed all commercial indoor tanning facilities (Brazil, Australia, and Iran).

Laws have become more restrictive regarding access to indoor tanning facilities by minors over time. Currently, nearly half of states and DC have enacted laws prohibiting all minors from using indoor tanning facilities without parental-involvement exceptions (2 states have medical exemptions). Under-18 bans were proposed in 19 states but failed. During a similar time period, 10 Canadian provinces, 25 European countries, and New Zealand also adopted under-18 bans and 4 Canadian provinces banned individuals aged younger than 19 years.[24] Supporters were able to inform legislators and overcome early opposition to ultimately enact bills with stringent restrictions. Sometimes this involved enacting a weaker bill and subsequently improving it and, in other cases, enacting more stringent bills after less stringent ones failed. Future advocacy may convert other failed efforts into enacted bills restricting minors in more states.

Most states without under-18 bans opted to enact laws that restrict children at ages younger than 18 years or require parental involvement (or both). These laws may be more acceptable to legislators who are concerned with parental rights or small business interests. Still, parental involvement provisions appear less effective at preventing indoor tanning by minors than under-18 bans.[9,10] Age-restrictions of all types may be undermined by suboptimal enforcement, poor compliance by facility operators or minors, and lack of awareness of indoor tanning laws and harms of indoor tanning by parents and adolescents. Stronger enforcement provisions might help but were weak in many bills. Enforcement may be strongest in states with under-18 bans,[25] which may be an added benefit of stringent age restrictions. Efforts to educate parents might improve compliance with indoor tanning laws by reducing parental permissiveness.[26,27] Future efforts should focus on increasing enforcement, compliance with indoor tanning laws (which we are studying separately), and educating families (and legislators) on the harms of indoor tanning.[26,27]

Finally, the broad definition of indoor tanning facilities is a favorable feature because many tanning beds outside of tanning salons, such as in gyms and

AJPH February 2025, Vol. 115, No. 2

fitness centers, apartment buildings, college campuses, or beauty salons and spas, fall within the scope of state laws. In non-salon facilities, compliance with parental consent laws can be low,[28] and high-frequency tanning has been reported,[29,30] potentially elevating risk of sunburns and developing melanoma. Home tanning beds are also used by some individuals, but, unfortunately, state laws do not apply to them.

Limitations

This analysis had strengths and limitations. The analysis of all bills proposed in the 50 states, DC, and Puerto Rico over the past 3 decades; an established coding protocol; and novel visual reporting format were major strengths. However, the study was limited to state legislation and did not include state regulatory actions or less-common local government laws, which were outside the aims of this research. It was conducted only in the US political system. The analysis did not examine the entire policy process, such as how bills came to be proposed, were considered, were approved by the executive, were implemented (including operator compliance and enforcement), and with what effect.[31] We are exploring these issues separately.[32]

Public Health Implications

Significant state legislative action addressing the risk posed by indoor tanning has occurred in the United States. Like any innovation, it took considerable time to adopt these health policies[33,34] and was subject to competing public health demands, such as state responses to COVID-19, which may explain the lack of indoor tanning laws enacted since 2020. In addition, COVID-19 may have had differential impact by state on the indoor tanning industry in terms of governmental loans, temporary shutdowns, or permanent facility closures, which could have affected legislative actions to restrict further indoor tanning facility use. The large proportion of under-18 bans in states across the political spectrum suggests a "tipping point"[34] has been achieved, which may motivate other states or the FDA to prohibit minors from using indoor tanning facilities. Some advocates contemplate expanding restrictions on indoor tanning.[35] New York recently considered, but did not enact, a ban on individuals aged younger than 21 years. Similar age restrictions on tobacco, alcohol, and gambling may make under-21 indoor tanning bans less controversial. Three countries outlawed all commercial indoor tanning facilities, as recommended by the World Health Organization,[23] but whether US legislators or the public would find this is acceptable is uncertain. Unless an FDA ban is finalized, further restrictions will be incremental, but the under-18 bans in almost half of US states may have laid the foundation for such efforts.[33] AJPH

ABOUT THE AUTHORS

David B. Buller, Julia Berteletti, and Irene Adjei are with Klein Buendel Inc, Golden, CO. Carolyn Heckman and Anna Mitarotondo are with the Rutgers Cancer Institute, Rutgers University, New Brunswick, NJ. Kevin R. J. Schroth is with the School of Public Health, Rutgers University, New Brunswick. Alan C. Geller is with the T. H. Chan School of Public Health, Harvard University, Cambridge, MA. Jerod L. Stapleton is with the College of Public Health, University of Kentucky, Lexington. Samantha R. Guild is with the AIM at Melanoma Foundation, Frisco, TX. Jeffrey E. Gershenwald is with the M D Andersen Cancer Center, University of Texas, Houston. Robert Dellavalle is with the Medical School, University of Minnesota, Minneapolis. Sherry Pagoto is with the Department of Allied Health Sciences, University of Connecticut, Storrs.

CORRESPONDENCE

Correspondence should be sent to David Buller, Klein Buendel Inc, 1667 Cole Blvd, Suite 220, Golden, CO 80401 (e-mail: dbuller@kleinbuendel.com). Reprints can be ordered at https://www.ajph.org by clicking the "Reprints" link.

PUBLICATION INFORMATION

Full Citation: Buller DB, Berteletti J, Heckman C, et al. Bills to restrict access to and harm from indoor tanning facilities in US state legislatures, 1992–2023. *Am J Public Health*. 2025;115(2):191–200.

Acceptance Date: September 30, 2024.

DOI: https://doi.org/10.2105/AJPH.2024.307894

ORCID iDs:

David B. Buller https://orcid.org/0000-0001-7902-9129

Julia Berteletti https://orcid.org/0000-0001-9193-8413

Carolyn Heckman https://orcid.org/0000-0003-1016-3965

Kevin R. J. Schroth https://orcid.org/0000-0002-9926-6639

Anna Mitarotondo https://orcid.org/0000-0002-4080-0307

Jeffrey E. Gershenwald https://orcid.org/0000-0003-4519-5369

Sherry Pagoto https://orcid.org/0000-0002-2462-8797

CONTRIBUTORS

D. B. Buller, C. Heckman, J. Berteletti, K. Schroth, A. C. Geller, and J. L. Stapleton conceptualized the study, designed methods, and secured extramural funding. D. B. Buller, J. Berteletti, C. Heckman, and A. Mitorotondo supervised project activities. J. Berteletti, I. Adjei, and A. Mitorotondo managed day-to-day study activities. J. Berteletti, I. Adjei, S. Guild, J. E. Gershenwald, R. Dellavalle, and S. Pagoto retrieved the documents. D. B. Buller, J. Berteletti, C. Heckman, and A. C. Geller analyzed the data. All authors reviewed and approved the article before submission.

ACKNOWLEDGMENTS

This research was supported by a grant from the National Cancer Institute (CA244370).

The results in this article were presented at the 6th International Conference on UV and Skin Cancer Prevention, Brisbane, Australia, September 13, 2024.

The authors thank the project consultants and advisory board members for their advice: Sophie Balk, MD, Donna Regen, BA, Karmen Hansen, MA, Maura Flynn, and John Antonishak.

CONFLICTS OF INTEREST

D. Buller discloses that his spouse is an owner of Klein Buendel Inc, and he receives a salary from Klein Buendel Inc.

HUMAN PARTICIPANT PROTECTION

All procedures were reviewed and approved by the WCG institutional review board (study 1336322). The research in this article was considered non–human participant research because it involved analysis of public documents.

REFERENCES

1. US Department of Health and Human Services. *The Surgeon General's Call to Action to Prevent Skin Cancer.* Washington, DC: Office of the Surgeon General; 2014.
2. Holman DM, Freeman MB, Shoemaker ML. Trends in melanoma incidence among non-Hispanic Whites in the United States, 2005 to 2014. *JAMA Dermatol.* 2018;154(3):361–362. https://doi.org/10.1001/jamadermatol.2017.5541
3. Lergenmuller S, Ghiasvand R, Robsahm TE, et al. Association of lifetime indoor tanning and subsequent risk of cutaneous squamous cell carcinoma. *JAMA Dermatol.* 2019;155(12):1350–1357. https://doi.org/10.1001/jamadermatol.2019.2681
4. O'Sullivan DE, Brenner DR, Demers PA, Villeneuve PJ, Friedenreich CM, King WD. Indoor tanning and skin cancer in Canada: a meta-analysis and attributable burden estimation. *Cancer Epidemiol.* 2019;59:1–7. https://doi.org/10.1016/j.canep.2019.01.004
5. Colantonio S, Bracken MB, Beecker J. The association of indoor tanning and melanoma in adults: systematic review and meta-analysis. *J Am Acad Dermatol.* 2014;70(5):847–857.e1–18. https://doi.org/10.1016/j.jaad.2013.11.050
6. Burgard B, Schöpe J, Holzschuh I, et al. Solarium use and risk for malignant melanoma: meta-analysis and evidence-based medicine systematic review. *Anticancer Res.* 2018;38(2):1187–1199. https://doi.org/10.21873/anticanres.12339
7. Bowers JM, Geller AC, Schofield E, Li Y, Hay JL. Indoor tanning trends among US adults, 2007–2018. *Am J Public Health.* 2020;110(6):823–828. https://doi.org/10.2105/AJPH.2020.305605
8. Holman DM, Jones SE, Qin J, Richardson LC. Prevalence of indoor tanning among US high school students from 2009 to 2017. *J Community Health.* 2019;44(6):1086–1089. https://doi.org/10.1007/s10900-019-00685-y
9. Qin J, Holman DM, Jones SE, Berkowitz Z, Guy GP Jr. State indoor tanning laws and prevalence of indoor tanning among US high school students, 2009–2015. *Am J Public Health.* 2018;108(7):951–956. https://doi.org/10.2105/AJPH.2018.304414
10. Guy GP Jr, Berkowitz Z, Jones SE, et al. State indoor tanning laws and adolescent indoor tanning. *Am J Public Health.* 2014;104(4):e69–e74. https://doi.org/10.2105/AJPH.2013.301850
11. Guy GPJ, Zhang Y, Ekwueme DU, Rim SH, Watson M. The potential impact of reducing indoor tanning on melanoma prevention and treatment costs in the United States: an economic analysis. *J Am Acad Dermatol.* 2017;76(2):226–233. https://doi.org/10.1016/j.jaad.2016.09.029
12. Food and Drug Administration. Code of federal regulations: sunlamp products and ultraviolet lamps intended for use in sunlamp products. 2018. Available at: https://www.accessdata.fda.gov/scripts/cdrh/cfdocs/cfcfr/CFRSearch.cfm?FR=1040.20. Accessed June 11, 2024.
13. Boyers LN, Karimkhani C, Guild SR, Dellavalle RP. Lessons from a legislative struggle to ban indoor tanning for children younger than 18. *Pediatr Dermatol.* 2015;32(4):553–556. https://doi.org/10.1111/pde.12491
14. Obayan B, Geller AC, Resnick EA, Demierre M-F. Enacting legislation to restrict youth access to tanning beds: a survey of advocates and sponsoring legislators. *J Am Acad Dermatol.* 2010;63(1):63–70. https://doi.org/10.1016/j.jaad.2009.09.019
15. Eskander A, Marqueen KE, Edwards HA, et al. To ban or not to ban tanning bed use for minors: a cost-effectiveness analysis from multiple US perspectives for invasive melanoma. *Cancer.* 2021;127(13):2333–2341. https://doi.org/10.1002/cncr.33499
16. Gordon LG, Rodriguez-Acevedo AJ, Køster B, et al. Association of indoor tanning regulations with health and economic outcomes in North America and Europe. *JAMA Dermatol.* 2020;156(4):401–410. https://doi.org/10.1001/jamadermatol.2020.0001
17. Reimann J, McWhirter JE, Cimino A, Papadopoulos A, Dewey C. Impact of legislation on youth indoor tanning behaviour: a systematic review. *Prev Med.* 2019;123:299–307. https://doi.org/10.1016/j.ypmed.2019.03.041
18. Simmons RG, Smith K, Balough M, Friedrichs M. Decrease in self-reported tanning frequency among Utah teens following the passage of Utah Senate Bill 41: an analysis of the effects of youth-access restriction laws on tanning behaviors. *J Skin Cancer.* 2014;2014:839601. https://doi.org/10.1155/2014/839601
19. Burris S, Wagenaar AC, Swanson J, Ibrahim JK, Wood J, Mello MM. Making the case for laws that improve health: a framework for public health law research. *Milbank Q.* 2010;88(2):169–210. https://doi.org/10.1111/j.1468-0009.2010.00595.x
20. Gosis B, Sampson BP, Seidenberg AB, Balk SJ, Gottlieb M, Geller AC. Comprehensive evaluation of indoor tanning regulations: a 50-state analysis, 2012. *J Invest Dermatol.* 2014;134(3):620–627. https://doi.org/10.1038/jid.2013.357
21. Diehl K, Lindwedel KS, Mathes S, Görig T, Gefeller O. Tanning bed legislation for minors: a comprehensive international comparison. *Children (Basel).* 2022;9(6):768. https://doi.org/10.3390/children9060768
22. Internal Revenue Service. Indoor tanning services tax center. 2023. Available at: https://www.irs.gov/businesses/small-businesses-self-employed/indoor-tanning-services-tax-center. Accessed June 11, 2024.
23. World Health Organization. Artificial tanning devices: public health interventions to manage sunbeds. 2017. Available at: https://www.who.int/publications/i/item/9789241512596. Accessed June 11, 2024.
24. Conte S, Aldien AS, Jetté S, et al. Skin cancer prevention across the G7, Australia and New Zealand: a review of legislation and guidelines. *Curr Oncol.* 2023;30(7):6019–6040. https://doi.org/10.3390/curroncol30070450
25. Williams MS, Buhalog B, Blumenthal L, Stratman EJ. Tanning salon compliance rates in states with legislation to protect youth access to UV tanning. *JAMA Dermatol.* 2018;154(1):67–72. https://doi.org/10.1001/jamadermatol.2017.3736
26. Buller DB, Pagoto S, Baker K, et al. Results of a social media campaign to prevent indoor tanning by teens: a randomized controlled trial. *Prev Med Rep.* 2021;22:101382. https://doi.org/10.1016/j.pmedr.2021.101382
27. Buller DB, Pagoto S, Henry KL, et al. Persisting effects of a social media campaign to prevent indoor tanning: a randomized trial. *Cancer Epidemiol Biomarkers Prev.* 2022;31(4):885–892. https://doi.org/10.1158/1055-9965.EPI-21-0059
28. Culley CA, Mayer JA, Eckhardt L, et al. Compliance with federal and state legislation by indoor tanning facilities in San Diego. *J Am Acad Dermatol.* 2001;44(1):53–60. https://doi.org/10.1067/mjd.2001.110063
29. Hillhouse J, Stapleton JL, Florence LC, Pagoto S. Prevalence and correlates of indoor tanning in nonsalon locations among a national sample of young women. *JAMA Dermatol.* 2015;151(10):1134–1136. https://doi.org/10.1001/jamadermatol.2015.1323
30. Pagoto SL, Nahar VK, Frisard C, et al. A comparison of tanning habits among gym tanners and other tanners. *JAMA Dermatol.* 2018;154(9):1090–1091. https://doi.org/10.1001/jamadermatol.2018.1779
31. Bullock HL, Lavis JN, Wilson MG, Mulvale G, Miatello A. Understanding the implementation of evidence-informed policies and practices from a policy perspective: a critical interpretive synthesis. *Implement Sci.* 2021;16(1):18. https://doi.org/10.1186/s13012-021-01082-7
32. Mitarotondo A, Berteletti J, Assan MA, Stapleton J, Heckman CJ, Buller DB. Indoor tanning (IT) policies are insufficient to protect young adults from skin cancer risks. Oral presentation at: Society of Behavioral Medicine 45th Annual Meeting & Scientific Sessions; March 15, 2024; Philadelphia, PA.
33. Sinclair CA, Makin JK, Tang A, Brozek I, Rock V. The role of public health advocacy in achieving an outright ban on commercial tanning beds in Australia. *Am J Public Health.* 2014;104(2):e7–e9. https://doi.org/10.2105/AJPH.2013.301703
34. Rogers EM. *Diffusion of Innovations.* New York, NY: Free Press; 2003.
35. McNoe BM, Reeder AI. 'Out of the frying pan, but not into the fire': quantifying commercial cosmetic tanning services in New Zealand to inform end-game regulation. *N Z Med J.* 2016;129(1446):84–88. Available at: https://pubmed.ncbi.nlm.nih.gov/27906923/. Accessed November 14, 2024.

Engaging Low-Wage Workers in Health and Well-Being Survey Research: Strategies From 5 Occupational Studies

Erika L. Sabbath, ScD, Meg Lovejoy, PhD, Daniel K. Schneider, PhD, Yaminette Diaz-Linhart, PhD, Grace DeHorn, MSW, and Susan E. Peters, PhD

Without perspectives of low-wage workers in studies of worker health and well-being, researchers cannot comprehensively assess occupational health and health equity impacts of workplace exposures and interventions. Researchers and practitioners have noted particular challenges in engaging low-wage workers in worksite-based health survey research, yet little scholarship has described strategies for improving their engagement and response rates.

To fill this gap, we present case examples from 5 occupational studies conducted between 2020 and 2024 in industries including health care, food service, and fulfillment centers. For each case, we describe how we identified barriers to worker engagement in surveys, explain specific strategies we used to address those barriers, and assess the effectiveness of these actions. Then, summarizing across case examples, we offer practical recommendations to researchers surveying low-wage populations, highlighting that high-touch recruitment, building trust with workers and managers, and obtaining manager support to take surveys during work time (for worksite-based studies) are critical for obtaining reliable, representative data.

Our work contributes to broader discussions on improving survey response rates in vulnerable worker populations and aims to support future researchers undertaking similar efforts. (*Am J Public Health*. 2025;115(2):201–208. https://doi.org/10.2105/AJPH.2024.307875)

AJPH February 2025, Vol. 115, No. 2

Work is an established social determinant of health.[1–4] In the United States, low-wage workers—those in the bottom 30% of the income distribution[5]—have higher rates of occupational illness and injury, less access to workplace benefits such as health insurance, and greater economic precarity.[6,7] Additionally, low-wage work is more common among those minoritized by race, ethnicity, and immigration status. Exposures and experiences associated with low-wage work may also amplify other health risks.[8]

To identify and address work-related health hazards and associated health outcomes, occupational health practitioners and researchers often collect survey data directly from workers to learn about their work experiences, exposures, and health. Although chemical and physical hazards can be measured environmentally, self-report surveys are critical tools for assessing how workers perceive their psychosocial work environment and measuring health outcomes such as pain, injury, sleep quality, mental health, and well-being.

Given the central role of organizational policies and practices in shaping health and well-being,[9,10] it is particularly important to conduct research on working conditions and health among workers from specific workplaces or employers rather than the broad working population. However, researchers have long noted challenges in recruiting workers for occupational health surveys, including survey overload, lack of perceived autonomy to respond during work time, and time pressures.[11–13] These challenges occur amid a long-term trend of declining survey response rates,[14,15] amplifying recruitment challenges.

In studies of mixed-wage or low-wage workforces, response rates may be disproportionately low among workers who have low literacy, high fears of retaliation, or unmanageable workloads—the very factors that may be associated with exposure to workplace health hazards.[16] The increasing use of e-mail–based survey recruitment for worksite-based studies may induce response bias by privileging white-collar workers (who regularly access work e-mail) over blue-, brown-, and pink-collar workers who do not have or use institutional e-mail accounts. To produce research that reflects the experiences of these vulnerable workers, researchers must carefully consider how to engage low-wage working populations in research.

Although some occupational health researchers describe innovative worker recruitment practices in their research articles,[17–19] a limited body of research focuses on strategies for improving response rates to occupational surveys specifically. Successful strategies, as reported in both occupational and nonoccupational surveys,[20] include monetary incentives, multiple response modality provision (e.g., paper, electronic), and prepaying monetary incentives at the time of recruitment (vs after completion).[11,12,21,22] Despite this concrete, data-driven guidance,[11,12,20–22] multiple knowledge gaps remain. Specifically, strategies may be most applicable to high- or moderate-wage workers with high literacy and jobs that involve regular e-mail access. Many strategies pertain to population-based, versus worksite-based, study designs. Finally, given rapidly changing technology norms, strategies from even 10 years ago (e.g., phone surveys) may be outdated.

Over the past 5 years, we have fielded multiple surveys of low-wage workers to assess determinants of worker health and well-being. These studies span multiple industries (e.g., fulfillment centers, health care, food service), encompass multiple employment and work arrangements, employ workers from diverse social and demographic groups, and include both employer–researcher partnerships and direct worker sampling. Through these studies, we have learned recruitment strategies that were particularly effective and those that were ineffective. Our goal in this analytic essay is to synthesize experiences from 5 research projects so that other researchers can apply our recommendations to more effectively recruit low-wage participants.

STRATEGIES TO IMPROVE RESPONSE RATES

We present the following case studies to improve response rates from low-wage workers in occupational health research:

1. High-touch recruitment: the Boston Hospital Workers Health Study (BHWHS),
2. Community-organizing approach: the Community Health Worker Study,
3. Social media engagement: the Shift Project,
4. Engaging workers in pressured environments: the Fulfillment Center Intervention Study, and
5. Overcoming low literacy and time constraints: the Work Organizational Health Study.

The Boston Hospital Workers Health Study

Study design and sample. The BHWHS is a longitudinal occupational cohort study of more than 27 000 hospital workers at 2 large academic medical centers in Boston, Massachusetts.[23] In periodic surveys of a random sample of workers, we measured working conditions, stressors, health, and well-being, with surveys directly linkable to administrative data.[24–26] In 2023, we expanded the cohort from our historical population of patient care workers (nurses, low-wage nursing assistants) to include low-wage service workers at the hospitals (environmental services, patient and materials transport).

Survey development and data collection. We conducted formative qualitative interviews with workers and managers from low-wage groups. Interviews informed survey content, built relationships and trust with managers, and identified potential barriers to participation (e.g., concerns with e-mailed surveys being mistaken for phishing).

We distributed the survey electronically to workers at their institutional e-mail address from June 2023 through January 2024. It was available in English, Spanish, Haitian Creole, and Portuguese and was designed to take 30 minutes or less. Respondents received a $20 Amazon claim code after completion, which was sent to their institutional e-mail address.

Challenges and strategies. The database linkage component of the BHWHS added methodological strength but presented barriers to survey response because a survey link unique to the workers' study identification number had to be sent by e-mail. Workers who did not regularly use work e-mail struggled to navigate their e-mail and the survey or did not understand certain questions, even in their preferred language. To address this, we reserved a conference room with institutional laptops, mirroring processes for mandatory hospital trainings. Managers helped us determine optimal times for our team to sit in the room, explain the study, and help workers access their e-mail. This strategy increased the response rate among environmental services workers by 5 percentage points, from 18% to 23%. By contrast, our initial approach of scheduled reminder e-mails to this group without accompanying team visits or support yielded an increase of less than 1 percentage point per reminder.

For unit-based workers (i.e., nurses, nursing assistants), study team members visited inpatient units (n = 149 units across the 2 hospitals) with flyers and study-branded candy to leave in break rooms, asking unit nurse directors to promote the survey to workers. During informal interactions with nursing assistants at these visits, the study team identified several barriers to response, even among those who reported receiving the survey: discomfort with navigating an online survey, literacy challenges, concern about permissibility of taking the survey on "work time," and the belief that as (self-perceived) peripheral workers, their responses were not valued.

To address these challenges, the study team transitioned away from our initial approach of leaving materials in break rooms and speaking with nurse directors to a high-touch approach. During visits, we asked the charge nurse on each unit to pull the on-duty nursing assistant off the floor so a study team member could help them access the survey; this provided available workers with implicit manager permission to take the survey at work. After each visit, we sent e-mails to unit directors inviting them to tell nursing assistants about the importance of taking the survey so their voice could be heard. These approaches boosted the response rate among nursing assistants from 33% to 46%, compared with increases of 1 to 2 percentage points with e-mail reminders but no accompanying visit. Overall, the study had responses from 2023 workers out of 4618 sampled (44%), with response rates of 49% among nurses, 46% among nursing assistants, 23% among environmental services workers, and 50% among patient and materials transport workers.

Community Health Worker Study

Study design and sample. Community health workers (CHWs) improve care quality for socially and medically complex communities.[27] The goal of the Community Health Worker Study was to understand how worker voice (i.e., ways that workers attempt to influence their work to meet individual and collective interests) may be associated with CHW health and well-being.[28,29] The study took place in Massachusetts from March through November 2021.

Recruitment. We initially hoped to partner with organizations employing CHWs, but although organizations expressed enthusiasm, none opted to formally partner. Instead, we proactively used community-organizing strategies for recruitment,[30] including engaging with CHWs before the launch of the study to codevelop research questions, and building partnerships with CHWs, CHW professional associations, and the employing organizations.

Challenges and strategies. We initially sent recruitment e-mails to hospitals, health centers, and community partner organizations, using publicly available contact information; we asked organizations to forward the e-mail to their CHWs. We quickly found that we could not rely on these organizations, so we developed a more grassroots recruitment approach. The primary investigator built trust with CHWs by volunteering to give invited talks at community meetings at which she shared findings from previous research on CHWs and discussed social service professionals' well-being.

At survey launch, many CHWs were exhausted from navigating the COVID-19 pandemic, and many felt oversurveyed. We established multiple systems to engage and support them. We sent recruited participants personalized e-mails (vs mass e-mails)—first to send them a unique survey link and then to offer support for survey completion. These strategies resulted in minimal missing data (94% had complete responses). We offered respondents a wide range of $40 incentive options: a Visa gift card, a gift card from any store they wanted (sent by postal mail or e-mail), or electronic payment. Personalized communication helped build relationships between worker and researcher, increasing trust and willingness to participate.

Overall, the study had a sample of CHWs who demographically mirrored the known population of CHWs across Massachusetts.[31] Of the 314 interested and eligible individuals, 220 responded (70% response rate), in contrast to a previous study of Massachusetts CHWs with a response rate of 36%.[31]

The Shift Project

Study design and sample. The Shift Project[32] is a repeated cross-sectional survey of hourly workers employed at

150 of the largest US service sector firms (i.e., fast food, casual dining, grocery, pharmacy, big-box stores, hardware, other retail, delivery, and fulfillment). We run the survey twice per year and since 2016 have collected 16 waves of data and accumulated surveys from 250 000 hourly workers.

Using surveys, the Shift Project measures workers' self-reported wages, work schedule stability and predictability, access to paid leave, exposure to surveillance and automation, respect, harassment, job security, and economic security, health, and well-being. These data are employer–employee linked, with workers nested in identifiable firms.

Data collection methods. No accessible sampling frames of hourly workers at large US service sector firms exist. Given relational, legal, and logistical challenges to survey workers associated with creating multiple employer–research partnerships, there are formidable barriers to using employer partnerships to construct employer–employee-matched survey data at scale. Thus, we developed a method to directly recruit workers at specific firms. We constructed a sampling frame using targeted advertising tools available through Meta to reach Facebook and Instagram users. Using the audience creation tool, we constructed employer-specific Meta "audiences" of workers at specific firms and then ran paid advertisements to each of these audiences, inviting users to complete the survey. We entered respondents into a drawing to receive a $500 gift card. Over the last 14 waves of data collection, we averaged advertising and incentive costs of $13 per "sufficient" survey response, defined as progressing sufficiently through the survey before breaking off to report on basic dimensions of job quality.

Challenges and strategies. We have honed multiple recruitment strategies on Facebook and Instagram. First, recruitment advertisements perform best when the audience characteristic, advertising design, and advertisement message align (e.g., Facebook and Instagram advertisements targeting Walmart workers containing a picture of a Walmart worker and a recruitment message of "survey for Walmart workers"). Advertisements missing any of these elements were less effective for recruiting target worker populations. For example, in April 2021, a set of recruitment advertisements was erroneously run that did not include employer-specific targeting but did include employer-specific recruitment language in the advertisement text, so the advertisement was shown to the general population on Meta platforms. After discovering the error, we fixed targeting and restarted data collection. Using this "natural experiment" to compare efficacy of targeting, we found that untargeted advertisements produced 17 responses (0.3% of clicks) versus 473 responses (10.0% of clicks) when correctly targeted.

Second, fraudulent, low-quality data are a concern in online data collection.[33] We assessed Internet protocol addresses and included "honeypot" questions to guard against bots; we have found no evidence of fraudulent responses across 16 waves of data collection. We also included basic attention checks; 91% of respondents pass checks, in excess of rates reported in online opt-in survey panels.[33] We, like other researchers,[34] have found that guaranteed incentives (vs random prize draws) attract fraudulent responses.

Beyond imperfect coverage of the sampling frame and low response rates, Meta's algorithm delivers recruitment advertisements nonrandomly. Nonrandom selection is a common problem in modern survey research and is often managed by poststratification and weighting.[35] Asking about core demographics upfront allows maximum preservation of sample size when weighting. Although we used a nonprobability sampling method, we benchmarked Shift data to gold standard sources (e.g., National Longitudinal Survey of Youth-97, Current Population Survey) to gauge representativeness. Before weighting, the shift sample was biased on univariate measures of gender, education, and race/ethnicity but not age, wages, or job tenure. However, the sample accurately represented bivariate associations (e.g., between job tenure and wages) as estimated in the National Longitudinal Survey of Youth-97 and the Current Population Survey.[36]

The Fulfillment Center Intervention Study

Study design and sample. The Fulfillment Center Intervention Study is a group-randomized controlled trial that compares participants in worksites randomized to a participatory intervention (health and well-being committees) with participants working for the same firm in control sites.[37] Health and well-being committees serve as a formal voice channel in which a small group of frontline workers and supervisors solicit workers' concerns and ideas about safety, the psychosocial environment, and work organization and then develop and implement improvement initiatives. In the study, we used an established research partnership with the supply chain division of a midsized, nonunionized US-based retailer. We randomized 16 fulfillment centers after matching on picking technology and building size.

Survey development and data collection. Survey measurement occurred at baseline, 6 months, and 12 months. At each time point, all current workers in each fulfillment center received a paper invitation to complete a Web-based survey. Survey packets included a survey ID number to track repeat participation and a treat (e.g., granola bars, fruit snacks). Letters contained a QR (quick response) code and link to the survey, allowing workers to take the survey electronically. We also sent hard copies to buildings if workers preferred. We distributed invitations at fulfillment centers during working hours; we encouraged building managers to provide workers with time off the floor to complete the survey. Upon survey completion, participants received a guaranteed incentive ($10–$15 as either a physical gift card sent to their home or an electronic card sent to their personal e-mail). We ran weekly raffles for each building during the 3-week–long survey periods, with prizes ranging from $25 to $150. During 3 waves of data collection, 4444 workers were eligible to participate; 63% participated in at least 1 survey (n = 2813). Response rates were 48% (wave 1), 47% (wave 2), and 55% (wave 3).

Challenges and strategies. Data collection coincided with COVID-19 pandemic–related restrictions (baseline recruitment started July 2021), which limited the research team's ability to be on-site to establish rapport and promote the survey. Instead, supervisors and managers announced the survey, which was a challenge, as they were managing COVID-19 pandemic challenges and regular work duties simultaneously. The research team designated a "survey point person" in each building to be an on-site contact to distribute and promote the survey. However, this reliance on management may have made workers skeptical, dampening participation. Once social-distancing rules were lifted, we encouraged town halls where everyone in the building was introduced to the study and given time to take surveys.

The organization of work and the incentive structure of the firm posed unique challenges. Time off the floor is frowned on in fulfillment centers, as managers perceive it as reducing productivity. Additionally, some sites use performance-based pay, which may have disincentivized workers from taking the survey while "on the clock" for fear of losing pay. Furthermore, the company launched their own engagement survey the same year as the study survey. The overlap created survey fatigue and difficulty for managers, who were recruiting workers for both surveys.

We adopted several strategies in response. First, regular updates on response rates were shared with our building contacts to create friendly competition for high participation; buildings that reached more than 50% participation received 3 additional $100 raffle prizes. To encourage participation and combat survey fatigue in the final survey wave, we increased guaranteed incentive amounts from $10 to $15. There were also 4 $25 to $150 raffles for participants in each site per wave. Finally, the research team extended survey timelines while in the field to maintain positive relationships with management, stagger with company-wide surveys, and avoid peak periods when time off the floor was especially challenging. We implemented all presented strategies between waves 1 and 3. The response rate increased by 6 percentage points between waves, from 48% (wave 1) to 54% (wave 3).

The Work Organizational Health Study

Study design and sample. The Work Organizational Health Study was a proof-of-concept cluster-randomized control trial among food service workers designed to test whether a multilevel participatory intervention targeting work organization and environment could be feasibly implemented and improve workers' safety, health, and well-being.[38,39] Collaborating with a large multinational food service organization, we worked with 10 cafeteria sites providing food service to contracted corporate clients in greater Boston. We randomized cafeterias to either intervention or control conditions. All food service workers were eligible to complete surveys. We collected baseline survey data July to August 2018, with follow-up in early 2020. Follow-up data collection was incomplete because of the COVID-19 pandemic.

Survey development and data collection. During intervention development, we conducted focus groups with workers and interviews with managers to learn about the worker population and work environment.[40] These data informed the intervention and alerted us to potential data collection barriers (e.g., literacy and language needs).

Because of managers' reports of low literacy among workers, surveys were conducted using an interviewer-administered protocol by 2 trained research assistants, 1 of whom was English–Spanish bilingual (16% of surveys were completed in Spanish). We hired experienced survey administrators who understood the importance of quickly establishing trust and rapport. We designed the survey to take 30 minutes or less. Survey respondents received a $25 Amazon gift card after completion. There was a 92% response rate (120/130 eligible workers).

Challenges and strategies. Some workers had low to no reading or spoken English literacy, so in addition to hiring the bilingual survey administrator, we also created Spanish versions of all materials (e.g., recruitment posters). We were invited to attend standing morning huddles with employees; we delivered prepared huddle scripts about the survey in both languages, emphasizing privacy of responses and voluntary participation. We learned from our project champion that communication and trust between managers and staff was strained. Accordingly, presurvey recruitment and study launch were driven by the research team, rather than managers, to communicate our independence.

Company management allowed surveys to be completed on work time; many workers had second jobs, making completion otherwise unfeasible. Because of already high workloads, we had difficulty accessing workers at times that they were able to complete the survey. The research team needed to be flexible to work around peak times and unexpected catering jobs. We spent many hours waiting for employees to be available to survey. We also returned for a "cleanup" day to offer the survey to staff who had been unable to complete the survey initially.

LESSONS LEARNED AND RECOMMENDATIONS

These studies affirm the necessity of several standard practices in survey data collection: conducting formative research, offering surveys in multiple languages and modalities, and providing incentives. Beyond these, cases yield a set of shared recommendations that may be specifically useful in future studies of low-wage working populations.

Recommendation 1: Build Trust

The 3 employer-engaged studies all worked with managers both before survey launch and while the survey was in the field. These collaborations did help generate specific recruitment ideas; for example, in the BHWHS, using the conference room for survey administration was a manager's idea. Conversations also built trust between the study team and managers. Because managers are often key linkage points with workers, management trust in the research team is necessary for managers to see the value of the study and encourage their workers to participate.

However, in some teams or organizations, manager–worker relationships are strained. The appearance of the study team being aligned with management may dampen response rates or lead to inaccurate responses owing to worker fear of confidentiality breaches. In such cases, trust is most effectively built with workers. The Shift Project's targeting of workers with social media advertisements is an example of how research teams can circumvent potentially untrusted managers. The Community Health Worker Study's primary investigator established trust with respondents by providing free webinars to workers before survey recruitment; this helped workers feel that she cared about their well-being instead of primarily valuing their survey responses.

Determining the appropriate trust-building activities for a given worksite or work group requires identifying, before survey deployment, whether a worksite has a project champion who workers trust or, conversely, whether worker–manager trust is fractured. In the Workplace Organizational Health Study, some sites had trusting worker–manager relationships; in these cases, managers were effective champions. In other sites, the research team communicated their independence from managers by providing information about the survey and fielding worker concerns regarding privacy.

Recommendation 2: Surveys During Work Time

All employer-engaged studies demonstrated the necessity of allowing workers to complete the survey during work time—thus increasing workers' likelihood of survey completion. Manager support for using work time to complete the survey was thus essential. However, permission may not correlate with uptake if not accompanied by reduction in duties to allow time to take the survey. Workers at all sites were busy. Some had productivity targets for a given shift (i.e., the Fulfillment Center Intervention Study) or time-sensitive catering jobs (i.e., the Work Organizational Health Study), dampening participation during work time even with manager permission. Some managers in the BHWHS scheduled extra workers for shifts when the study team would be on-site assisting with survey administration so that workers could complete the survey without affecting the team's overall workload. In addition to providing time to complete the survey, such scheduling signaled to workers that their managers thought the study

AJPH February 2025, Vol. 115, No. 2

was important. In multisite trials or observational studies, response rates might be higher at sites with managers who undertake these practices, with implications for bias.

Recommendation 3: High-Touch Recruitment

No worker groups in the studies regularly accessed e-mail as part of daily job duties. Therefore, even if workers had an institutional e-mail address as part of their employment (many do not), survey invitations may be missed. In study designs in which e-mail is unavoidable (e.g., the BHWHS), in-person wraparound recruitment helped overcome this barrier; researchers were on-site to help workers navigate their e-mail and find the survey. Non–e-mail modalities, such as social media recruitment (i.e., the Shift Project), QR codes to take the survey on participants' own devices (i.e., the Fulfillment Center Intervention Study), or interviewer-administered protocols (i.e., the Work Organizational Health Study) were all effective. Regardless of modality, a high-touch approach was essential for both recruitment and survey completion.

Recommendation 4: In-Person Data Collection

Two studies (the Fulfillment Center Study and the Community Health Worker Study) undertook some or all of their data collection early in the COVID-19 pandemic, when social-distancing rules prohibited nonessential personnel (e.g., study team members) from entering worksites. These studies navigated remote data collection through close partnerships with managers, who served as their proxies (see recommendation 1 for potential downsides of this relationship). In some cases (e.g., the BHWHS), remote recruitment was ineffective.

Across most studies, in-person recruitment occurred in the evenings, late at night, on weekends, early in the morning, and at other nonstandard times to reach workers during times that they might be available to complete the survey. Off-hour recruitment sessions were especially important for capturing the perspectives of workers on nonstandard shift schedules.

CONCLUSIONS

We hope that future research projects benefit from the strategies and principles described here. We also hope that this analytic essay augments broad scholarship on methods for promoting survey response by describing specific needs of low-wage worker research participants. Although many empirical articles provide general descriptions of recruitment methods, we encourage low-wage workforce researchers to use methods sections in their articles to additionally describe specific survey recruitment activities and strategies, as we have done in these case studies. Doing so will allow others to learn from data collection processes as well as scientific findings. AJPH

ABOUT THE AUTHORS

Erika L. Sabbath is with the Boston College School of Social Work, Chestnut Hill, MA. Meg Lovejoy is with the Harvard Center for Population and Development Studies, Harvard University, Cambridge, MA. Daniel K. Schneider is with the Harvard Kennedy School, Harvard University, Cambridge, MA. Yaminette Diaz-Linhart and Grace DeHorn are with the Institute for Work and Employment Research, Massachusetts Institute of Technology Sloan School of Management, Cambridge. Susan E. Peters is with the Department of Social and Behavioral Sciences, Harvard T. H. Chan School of Public Health, Boston, MA.

CORRESPONDENCE

Correspondence should be sent to Erika L. Sabbath, Boston College School of Social Work, 140 Commonwealth Ave, Chestnut Hill, MA 02467 (e-mail: erika.sabbath@bc.edu). Reprints can be ordered at https://www.ajph.org by clicking the "Reprints" link.

PUBLICATION INFORMATION

Full Citation: Sabbath EL, Lovejoy M, Schneider DK, Diaz-Linhart Y, DeHorn G, Peters SE. Engaging low-wage workers in health and well-being survey research: strategies from 5 occupational studies. *Am J Public Health*. 2025;115(2):201–208.

Acceptance Date: September 18, 2024.

DOI: https://doi.org/10.2105/AJPH.2024.307875

ORCID iDs:

Erika L. Sabbath https://orcid.org/0000-0002-7866-7812

Meg Lovejoy https://orcid.org/0000-0002-6362-1520

Daniel K. Schneider https://orcid.org/0000-0001-6786-0302

Yaminette Diaz-Linhart https://orcid.org/0000-0003-1380-713X

Grace DeHorn https://orcid.org/0009-0006-6690-5736

Susan E. Peters https://orcid.org/0000-0002-2705-643X

CONTRIBUTORS

E. L. Sabbath drafted the overall article. E. L. Sabbath and S. E. Peters developed the concept for the article and convened the author group. All authors drafted narratives for the studies they led and edited the article.

ACKNOWLEDGMENTS

This work was supported by the Harvard Center for Work, Health, and Well-Being (grant U19 OH008861).

We thank the Boston-Area Work, Well-Being, and Equity Network for the conversation that led to this article and Maggie Woodlock for research assistance.

Note. The content of this essay is solely the responsibility of the authors and does not necessarily represent the official views of the funders.

CONFLICTS OF INTEREST

The authors have no conflicts of interest to declare.

HUMAN PARTICIPANT PROTECTION

Human participants approval was provided by institutional review boards at Mass General Brigham (Boston Hospital Workers Health Study), Brandeis University (Community Health Worker Study), the Harvard Kennedy School (Shift Project), Massachusetts Institute of Technology (Fulfillment Center Intervention Study), and the Harvard T. H. Chan School of Public Health (Work Organizational Health Study).

REFERENCES

1. Lipscomb HJ, Loomis D, McDonald MA, Argue RA, Wing S. A conceptual model of work and health disparities in the United States. *Int J Health Serv.* 2006;36(1):25–50. https://doi.org/10.2190/BRED-NRJ7-3LV7-2QCG
2. Krieger N. Workers are people too: societal aspects of occupational health disparities—an ecosocial perspective. *Am J Ind Med.* 2010;53(2):104–115. https://doi.org/10.1002/ajim.20759
3. Landsbergis PA, Grzywacz JG, LaMontagne AD. Work organization, job insecurity, and occupational health disparities. *Am J Ind Med.* 2014;57(5):495–515. https://doi.org/10.1002/ajim.22126
4. Ahonen EQ, Fujishiro K, Cunningham T, Flynn M. Work as an inclusive part of population health inequities research and prevention. *Am J Public Health.* 2018;108(3):306–311. https://doi.org/10.2105/AJPH.2017.304214
5. Fusaro VA, Shaefer HL. How should we define "low-wage" work? An analysis using the Current Population Survey. October 2016. Available at: https://www.bls.gov/opub/mlr/2016/article/how-should-we-define-low-wage-work.htm. Accessed June 11, 2024.
6. Leigh JP, De Vogli R. Low wages as occupational health hazards. *J Occup Environ Med.* 2016;58(5):444–447. https://doi.org/10.1097/JOM.0000000000000717
7. Hajat A, Andrea SB, Oddo VM, Winkler MR, Ahonen EQ. Ramifications of precarious employment for health and health inequity: emerging trends from the Americas. *Annu Rev Public Health.* 2024;45(1):235–251. https://doi.org/10.1146/annurev-publhealth-071321-04243
8. Rosemberg M-AS, Boutain DM, Hsin-Chun Tsai J. Occupational health research beyond the work setting: inclusive inquiry with ethnic minority and immigrant workers. *Ethn Health.* 2021;26(8):1242–1260. https://doi.org/10.1080/13557858.2019.1612517
9. Sorensen G, Dennerlein JT, Peters SE, Sabbath EL, Kelly EL, Wagner GR. The future of research on work, safety, health and wellbeing: a guiding conceptual framework. *Soc Sci Med.* 2021;269:113593. https://doi.org/10.1016/j.socscimed.2020.113593
10. Lovejoy M, Kelly EL, Kubzansky LD, Berkman LF. Work redesign for the 21st century: promising strategies for enhancing worker well-being. *Am J Public Health.* 2021;111(10):1787–1795. https://doi.org/10.2105/AJPH.2021.306283
11. VanGeest JB, Johnson TP, Welch VL. Methodologies for improving response rates in surveys of physicians: a systematic review. *Eval Health Prof.* 2007;30(4):303–321. https://doi.org/10.1177/0163278707307899
12. VanGeest J, Johnson TP. Surveying nurses: identifying strategies to improve participation. *Eval Health Prof.* 2011;34(4):487–511. https://doi.org/10.1177/0163278711399572
13. Rogelberg SG, Stanton JM, Stanton JM. Introduction: understanding and dealing with organizational survey nonresponse. *Organ Res Methods.* 2007;10(2):195–209. https://doi.org/10.1177/109442810629469
14. Wu MJ, Zhao K, Fils-Aime F. Response rates of online surveys in published research: a meta-analysis. *Comput Hum Behav Rep.* 2022;7:100206. https://doi.org/10.1016/j.chbr.2022.100206
15. Eggleston J. Frequent survey requests and declining response rates: evidence from the 2020 Census and Household Surveys. *J Surv Stat Methodol.* [Published: April 26, 2024]. https://doi.org/10.1093/jssam/smae022
16. Clark MA, Roman A, Rogers ML, Tyler DA, Mor V. Surveying multiple health professional team members within institutional settings: an example from the nursing home industry. *Eval Health Prof.* 2014;37(3):287–313. https://doi.org/10.1177/0163278714521633
17. Williams JAR, Vriniotis MG, Gundersen DA, et al. How to ask: surveying nursing directors of nursing homes. *Health Sci Rep.* 2021;4(2):e304. https://doi.org/10.1002/hsr2.304
18. Collins JE, Boden LI, Gundersen DA, et al. Workplace integrated safety and health program uptake in nursing homes: associations with ownership. *Int J Environ Res Public Health.* 2021;18(21):11313. https://doi.org/10.3390/ijerph182111313
19. Anderson NJ, Smith CK, Foley MP. Work-related injury burden, workers' compensation claim filing, and barriers: results from a statewide survey of janitors. *Am J Ind Med.* 2022;65(3):173–195. https://doi.org/10.1002/ajim.23319
20. Phillips AW, Reddy S, Durning SJ. Improving response rates and evaluating nonresponse bias in surveys: AMEE guide no. 102. *Med Teach.* 2016;38(3):217–228. https://doi.org/10.3109/0142159X.2015.1105945
21. Avemegah E, Gu W, Abulbasher A, et al. An examination of best practices for survey research with agricultural producers. *Soc Nat Resour.* 2021;34(4):538–549. https://doi.org/10.1080/08941920.2020.1804651
22. Cho YI, Johnson TP, VanGeest JB. Enhancing surveys of health care professionals: a meta-analysis of techniques to improve response. *Eval Health Prof.* 2013;36(3):382–407. https://doi.org/10.1177/0163278713496425
23. Sabbath EL, Hashimoto D, Boden LI, et al. Cohort profile: the Boston Hospital Workers Health Study (BHWHS). *Int J Epidemiol.* 2018;47(6):1739–1740. https://doi.org/10.1093/ije/dyy164
24. Sabbath EL, Boden LI, Williams JA, Hashimoto D, Hopcia K, Sorensen G. Obscured by administrative data? Racial disparities in occupational injury. *Scand J Work Environ Health.* 2017;43(2):155–162. https://doi.org/10.5271/sjweh.3611
25. Sabbath EL, Yang J, Dennerlein JT, Boden LI, Hashimoto D, Sorensen G. Paradoxical impact of a patient-handling intervention on injury rate disparity among hospital workers. *Am J Public Health.* 2019;109(4):618–625. https://doi.org/10.2105/AJPH.2018.304929
26. Sabbath EL, Williams JA, Boden LI, et al. Mental health expenditures: association with workplace incivility and bullying among hospital patient care workers. *J Occup Environ Med.* 2018;60(8):737–742. https://doi.org/10.1097/JOM.0000000000001322
27. Rodriguez NM. Community health workers in the United States: time to expand a critical workforce. *Am J Public Health.* 2022;112(5):697–699. https://doi.org/10.2105/AJPH.2022.306775
28. Linhart YD, Bishop C. Designing work for complex care management programs: what works for the workers? Paper presented at: 72nd Annual Labor and Employment Relations Association Meeting. Virtual; June 2020.
29. Diaz-Linhart Y. It may not be rainbows and sunshine every day, but I know I made a difference: voice as a resource for well-being at work. August 2022. Available at: https://scholar.google.com/citations?view_op=view_citation&hl=en&user=eo1PzOwAAAAJ&sortby=pubdate&citation_for_view=eo1PzOwAAAAJ:2P1L_qKh6hAC. Accessed June 6, 2024.
30. Staples L. *Roots to Power: A Manual for Grassroots Organizing.* 3rd ed. Santa Barbara, CA: Praeger; 2016.
31. Nielsen VM, Ursprung WWS, Song G, et al. Evaluating the impact of community health worker certification in Massachusetts: design, methods, and anticipated results of the Massachusetts Community Health Worker Workforce survey. *Front Public Health.* 2023;10:1043668. https://doi.org/10.3389/fpubh.2022.1043668
32. Schneider D, Harknett K. The Shift Project. Available at: https://shift.hks.harvard.edu. Accessed June 6 2024.
33. Peer E, Rothschild D, Gordon A, Evernden Z, Damer E. Data quality of platforms and panels for online behavioral research. *Behav Res Methods.* 2022;54(4):1643–1662. https://doi.org/10.3758/s13428-021-01694-3
34. Data@Urban. How to tackle fraudulent survey responses. September 28, 2023. Available at: https://urban-institute.medium.com/how-to-tackle-fraudulent-survey-responses-4427f271a194. Accessed October 23, 2024.
35. Cornesse C, Blom AG, Dutwin D, et al. A review of conceptual approaches and empirical evidence on probability and nonprobability sample survey research. *J Surv Stat Methodol.* 2020;8(1):4–36. https://doi.org/10.1093/jssam/smz041
36. Schneider D, Harknett K. What's to like? Facebook as a tool for survey data collection. *Sociol Methods Res.* 2022;51(1):108–140. https://doi.org/10.1177/0049124119882477
37. Kelly EL, Siebach KF, DeHorn G, Lovejoy M. The Fulfillment Center Intervention Study: protocol for a group-randomized control trial of a participatory workplace intervention. *PLoS One.* 2024;19(7):e0305334. https://doi.org/10.1371/journal.pone.0305334
38. Sorensen G, Peters S, Nielsen K, et al. Improving working conditions to promote worker safety, health, and well-being for low-wage workers: the Workplace Organizational Health Study. *Int J Environ Res Public Health.* 2019;16(8):1449. https://doi.org/10.3390/ijerph16081449
39. Sorensen G, Peters SE, Nielsen K, et al. Implementation of an organizational intervention to improve low-wage food service workers' safety, health and wellbeing: findings from the Workplace Organizational Health Study. *BMC Public Health.* 2021;21(1):1869. https://doi.org/10.1186/s12889-021-11937-9
40. Peters SE, Nielsen KM, Nagler EM, Revette AC, Madden J, Sorensen G. Ensuring organization–intervention fit for a participatory organizational intervention to improve food service workers' health and wellbeing: Workplace Organizational Health Study. *J Occup Environ Med.* 2020;62(2):e33–e45. https://doi.org/10.1097/JOM.0000000000001792

Influenza Vaccination, Household Composition, and Race-Based Differences in Influenza Incidence: An Agent-Based Modeling Study

Katherine V. Williams, MD, MPH, Mary G. Krauland, PhD, Lee H. Harrison, MD, John V. Williams, MD, Mark S. Roberts, MD, MPP, and Richard K. Zimmerman, MD, MPH

Objectives. To estimate the effect of influenza vaccination disparities.

Methods. We compared symptomatic influenza cases between Black and White races in 2 scenarios: (1) race- and age-specific vaccination coverage and (2) equal vaccination coverage. We also compared differences in household composition between races. We used the Framework for Reconstructing Epidemiological Dynamics, an agent-based model that assigns US Census–based age, race, households, and geographic location to agents (individual people), in US counties of varying racial and age composition.

Results. Influenza cases were highest in counties with higher proportions of children. Cases were up to 30% higher in Black agents with both race-based and race-equal vaccination coverage. Compared with corresponding categories of White households, cases in Black households without children were lower and with children were higher.

Conclusions. Racial disparities in influenza cases persisted after equalizing vaccination coverage. The proportion of children in the population contributed to the number of influenza cases regardless of race. Differences in household composition may provide insight into racial differences and offer an opportunity to improve vaccination coverage to reduce influenza burden for both races. (*Am J Public Health*. 2025;115(2):209–216. https://doi.org/10.2105/AJPH.2024.307878)

AJPH February 2025, Vol. 115, No. 2

Influenza vaccination prevents millions of influenza illnesses and medical visits, up to 100 000 influenza-associated hospitalizations, and thousands of influenza-associated deaths in a single season, as the Centers for Disease Control and Prevention (CDC) estimates.[1] Compared with White Americans, Black Americans average 10% lower influenza vaccination coverage and twice the number of hospitalizations for every age group from birth to 64 years.[2] While comorbid conditions,[3] health care use,[4] and other social determinants of health[5] may contribute to hospitalization disparities, a better understanding of the impact of race-based vaccination coverage on influenza cases may help focus vaccination efforts.

In addition to differences in vaccination coverage by age and race, variable population age distributions may contribute to the spreading of infectious diseases. Sociodemographic differences are particularly interesting for influenza, as children carry a significant portion of the annual symptomatic influenza burden and can be an important source of influenza transmission,[6,7] yet significant infections also occur in older adults. The Framework for Reconstructing Epidemiological Dynamics (FRED) is an agent-based modeling platform that uses census-based synthetic populations to spread infectious conditions via interactions in specific locations (schools, workplaces, neighborhoods, and households), as detailed in the Appendix, Section 1, "Overview" (available as a supplement to the online version of this article at https://ajph.org).

FRED addresses the weaknesses of other infectious disease modeling by assigning census-based age, race, and household characteristics to individual people (agents) geographically across the United States.[8] Its findings can be used to address social inequities.[9] Thus, FRED can examine the role of race, age distribution, and vaccination coverage strategies on influenza cases in ways that cannot be readily assessed in the population at large.[10–16]

In an effort to further examine the interplay of population-level race and age distributions and vaccination coverage on influenza disease in 8 large US counties, we used FRED's capabilities to account for individual characteristics. We selected these counties because they represented a wide array of distributions of sociodemographic factors. We assessed symptomatic influenza cases by assigning race-specific vaccination coverage to Black and White races in 2 different scenarios: (1) documented race-specific vaccination coverage and (2) equalized vaccination coverage in Black and White agents, accounting for population composition by race, age, and household makeup.

METHODS

FRED has been used to model influenza and other diseases and conditions as described in detail previously.[8,10–18] In FRED, diseases such as influenza are defined as a series of health states through which individuals can progress (susceptible, exposed, infected, recovered [SEIR]) based on probabilities and time periods to evaluate state changes (Appendix Table A). In this study, we used a modified SEIR model to describe influenza (Appendix Figure A).[14] Presymptomatic and asymptomatic influenza conditions, behavioral factors such as staying home for illness (half of symptomatic individuals), and seasonal breaks from school (winter and spring) were also incorporated.

The base model simulated race-based influenza vaccination coverage per CDC 2021–2022 reporting by race and age, including 4 age categories for children (Appendix Table B).[19] We chose the 2021–2022 season for vaccination coverage because the information was the most recent set of complete data on vaccination coverage at the time of analysis that began in 2023 and was ongoing through March 2024. Agents were assigned vaccination coverage as defined by their race in FRED as Black alone, White alone, or "not Black alone or White alone." Agents who were not designated as Black alone or White alone represented a smaller proportion of a mix of races in FRED population counts and were assigned vaccination coverage based on the average of the US population by age. Within age and race definitions, agents were randomly chosen for application of vaccination and received 1 influenza vaccine dose beginning September 1 over a mean of 45 days with a standard deviation of 14 days.

A single influenza season was modeled from August 15 through May 31 and started by seeding 50 cases into the population on October 15, a standard seeding size within FRED for populations of the size studied, resulting in mid-February peak cases. In FRED, the reproduction number is not fixed but a product of the model transmissibility parameter, the characteristics of the infection (e.g., infectious period), and the characteristics of the population, such as prior immunity, age structure, and vaccination-induced immunity. The effective reproductive rate across the counties ranged from 1.27 in county G to 1.48 in county A (mean ±SD across counties: 1.36 ±0.07). The simulation included a single strain of influenza, similar to type A(H1N1), one of the most commonly circulating strains in the past 10 years, in terms of burden. We calibrated symptomatic influenza cases to CDC age-group estimates (Appendix Tables C and D) and reported them by total cases in each county's population. We considered symptomatic agents fully infectious and asymptomatic individuals half as infectious.

At the start of the model, we assigned agents a susceptibility of 1 across all age groups. To account for immunity from previous influenza infection, we used the estimated percentage of age-based symptomatic influenza infections in the US population in a representative past season (2019–2020)[20] to assign reduced susceptibility by 50% in the corresponding percentage of agents by age in FRED (Appendix Table A). For vaccination, we set baseline vaccine effectiveness at 40% (i.e., a 40% reduction in susceptibility to infection) for all ages 2 weeks after vaccination based on reported vaccine effectiveness in 2004–2005 to 2019–2020 seasons (mean 40%; range = 10%–60%).[21] We set waning of vaccine protection at 7% per month for age younger than 65 years and 10% per month for age 65 years and older.[22,23] After infection, susceptibility for all agents was reduced to 0 and then increased by 3% per month to account for waning.[24] Because FRED models are stochastic, we ran each model 100 times per scenario for 8 counties (1600 total simulations) to produce mean values and 95% confidence intervals (CIs) for cases.

For this study, FRED tracked populations from a range of metropolitan (urban and suburban) counties

(Appendix Table E) based on a minimum population of at least 550 000 agents and a range of

1. representation of children (e.g., county A had the highest proportion of children),
2. older age (counties B and C had the 2 highest proportions of adults aged ≥ 65 years);
3. an overall mix of Black and White race and age representations in Midwestern (county D), Southern (county E), and Northeastern (counties F and G) geographic regions; and
4. high Black resident representation (county H had 63.7% Black residents; Figure 1).

Black-only or White-only races in chosen counties ranged from 83% (county F) to 93% (county B) of the population; the remaining agents were classified as "not Black or White." County A was included to represent high proportions of children, not for the representation of Black agents (1.4%). Hispanic ethnicity was not available in the current version of the FRED population.

RESULTS

With race-based vaccination coverage, symptomatic influenza cases per 100 000 were highest for White and Black agents in county A where children were highly represented and lowest for White agents and Black agents in counties F and G, respectively, both counties where a mix of ages and races were represented (Table 1). The ratio of symptomatic cases per 100 000 in Black agents compared with White agents was greater than 1 in all counties, ranging from as high as 1.45 (95% CI = 1.41, 1.48) in county F to 1.13 in county H (Table 1). The excess number of cases in Black agents compared with White agents varied by county (Appendix Figure B). County F, despite having the lowest number of cases per 100 000 for White agents, had the greatest excess cases for Black agents compared with White agents at 4992 cases per 100 000 or 45% greater (Appendix Figure B). Counties D and H had the lowest excess cases among Black agents at 13.5% and 13.1%, respectively.

When vaccination coverage in Black agents was increased to equal that of White agents, symptomatic influenza cases per 100 000 for both Black and White agents decreased (Table 1).

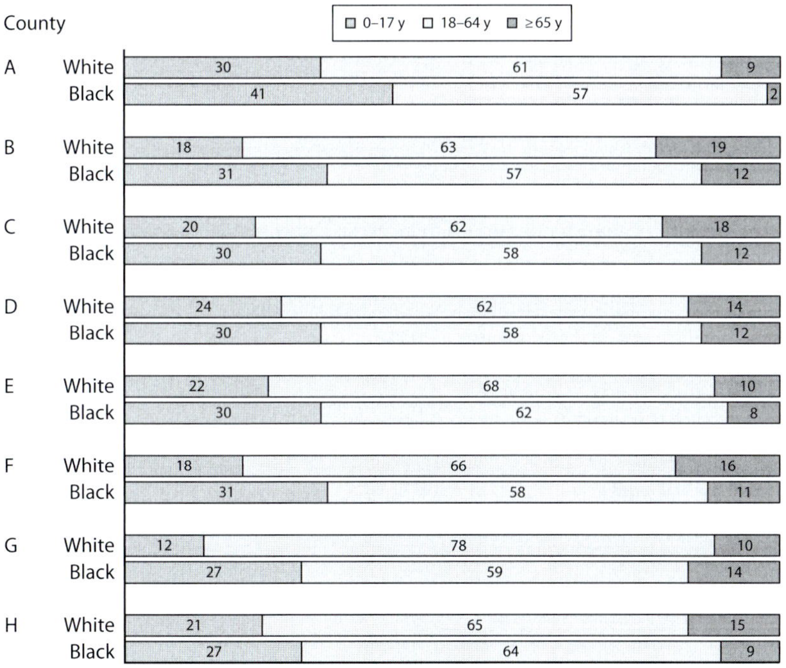

Race	Total Population (%)	Ratio of Black-to-White[a] Overall	Age < 18 y	Age 18–64 y	Age ≥ 65 y
White	86.3	0.02	1.37	0.93	0.22
Black	1.4				
White	80.5	0.15	1.72	0.90	0.63
Black	12.2				
White	64.6	0.43	1.50	0.94	0.67
Black	28.0				
White	53.5	0.73	1.25	0.94	0.86
Black	38.8				
White	46.0	0.92	1.36	0.91	0.80
Black	42.2				
White	40.7	1.04	1.72	0.88	0.69
Black	42.2				
White	35.8	1.41	2.25	0.76	1.40
Black	50.5				
White	21.2	3.00	1.29	0.98	0.60
Black	63.7				

FIGURE 1— Age Distribution by Race for 8 US Counties in Synthetic Framework for Reconstructing Epidemiological Dynamics (FRED) Populations: 2010 Census-Based Population

Note. Each bar represents the percentage distribution of the total county population in FRED by White and Black race for 3 age groups: children, adults aged 18 to 64 years, and adults aged 65 years and older.
[a]To calculate the Black-to-White ratio for the county overall and each age group, the percentage of Black agents for a given county was divided by the percentage of White agents in that group.

TABLE 1— Symptomatic Cases Simulated Across 8 US Counties With Race-Based Actual Vaccination Coverage or Equal Vaccination Coverage: 2021–2022

	Race-Based Vaccination, Symptomatic Cases/100 000 (95% CI)		Equal Vaccination Symptomatic Cases/100 000 (95% CI)		Black-to-White Case Ratio by Vaccination Scenario (95% CI)	
County	White	Black	White	Black	Race-Based	Equal
A	18 300 (18 280, 18 319)	21 893 (21 828, 21 959)	18 233 (17 628, 18 838)	21 420 (21 381, 22 459)	1.20 (1.17, 1.22)	1.17 (1.02, 1.35)
B	12 076 (11 007, 13 146)	15 726 (14 731, 16 722)	11 966 (11 261, 12 671)	15 370 (14 670, 16 071)	1.30 (1.27, 1.33)	1.28 (1.11, 1.49)
C	12 496 (12 448, 12 544)	16 083 (16 045, 16 121)	12 313 (11 819, 2 806)	15 603 (15 174, 16 032)	1.29 (1.26, 1.32)	1.27 (1.06, 1.52)
D	15 136 (15 114, 15 159)	17 181 (17 162, 17 201)	14 990 (14 727, 15 252)	16 680 (16 211, 17 149)	1.14 (1.11, 1.16)	1.11 (0.90, 1.38)
E	14 961 (14 580, 15 342)	17 492 (16 751, 18 233)	14 652 (14 011, 15 293)	16 908 (16 113, 17 704)	1.17 (1.14, 1.19)	1.15 (1.00, 1.34)
F	11 174 (10 854, 11 493)	16 165 (15 828, 16 503)	10 910 (10 508, 11 312)	15 604 (15 173, 16 035)	1.45 (1.41, 1.48)	1.43 (1.18, 1.73)
G	12 467 (11 713, 13 221)	14 916 (14 464, 15 369)	12 009 (11 201, 12 817)	14 365 (13 929, 14 800)	1.20 (1.17, 1.23)	1.20 (1.01, 1.41)
H	14 986 (14 650, 15 322)	16 950 (16 598, 17 302)	14 578 (14 184, 14 971)	16 199 (15 795, 16 603)	1.13 (1.11, 1.16)	1.11 (0.91, 1.35)

Note. CI = confidence interval. Counties were selected because they represented a wide array of distributions of sociodemographic factors.

Despite this reduction in overall cases with equalization of vaccination coverage, the ratio of cases per 100 000 in Black agents to White agents declined by only a nominal amount (Table 1), remaining as high as 1.43 (95% CI = 1.18, 1.73) in county F and greater than 1 in all counties. However, in counties D and H, counties that also had the lowest excess cases in influenza cases with race-based vaccination, the 95% CI included 1, suggesting that race-based differences in influenza cases in these populations were no longer significant after equalizing vaccination coverage. For the overall population by county (Appendix Figure C), equalizing vaccination coverage decreased cases per 100 000 overall by 0.4% (county A) to 3.7% (county H) and correspondingly decreased cases per 100 000 in Black agents by a range of 2.2% (county A) to 4.4% (county H). The maximum reduction in Black agents was found in county H at 751 cases per 100 000. These percentage reductions show some consistency with the proportion of Black and White agents represented in each county, but age composition by age and race when comparing across the counties also varied.

To explore differences in age by race between the counties, we calculated the percentage of the Black and White populations in age groups of children, adults aged 18 to 64 years, and adults aged 65 years or older, and we compared the ratio of the percentage of Black-to-White agents in each group (Figure 1). Correspondingly, county A had the highest percentage of children, predominantly White, and the most influenza cases per 100 000 population. In contrast, the counties with the highest representation of agents aged 65 years or older (counties B, C, and F) had some of the lowest cases for the White agents. Still, cases remained higher in Black agents in these counties. In all counties, the Black population tended to be younger, with the ratio of the percentage representation in Black-to-White agents by age being greater than 1 for children and correspondingly less than 1 for all other age groups (Figure 1). The lowest ratio of Black-to-White children was in county D (1.25) and county H (1.29); both were counties that also had the lowest ratio of excess cases of influenza in Black agents to White agents (1.14 and 1.13, respectively, Table 1). Some exceptions to the race-by-age county population distribution patterns existed but did not have a clear distinguishing impact on influenza cases. For example, county G had the highest Black-to-White ratio for children (2.25) and adults aged 65 years or older (1.40) and the lowest ratio for adults aged 18 to 65 years (0.76). However, symptomatic influenza cases per 100 000 and elevated Black-to-White case ratios were similar to other counties (Table 1).

In addition to race-based differences in age distribution by county, variability by race in household characteristics defined by no children, 1 or 2 children, or 3 or more children also existed (Figure 2). The ratio of Black-to-White agents living in households without children was lower in all counties (Figure 2). In 75% of the counties, more than half of White agents lived in households with no children. County A, which was predominantly White (86.9% of households), had the lowest percentage of agents in households without children (38.8% for White and 29.9% for Black), followed by county F with 39.3% for Black agents. County G had the highest percentage of households without children (73.6% for White agents).

The impact of varying representation of children in households by race could affect differences in cases among counties and race and was examined in the next set of analyses for the scenario of equal vaccination coverage for Black or White agents (Table 2). In households with no children, though less common for Black agents (Figure 2), the corresponding symptomatic cases of influenza per 100 000 for Black agents were similar or lower than for White agents (Table 2). Overall, symptomatic cases per 100 000 increased for all agents as children in the household increased. Exceptions were county A, where the Black agent population was particularly low (1.4%) and the Black-to-White case ratio based on household children was only greater than 1 for households with 3 or more children, and county H, where the ratio of Black-to-White agents living in a household of 3 or more children was only 1.06. In those counties, increasing household children from 1 or 2 to 3 or more children did not substantially increase the racial differences in influenza cases.

DISCUSSION

Racial disparities in influenza cases can be accounted for and simulated across diverse geographic populations in our agent-based model, FRED. When we used lower vaccination rates for the Black population,[19] symptomatic cases per 100 000 were higher in Black agents than in White agents. Increasing vaccination coverage in Black agents to equal that of White agents decreased symptomatic influenza cases per 100 000 but did not eliminate racial disparities in influenza burden. Among counties, cases varied relative to the representation of children, as demonstrated by the

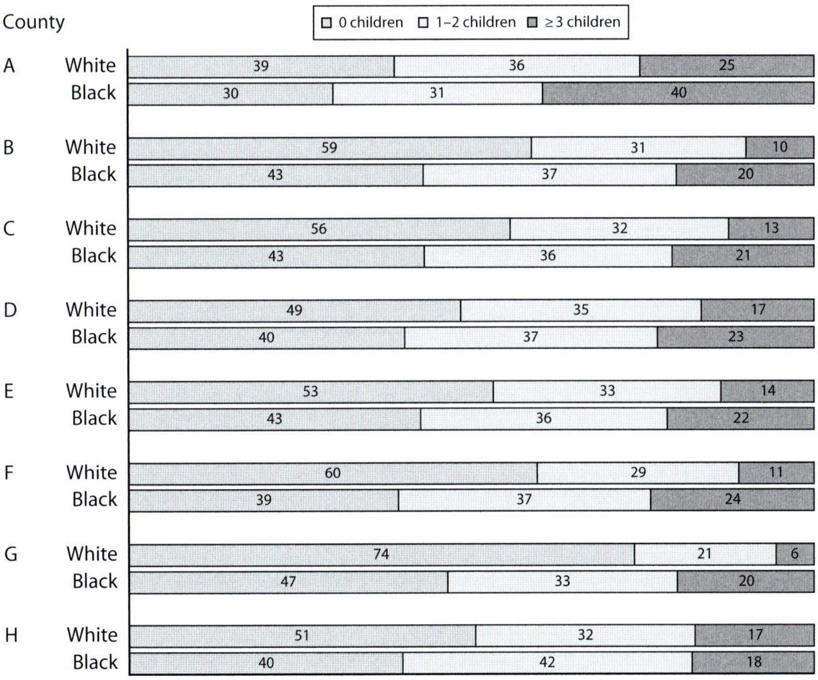

Race	Total Population (%)	Ratio of Black-to-White Households[a]: Overall	0 Children	1–2 Children	≥3 Children
White	86.9	0.02	0.77	0.85	1.55
Black	1.4				
White	82.6	0.15	0.73	1.18	2.00
Black	12.5				
White	65.8	0.43	0.78	1.13	1.66
Black	28.5				
White	53.9	0.73	0.83	1.05	1.39
Black	39.1				
White	47.4	0.92	0.80	1.08	1.58
Black	43.4				
White	42.0	1.04	0.66	1.25	2.15
Black	43.5				
White	37.9	1.41	0.63	1.61	3.57
Black	53.4				
White	21.6	3.01	0.79	1.32	1.03
Black	65.0				

FIGURE 2— Household Size Distribution by Race for 8 US Counties in Synthetic Framework for Reconstructing Epidemiological Dynamics (FRED) Populations: 2010 Census-Based Population

Note. Each bar represents the percentage distribution of the total county population in FRED by White and Black household distributions for 3 groups: no children, 1 or 2 children, and 3 or more children.
[a]To calculate the Black-to-White ratio for the county overall and each household group, the percentage of Black agents for a given county were divided by the percentage of White agents in that group.

TABLE 2— Symptomatic Cases by the Number of Children in the Household Simulated With Equal Vaccination Rates by Race: United States, 2021–2022

Household Children	Symptomatic Cases/100 000 (95% CI)		Ratio of Black-to-White, (95% CI)
	White	Black	
County A			
0	12 908 (12 612, 13 205)	13 062 (11 969, 14 155)	1.01 (0.99, 1.04)
1 or 2	21 120 (20 355, 21 885)	23 047 (21 447, 24 647)	1.09 (1.07, 1.11)
≥ 3	26 682 (25 410, 27 955)	28 093 (26 223, 29 962)	1.05 (1.04, 1.07)
County B			
0	7 679 (7 017, 8 340)	7 438 (6 731, 8 146)	0.97 (0.94, 1.00)
1 or 2	16 877 (16 073, 17 682)	18 871 (18 120, 19 622)	1.12 (1.10, 1.14)
≥ 3	21 781 (20 883, 22 680)	25 923 (24 943, 26 902)	1.19 (1.17, 1.21)
County C			
0	7 693 (7 205, 8 182)	7 436 (7 042, 7 831)	0.97 (0.94, 1.00)
1 or 2	16 869 (16 288, 17 449)	19 246 (18 653, 19 839)	1.14 (1.12, 1.16)
≥ 3	21 278 (20 634, 21 921)	26 262 (25 501, 27 017)	1.23 (1.21, 1.26)
County D			
0	8 363 (8 100, 8 625)	7 142 (6 955, 7 329)	0.85 (0.83, 0.88)
1 or 2	19 242 (18 851, 19 634)	20 080 (19 430, 20 731)	1.04 (1.02, 1.06)
≥ 3	25 442 (24 814, 26 070)	27 976 (27 004, 28 948)	1.10 (1.08, 1.12)
County E			
0	10 365 (9 647, 11 083)	9 085 (8 530, 9 640)	0.88 (0.85, 0.90)
1 or 2	18 007 (17 242, 18 772)	19 916 (18 843, 20 990)	1.11 (1.08, 1.13)
≥3	23 198 (22 189, 24 207)	27 378 (25 736, 29 109)	1.18 (1.16, 1.20)
County F			
0	7 761 (7 326, 8 196)	7 066 (6 702, 7 429)	0.91 (0.88, 0.94)
1 or 2	13 994 (13 523, 14 466)	18 206 (17 694, 18 717)	1.30 (1.27, 1.33)
≥ 3	19 635 (18 975, 20 294)	25 611 (24 849, 26 374)	1.30 (1.28, 1.33)
County G			
0	11 130 (10 249, 12 011)	7 301 (6 799, 7 802)	0.66 (0.64, 0.68)
1 or 2	13 657 (12 923, 14 390)	17 477 (16 812, 18 141)	1.28 (1.25, 1.31)
≥ 3	17 430 (16 289, 18 571)	25 551 (24 355, 26 748)	1.47 (1.44, 1.49)
County H			
0	10 010 (9 555, 10 465)	10 177 (9 754, 10 601)	1.02 (0.99, 1.05)
1 or 2	17 420 (16 805, 18 035)	18 600 (18 059, 19 141)	1.07 (1.05, 1.09)
≥ 3	22 585 (21 795, 23 376)	23 940 (23 199, 24 682)	1.06 (1.04, 1.08)

Note. CI = confidence interval. Counties were selected because they represented a wide array of distributions of sociodemographic factors.

highest number of cases in county A in both Black and White agents. Between races, household size and composition differed and, through FRED, were explored as a potential source of persistent racial differences based on the race of each specific agent in the household. For agents in households with no children, cases were lower for Black than White agents. As the number of household children increased to 1 or 2 children and 3 or more children, Black agents within those households had progressively more cases than White agents.

In this model, vaccination using 2021–2022 age- and race-specific estimates resulted in a 12% to 31% excess of symptomatic influenza cases in Black agents compared with equalizing vaccination for Black and White agents. The results of this study suggest that increased vaccination coverage for Black agents decreased cases by 2.3% to 4.4%, which, if implemented, could result in fewer influenza-related hospitalizations.[2] Additional variables such as comorbid conditions, access to care, and disease severity may determine if a symptomatic case leads to hospitalization.

Previous studies have shown that small increases of 5% in vaccine effectiveness or vaccination coverage can significantly affect the influenza burden in the United States.[25] Given that strategies to promote vaccination are challenging, incorporating factors of race, age, and household size, regardless of race, may optimize their impact. For example, the youngest children have high vaccination coverage, which declines throughout childhood.[19] Sustaining high levels of influenza vaccine coverage among children may benefit from increasing access and convenience, such as offering school vaccination or non–working-hour vaccine clinics for parents.[26] Vaccination coverage was assigned based on 2021–2022 estimates, which were already relatively high in White children aged 0.5 to 1 year (71.3%) and White adults aged 65 years and older (75.7%). Influenza vaccination coverage is typically lower in Black compared with White adults annually but can vary across years in children.[27]

Because household size varied by race, we explored whether symptomatic cases differed by household size by race. Although equalizing vaccination coverage reduced symptomatic cases in both races, racial disparities did not resolve with equal Black and White agent vaccination coverage in FRED where census-based households are represented by both age and race. In households without children, Black agents tended to have lower cases than White agents. Children alone may not be the sole source of these differences, as household agents without children may be older and may not have workplace influenza exposure, and their household size may be smaller overall than households with children. Racial differences in household structure are beyond the scope of this work and were not factored into the model (e.g., household income, crowding, education, access to health care). However, our results demonstrated significant disparities without consideration of these important factors.

Strengths and Limitations

This study had several strengths, including the ability of FRED to (1) report symptomatic influenza cases by race using census-based populations by age, race, household, and geographic region; (2) incorporate estimates of prior immunity, vaccination coverage, vaccine effectiveness, waning immunity, school breaks, and a proportion of agents staying home when ill; and (3) provide some insight into census-based social factors related to household size and composition by race.

Limitations included that (1) actual symptomatic and asymptomatic cases by age and race were unknown; (2) because of the variable mix of small numbers of agents of non-Black, non-White race, this group was assigned average vaccination coverage for the entire population by age thereby potentially overestimating actual vaccination coverage in this group; and (3) vaccination was assigned stochastically across the population but may instead vary by household, although data on vaccination coverage by household by race are not available. Annual vaccine effectiveness varies, and we used a single mean vaccine effectiveness value of 40%[21] in our model because the primary focus was on racial differences in vaccinations. We chose the counties studied based on combinations of race and age from the 2010 census because of the time required to convert 2020 census populations to FRED populations, which would excessively delay analysis. Had 2020 data been available, different counties for age and race representation may have been chosen.

Public Health Implications

Vaccination coverage by race and age contributed to racial disparities in influenza burden. Equalizing vaccination for Black and White agents decreased symptomatic influenza cases for Black and White agents but did not eliminate racial disparity in influenza burden. Demographic factors such as household size and structure should be considered when assessing influenza cases and implementing vaccination strategies. AJPH

ABOUT THE AUTHORS

Katherine V. Williams and Richard K. Zimmerman are with the Department of Family Medicine, University of Pittsburgh School of Medicine, Pittsburgh, PA. Mary G. Krauland and Mark S. Roberts are with the Department of Health Policy and Management and Public Health Dynamics Laboratory, School of Public Health, University of Pittsburgh. Lee H. Harrison is with the Center for Genomic Epidemiology, Division of Infectious Diseases, University of Pittsburgh School of Medicine. John V. Williams is with the Department of Pediatrics, Division of Pediatric Infectious Disease, University of Pittsburgh School of Medicine.

CORRESPONDENCE

Correspondence should be sent to Katherine V. Williams, MD, MPH, Department of Family Medicine, 4420 Bayard St, Suite 520, Pittsburgh, PA 15213 (e-mail: kvw3@pitt.edu). Reprints can be ordered at https://www.ajph.org by clicking the "Reprints" link.

PUBLICATION INFORMATION

Full Citation: Williams KV, Krauland MG, Harrison LH, Williams JV, Roberts MS, Zimmerman RK. Influenza vaccination, household composition, and race-based differences in influenza incidence: an agent-based modeling study. *Am J Public Health*. 2025;115(2):209–216.

Acceptance Date: September 19, 2024.

DOI: https://doi.org/10.2105/AJPH.2024.307878

ORCID iDs:

Katherine V. Williams https://orcid.org/0000-0002-1633-2283

Mary G. Krauland https://orcid.org/0000-0002-1548-6221

John V. Williams https://orcid.org/0000-0001-8377-5175

Richard K. Zimmerman https://orcid.org/0000-0001-5941-6092

CONTRIBUTORS

K. V. Williams conceptualized the study, performed the formal analysis, and drafted the article. M. G. Krauland and M. S. Roberts provided oversight and critique on the data analysis and project supervision. R. K. Zimmerman, J. V. Williams, and L. H. Harrison contributed to the data presentation and summarization and provided important intellectual content. All authors read, critically reviewed, and approved the final version of the article.

ACKNOWLEDGMENTS

This research was funded by the Centers for Disease Control and Prevention (U01-IP001141-01).

An early version of this work was presented in poster format at the annual Society for Medical Decision Making conference in Philadelphia, PA, held October 22–25, 2023.

The authors acknowledge Mary Patricia Nowalk, PhD, RD, professor, University of Pittsburgh Department of Family Medicine, for her editorial assistance in the final manuscript presentation.

Note. The funder had no role in the study's design; in the collection, analyses, or interpretation of data; in the writing of the manuscript; or in the decision to publish the results.

CONFLICTS OF INTEREST

L. H. Harrison has consulted with Sanofi Pasteur, GSK, Pfizer, and Merck without compensation. R. K. Zimmerman has investigator-initiated research grant funding to the University of Pittsburgh from Sanofi Pasteur.

HUMAN PARTICIPANT PROTECTION

The University of Pittsburgh institutional review board determined that this study was not human participant research.

REFERENCES

1. Centers for Disease Control and Prevention. Past seasons estimated influenza disease burden prevented by vaccination. December 29, 2023. Available at: https://www.cdc.gov/flu/vaccines-work/past-burden-prevented-est.html. Accessed May 5, 2024.
2. Black CL, O'Halloran A, Hung MC, et al. Vital Signs: Influenza hospitalizations and vaccination coverage by race and ethnicity—United States, 2009–10 through 2021–22 influenza seasons. *MMWR Morb Mortal Wkly Rep.* 2022;71(43):1366–1373. https://doi.org/10.15585/mmwr.mm7143e1
3. Zimmerman RK, Lauderdale DS, Tan SM, Wagener DK. Prevalence of high-risk indications for influenza vaccine varies by age, race, and income. *Vaccine.* 2010;28(39):6470–6477. https://doi.org/10.1016/j.vaccine.2010.07.037
4. Dickman SL, Gaffney A, McGregor A, et al. Trends in health care use among Black and White persons in the US, 1963–2019. *JAMA Netw Open.* 2022;5(6):e2217383. https://doi.org/10.1001/jamanetworkopen.2022.17383
5. Chandrasekhar R, Sloan C, Mitchel E, et al. Social determinants of influenza hospitalization in the United States. *Influenza Other Respir Viruses.* 2017;11(6):479–488. https://doi.org/10.1111/irv.12483
6. Centers for Disease Control and Prevention. Past seasons estimated influenza disease burden. February 28, 2024. Available at: https://www.cdc.gov/flu/about/burden/past-seasons.html. Accessed May 5, 2024.
7. Nayak J, Hoy G, Gordon A. Influenza in children. *Cold Spring Harb Perspect Med.* 2021;11(1):a038430. https://doi.org/10.1101/cshperspect.a038430
8. Grefenstette JJ, Brown ST, Rosenfeld R, et al. FRED (a Framework for Reconstructing Epidemic Dynamics): an open-source software system for modeling infectious diseases and control strategies using census-based populations. *BMC Public Health.* 2013;13(1):940. https://doi.org/10.1186/1471-2458-13-940
9. Zelner J, Masters NB, Naraharisetti R, Mojola SA, Chowkwanyun M, Malosh R. There are no equal opportunity infectors: epidemiological modelers must rethink our approach to inequality in infection risk. *PLOS Comput Biol.* 2022;18(2):e1009795. https://doi.org/10.1371/journal.pcbi.1009795
10. Krauland MG, Zimmerman RK, Williams KV, et al. Agent-based model of the impact of higher influenza vaccine efficacy on seasonal influenza burden. *Vaccine X.* 2023;13:100249. https://doi.org/10.1016/j.jvacx.2022.100249
11. Williams KV, Krauland MG, Harrison LH, Williams JV, Roberts MS, Zimmerman RK. Can a two-dose influenza vaccine regimen better protect older adults? An agent-based modeling study. *Vaccines (Basel).* 2022;10(11):1799. https://doi.org/10.3390/vaccines10111799
12. Lee K, Jalal H, Raviotta JM, et al. Estimating the impact of low influenza activity in 2020 on population immunity and future influenza seasons in the United States. *Open Forum Infect Dis.* 2021;9(1):ofab607. https://doi.org/10.1093/ofid/ofab607
13. Sinclair DR, Grefenstette JJ, Krauland MG, et al. Forecasted size of measles outbreaks associated with vaccination exemptions for schoolchildren. *JAMA Netw Open.* 2019;2(8):e199768. https://doi.org/10.1001/jamanetworkopen.2019.9768
14. Krauland MG, Galloway DD, Raviotta JM, Zimmerman RK, Roberts MS. Impact of low rates of influenza on next-season influenza infections. *Am J Prev Med.* 2022;62(4):503–510. https://doi.org/10.1016/j.amepre.2021.11.007
15. DePasse JV, Smith KJ, Raviotta JM, et al. Does choice of influenza vaccine type change disease burden and cost-effectiveness in the United States? An agent-based modeling study. *Am J Epidemiol.* 2017;185(9):822–831. https://doi.org/10.1093/aje/kww229
16. DePasse JV, Nowalk MP, Smith KJ, et al. Does cost-effectiveness of influenza vaccine choice vary across the US? An agent-based modeling study. *Vaccine.* 2017;35(32):3974–3981. https://doi.org/10.1016/j.vaccine.2017.05.093
17. Kumar S, Grefenstette JJ, Galloway D, Albert SM, Burke DS. Policies to reduce influenza in the workplace: impact assessments using an agent-based model. *Am J Public Health.* 2013;103(8):1406–1411. https://doi.org/10.2105/AJPH.2013.301269
18. Kumar S, Piper K, Galloway DD, Hadler JL, Grefenstette JJ. Is population structure sufficient to generate area-level inequalities in influenza rates? An examination using agent-based models. *BMC Public Health.* 2015;15(1):947. https://doi.org/10.1186/s12889-015-2284-2
19. Centers for Disease Control and Prevention. Influenza vaccination coverage by race and age based on the United States 2021–2022 influenza season. Available at: https://www.cdc.gov/flu/fluvaxview/coverage-2022estimates.htm. Accessed May 5, 2024.
20. Centers for Disease Control and Prevention. Estimated flu disease burden, by age group—United States, 2019–2020 flu season. July 28, 2022. Available at: https://www.cdc.gov/flu/about/burden/2019-2020.html. Accessed July 28, 2022.
21. Centers for Disease Control and Prevention. Influenza (flu), vaccine effectiveness studies. February 8, 2024. Available at: https://www.cdc.gov/flu/vaccines-work/past-seasons-estimates.html. Accessed February 8, 2024.
22. Ferdinands JM, Fry AM, Reynolds S, et al. Intraseason waning of influenza vaccine protection: evidence from the US Influenza Vaccine Effectiveness Network, 2011–12 through 2014–15. *Clin Infect Dis.* 2017;64(5):544–550. https://doi.org/10.1093/cid/ciw816
23. Ferdinands JM, Gaglani M, Martin ET, et al. Waning vaccine effectiveness against influenza-associated hospitalizations among adults, 2015–2016 to 2018–2019, United States Hospitalized Adult Influenza Vaccine Effectiveness Network. *Clin Infect Dis.* 2021;73(4):726–729. https://doi.org/10.1093/cid/ciab045
24. Patel MM, York IA, Monto AS, Thompson MG, Fry AM. Immune-mediated attenuation of influenza illness after infection: opportunities and challenges. *Lancet Microbe.* 2021;2(12):e715–e725. https://doi.org/10.1016/S2666-5247(21)00180-4
25. Hughes MM, Reed C, Flannery B, et al. Projected population benefit of increased effectiveness and coverage of influenza vaccination on influenza burden in the United States. *Clin Infect Dis.* 2020;70(12):2496–2502. https://doi.org/10.1093/cid/ciz676
26. de Lusignan S, Correa A, Ellis J, Pebody R. Influenza vaccination: in the UK and across Europe. *Br J Gen Pract.* 2016;66(650):452–453. https://doi.org/10.3399/bjgp16X686677
27. Centers for Disease Control and Prevention. Flu vaccination coverage, United States, 2021–22 influenza season. October 28, 2022. Available at: https://www.cdc.gov/flu/fluvaxview/coverage-2022estimates.htm#figure3. Accessed May 5, 2024.

HIV Trends in Metropolitan US Cities From 2014 to 2021: Baseline Data for the Ending the HIV Epidemic Initiative

Ribhav Gupta, MS, and Sten H. Vermund, MD, PhD

Objective. To examine baseline trends for the 2019 Ending the HIV Epidemic in the United States (EHE), which aims to reduce HIV incidence by 90% by 2030 in the 57 counties and states responsible for half of incident infections, and to provide a counterfactual comparator for future evaluation of the initiative's midpoint.

Methods. We used 2014–2021 metropolitan statistical area (MSA) data to compare HIV diagnostic rate trends between MSAs subsuming EHE regions (n = 46) and other MSAs (n = 76). A difference-in-difference analysis illustrated potential early-stage programmatic effects.

Results. From 2014 to 2021 across 122 MSAs, 305 413 HIV cases were diagnosed with a mean annual MSA-level diagnostic rate change of –6.7% (range = –66.1–466.7%). MSA-level diagnostic rate changed by –21.3% (range = –50.8%–14.8%) amongst MSAs including EHE regions and by 2.1% (range = –66.1%–466.7%) in other MSAs. In a difference-in-difference analysis, the HIV diagnostic rate change from 2020 to 2021 was 3.1 cases per 100 000 people-years (P = .03) greater in EHE regions compared to the baseline HIV diagnostic rate change of –0.8 cases per 100 000 people-years (P < .01) across all MSAs.

Conclusions. Although MSAs including EHE regions experienced greater reductions in HIV diagnoses from 2014 to 2021, high interregional variability requires exploration. These trends provide a baseline for subsequent EHE programmatic evaluations. (*Am J Public Health*. 2025;115(2):217–220. https://doi.org/10.2105/AJPH.2024.307890)

AJPH February 2025, Vol. 115, No. 2

HIV remains a serious endemic concern in the United States with nearly 31 800 new cases diagnosed in 2022 alone.[1] In the State of the Union address of February 2019, then–President Trump announced a new initiative—Ending the HIV Epidemic in the United States (EHE).[2] EHE engaged the Centers for Disease Control and Prevention (CDC) and Health Resources and Services Administration, along with other agencies of the US Public Health Service, allocating additional funding and resources to 50 counties (or county equivalents) and 7 states that accounted for more than half of all newly reported HIV cases (i.e., had the highest burden of HIV transmission).[3,4] Resources are allocated according to health department–generated EHE plans, including funding proposals, to support their needs and goals.[5] The EHE goal was to reduce incident HIV cases by 75% by 2025 and by 90% by 2030.[2]

We sought to analyze HIV diagnostic rate trends comparing the metropolitan statistical areas (MSAs) targeted by the EHE program with all other MSAs in a period during which early EHE investments were unlikely to have had an impact on HIV incidence. Our baseline ecological analysis may be useful in the future with counterfactual comparisons considered for broad-stroke evaluation of EHE implementation success and possible impact after 2021 and 2022 funding surges for EHE from Congress and the Biden administration.[6,7]

METHODS

We assembled annual HIV diagnostic rates for MSA level from 2014 through 2021 from CDC *HIV Surveillance Reports* (also available on the America's HIV Epidemic Analysis Dashboard) for 122 MSAs (including subdivisions where available).[1,8] We mapped MSAs to the counties they covered and stratified them as EHE and non-EHE regions as designated in 2019. Of the 122 MSAs included in reports, 46 MSAs were identified that subsumed the 57 EHE target regions (i.e., all the counties and states deemed EHE priority regions, termed "EHE regions"). The remaining 76 MSAs were in areas not deemed EHE priority areas (termed "other regions").

We performed a difference-in-difference analysis based on a Gaussian linear regression model (equation 1) and fit the model to measure the annual change in the MSA-level HIV diagnostic rates (per 100 000 people-years) in current EHE regions versus other regions from 2015 through 2021. Assuming a lag period of 1 year before any plausible initial impact from the enactment of phase 1 of the EHE program in 2020, EHE venues are unlikely to have experienced an impact of the EHE investments, though any MSA in EHE or other regions might have been influenced by other programs during our study period.

We calculated descriptive epidemiological statistics—cumulative HIV cases, annual HIV diagnostic rates (per 100 000 people-years), and change in HIV diagnostic rates:

$$(1) \qquad Y_{m,t} = \alpha + B_1 t + B_2 D + I_1 t D$$

where $Y_{m,t}$ = HIV incidence rate (per 100 000 people-years); t = time index (i.e., number of years since the study period started); m = MSA; D = binary term for whether EHE is now extant in the particular MSA; B_1 = baseline change to incidence over time; B_2 = baseline difference in incidence between MSAs included in EHE jurisdictions; I_1 = interaction term of EHE intervention over time; and α = intercept.

We did our analyses with R version 3.6.2 (R Foundation for Statistical Computing, Vienna, Austria); analytic files are available online.[9]

RESULTS

From 2014 through 2021, 305 413 cases of HIV were diagnosed among individuals living in 122 US metropolitan areas. The mean MSA-level diagnostic rate of HIV (per 100 000 people-years) decreased by 20% from 14.0 cases in 2014 to 11.2 cases in 2021. Ranges in 2014 were from 0.6 cases (Provo-Orem, UT) to 49.9 cases (Miami, FL), and in 2021 were from 2.3 (Ogden-Clearfield, UT) to 35.2 cases (Miami, FL). The mean difference in MSA-level HIV diagnostic rate (per 100 000 people-years) from 2014 to 2021 was –6.7% (range across the 122 MSAs = –66.1% to 466.7%). There was a difference in HIV diagnostic rates of 17.5 cases per 100 000 people-years (SE = 10.8) at baseline (2014) between MSAs that eventually included EHE regions and other regions, though the difference may have been attributable to chance (Figure 1; $P = .10$).

The mean MSA-level HIV diagnostic rate (per 100 000 people-years) in EHE regions (n = 46) decreased by 25.6% from 21.2 cases in 2014 (range = 8.3–49.9 cases) to 15.8 cases in 2021 (range = 8.2–35.2 cases). The mean difference in MSA-level HIV diagnostic rates (per 100 000 people-years) amongst EHE regions from 2014 to 2021 was –21.3% (range = –50.8%–14.8%).

The mean MSA-level diagnostic rate of HIV (per 100 000 people-years) in other regions (n = 76) decreased by 12.6% from 9.6 cases in 2014 (range = 0.6–25.6 cases) to 8.4 cases in 2021 (range = 2.3–19.8 cases). The mean difference in MSA-level HIV diagnostic rates (per 100 000 people-years) in other regions from 2014 to 2021 was 2.1% (range = –66.1%–466.7%). Comparing 2014 with 2021, there was a significant reduction in HIV diagnostic rates over time of 0.8 cases per 100 000 people-years (SE = 0.1; $P < .001$) annually in other regions.

Based on a Gaussian linear regression model for the difference-in-difference analysis (Table A, available as a supplement to the online version of this article at https://ajph.org), the change in HIV diagnostic rate from 2020 to 2021 was 3.1 cases per 100 000 people-years (I_1; SE = 1.4 cases; $P = .031$) greater in EHE regions relative to the baseline annual change in HIV diagnostic rate of –0.8 cases per 100 000 people-years (B_2; SE = 0.1; $P < .01$) across all 122 MSAs. These findings were robust to a sensitivity analysis varying the analysis time period (base case of 2015 to 2021) to include 2014 to 2021 and 2016 to 2021 case data.

DISCUSSION

The diagnostic rate of HIV across the metropolitan United States decreased on average from 2014 through 2021 with a high variability in trends by MSA. At the advent of the EHE initiative, EHE regions had a much higher HIV diagnostic rate compared to other targets, as intended by White House planners. Decreases in HIV diagnostic rate were greater in EHE regions that had started with higher baselines, with a minor increase in diagnostic rate noted in other regions. Though EHE and other regions both experienced decreases in HIV diagnostic rate during the study period, the range extremes were more pronounced across the other regions. Although trends in HIV diagnostic rate for EHE and other regions broadly follow the national-level decline, the mean HIV diagnostic rate remained notably higher in EHE regions and lower in

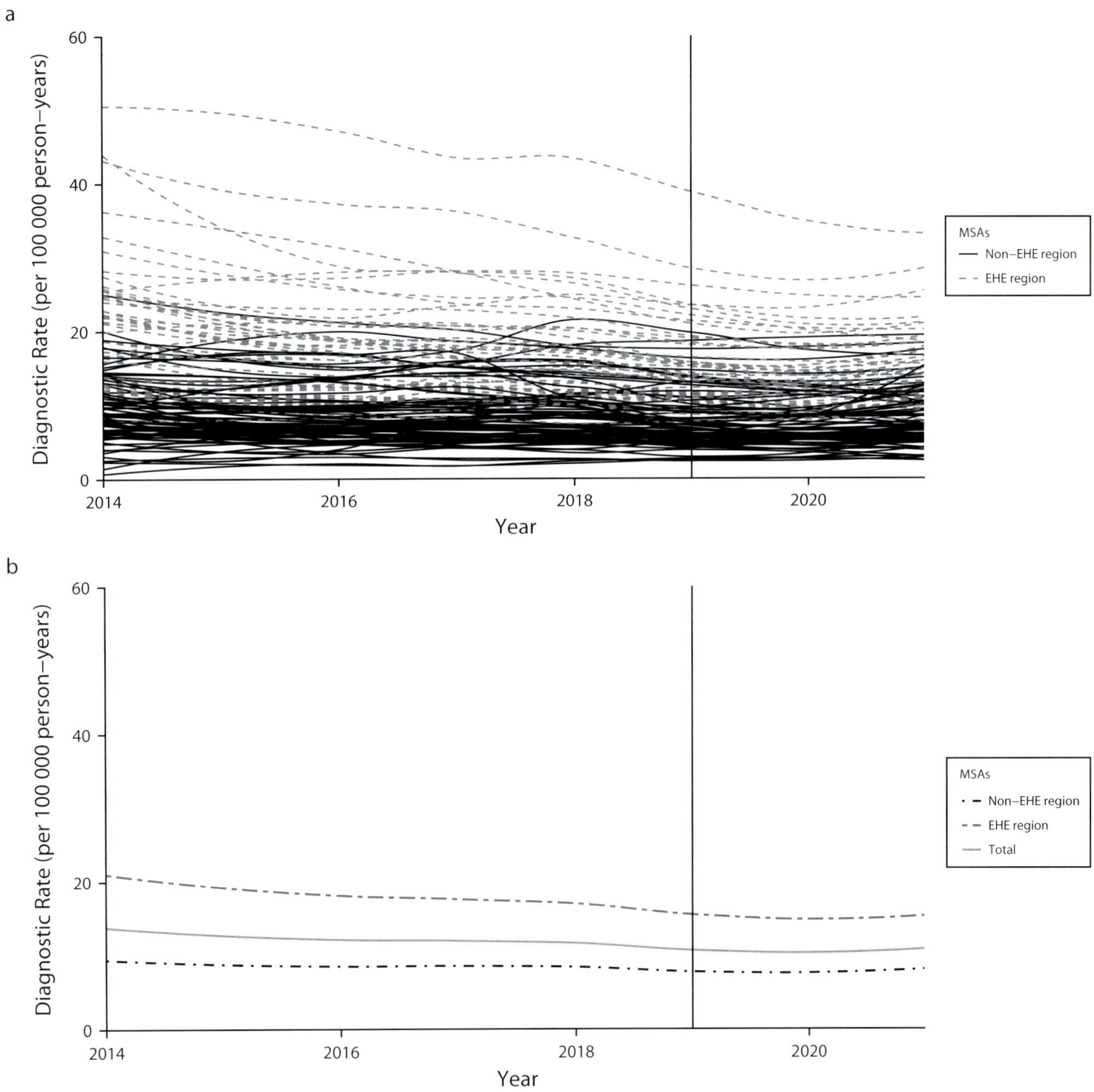

FIGURE 1— Metropolitan Statistical Area (MSA)–Level HIV Diagnostic Rates by Ending the HIV Epidemic in the United States (EHE) Classification for (a) All MSAs and (b) Mean per EHE Exclusion Group: United States, 2014–2021

Note. Vertical line represents the year the EHE initiative was introduced nationally (2019), although we anticipate full enactment and potential impacts required an additional year.

other regions when compared to national-level metrics at the study end.[1] All regions could benefit from shared monitoring and intervention programs being ramped up in the EHE regions. Trends may be partially explained by reduced testing and reported transmission during the COVID-19 pandemic.[10] Programmatic research on EHE implementation can optimize lessons learned and inform resource allocations for each region's unique needs.[7,11] Our study is only illustrative of the EHE program's early impact (first 2 years) and future potential.

Though EHE regions, on average, experienced larger reductions in HIV diagnostic rate compared to other regions, high interregion variability in trends indicates a need for careful study of program implementation and resource allocation at a local level as the EHE progresses. We present these pre-EHE trends to aid future assessments of EHE program impact; our findings can serve as counterfactual data for future ecological analyses. AJPH

ABOUT THE AUTHORS

Ribhav Gupta is with Department of Medicine at the University of Minnesota School of Medicine in Minneapolis and the Department of Epidemiology of Microbial Disease at the Yale School of Public Health in New Haven, CT. Sten H. Vermund is with the Department of Epidemiology of Microbial Disease at the Yale School of Public Health and the Department of Pediatrics at the Yale School of Medicine in New Haven.

CORRESPONDENCE

Correspondence should be sent to Ribhav Gupta, MS, Department of Medicine, University of Minnesota School of Medicine, 420 Delaware St SE, Minneapolis, MN 55455 (e-mail: gupta132@umn.edu). Reprints can be ordered at https://www.ajph.org by clicking the "Reprints" link.

PUBLICATION INFORMATION

Full Citation: Gupta R, Vermund SH. HIV trends in metropolitan US cities from 2014 to 2021: baseline data for the ending the HIV epidemic initiative. *Am J Public Health*. 2025;115(2):217–220.

Acceptance Date: September 29, 2024.

DOI: https://doi.org/10.2105/AJPH.2024.307890

ORCID iDs:

Ribhav Gupta https://orcid.org/0000-0002-4872-0774

Sten H. Vermund https://orcid.org/0000-0001-7289-8698

CONTRIBUTORS

R. Gupta and S. H. Vermund contributed equally to the design of the study and to drafting and reviewing the article. R. Gupta implemented the study and performed the analysis.

ACKNOWLEDGMENTS

This work was supported in part by the National Institutes of Health (NIH) with a supplement grant to the Third Coast Center for AIDS Research (P30 AI117943; PIs: Mustanski and D'Aquila; supplement PIs: Mustanski and Benbow) and by the Center for Interdisciplinary Research on AIDS at Yale University (P30MH062294; PI: Kershaw).

Note. The content is solely the responsibility of the authors and does not necessarily represent the official views of the NIH.

CONFLICTS OF INTEREST

The authors have no conflicts of interest to disclose.

HUMAN PARTICIPANT PROTECTION

This study did not involve human participants and was performed in accordance with guidelines of the University of Minnesota institutional review board.

REFERENCES

1. Division of HIV Prevention, National Center for HIV, Viral Hepatitis, STD, and TB Prevention, Centers for Disease Control and Prevention. *HIV Surveillance Reports*. Available at: https://www.cdc.gov/hiv-data/nhss/index.html. Accessed November 28, 2023.
2. Fauci AS, Redfield RR, Sigounas G, Weahkee MD, Giroir BP. Ending the HIV epidemic: a plan for the United States. *JAMA*. 2019;321(9):844–845. https://doi.org/10.1001/jama.2019.1343
3. Pitasi MA, Delaney KP, Brooks JT, DiNenno EA, Johnson SD, Prejean J. HIV testing in 50 local jurisdictions accounting for the majority of new HIV diagnoses and seven states with disproportionate occurrence of HIV in rural areas, 2016–2017. *MMWR Morb Mortal Wkly Rep*. 2019;68(25):561–567. https://doi.org/10.15585/mmwr.mm6825a2
4. Office of Infectious Disease and HIV/AIDS Policy. Ending the HIV Epidemic. Counties, territories and states. US Department of Health and Human Services. 2019. Available at: https://files.hiv.gov/s3fs-public/Ending-the-HIV-Epidemic-Counties-and-Territories.pdf. Accessed March 20, 2024.
5. Centers for Disease Control and Prevention. Notice of funding opportunity (NOFO) PS19-1906: Strategic partnerships and planning to support ending the HIV epidemic in the United States. Component B: Accelerating state and local HIV planning to end the HIV epidemic. Available at: https://www.cdc.gov/hiv/pdf/funding/announcements/ps19-1906/cdc-hiv-PS19-1906-component-B-program-guidance.pdf. Accessed September 1, 2024.
6. Centers for Disease Control and Prevention. Ending the HIV Epidemic in the US funding. 2023. Available at: https://www.cdc.gov/endhiv/about-ehe/funding.html. Accessed March 20, 2024.
7. Mustanski B, Smith JD, Keiser B, Li DH, Benbow N. Supporting the growth of domestic HIV implementation research in the United States through coordination, consultation, and collaboration: how we got here and where we are headed. *J Acquir Immune Defic Syndr*. 2022;90(suppl 1):S1–S8. https://doi.org/10.1097/QAI.0000000000002959
8. Sullivan PS, Woodyatt CR, Kouzouian O, et al. America's HIV epidemic analysis dashboard: protocol for a data resource to support ending the HIV epidemic in the United States. *JMIR Public Health Surveill*. 2022;8(2):e33522. https://doi.org/10.2196/33522
9. Gupta R. rgupta97/HIV_EHE. 2023. https://github.com/rgupta97/HIV_EHE. Accessed March 23, 2024.
10. DiNenno EA, Delaney KP, Pitasi MA, et al. HIV testing before and during the COVID-19 pandemic—United States, 2019–2020. *MMWR Morb Mortal Wkly Rep*. 2022;71(25):820–824. https://doi.org/10.15585/mmwr.mm7125a2
11. Jacobson EU, Hicks KA, Carrico J, et al. Optimizing HIV prevention efforts to achieve EHE incidence targets. *J Acquir Immune Defic Syndr*. 2022;89(4):374–380. https://doi.org/10.1097/QAI.0000000000002885

No-Test Telehealth Medication Abortion Services Provided by US-Based Clinicians in 21 States and the District of Columbia, 2020–2022

Emily M. Godfrey, MD, MPH, Anna E. Fiastro, PhD, MPH, MEM, Erin K. Thayer, MPH, Rebecca Gomperts, MD, Sophia M. Orlando, and Caitlin K. Myers, PhD

See also Janiak, p. 110.

Objectives. To evaluate the association between distance from closest abortion facility and number of fulfilled requests through no-test telehealth medication abortion (NTMA) asynchronous service.

Methods. Using deidentified 2020–2022 electronic medical record data from Aid Access users in US states where NTMA is prescribed by US-based clinicians, we describe individual user demographics and their resident county characteristics. We conducted a county-level geospatial analysis of distance to abortion facility (Myers Abortion Facility Database) on fulfilled requests using Poisson regression.

Results. US-based clinicians fulfilled NTMA requests to 8411 individuals in 21 states and the District of Columbia. Each 100-mile increase in distance to an abortion facility increased per-capita NTMA by 61% (95% confidence interval [CI] = 26%, 86%). Most individuals were aged 20 to 29 years (54%), had no living children (57%), were less than 6 weeks' gestation (62%), and lived in urban areas (65%). Almost half (49%) lived in higher socially vulnerable counties compared with 17% in less socially vulnerable counties.

Conclusions. In the United States, telehealth medication abortion is a critically important service for individuals who are young, socially vulnerable, and living in counties far from abortion care facilities.

Public Health Implications. With abortion now banned or highly restricted in 22 US states, telehealth abortion services are necessary to maintain essential reproductive health services. (*Am J Public Health*. 2025;115(2):221–231. https://doi.org/10.2105/AJPH.2024.307892)

AJPH February 2025, Vol. 115, No. 2

The number of medication abortions by telehealth continues to rise and now accounts for 20% of all abortions provided in the United States.[1] US-based licensed clinicians providing "direct-to-individual" telehealth medication abortions using mifepristone, the first drug of a medication abortion, took hold in the United States only as recently as 2020, more than 2 decades after mifepristone was approved by the US Food and Drug Administration (FDA). This particular care model does not require laboratory and imaging tests and allows patients to receive care and have medications directly shipped to a place of their choosing, including their own home (i.e., no-test telehealth medication abortion [NTMA]).[2] Previously, telehealth abortion and prescription of mifepristone by US-based licensed clinicians was restricted to "site-to-site," in which individuals had to travel in person to specialized or high-volume abortion clinics for preabortion testing and abortion medications because of FDA restrictions.[3] NMTA is also different from hybrid telehealth models in which individuals receive ultrasound testing either before or after abortion medications.[3,4] NTMA is safe and effective and even potentially preferred by patients, compared with in-person medication abortion.[5,6]

Although US residents could obtain NTMA through Aid Access starting in 2018, this service was considered outside the FDA because doctors unlicensed in the United States provided the service and shipped medications from India. But in 2020, an opportunity to change to direct-to-individual telehealth under the FDA came when international air distribution networks transporting mifepristone from India stopped because of COVID-19. Halted shipments coincided with a temporary COVID-19–related injunction on the FDA mifepristone Risk Evaluation and Mitigation Strategy (REMS) program, which, at that time, required US licensed clinicians to dispense mifepristone in person from a clinic or hospital. In addition, in 2020, US-based professional organizations made no-test protocols the standard of care.[7] By mid-2020, several US-based primary care clinicians joined Aid Access and responded to requests for medication abortion from individuals in states where they were licensed to practice.[8] They demonstrated that NTMA is feasible, even in low-volume primary care settings.

NTMA provides an important alternative for US residents with difficulty accessing in-clinic care, who cannot afford in-clinic services or live far from an abortion facility.[9–11] Distance to nearest abortion clinic is a key predictor of an individual's ability to travel to a brick-and-mortar facility.[12,13] Previous research evaluating Aid Access services provided by non–US-based clinicians suggests NTMA fills a gap for persons living far from abortion clinics.[9] With the change in Aid Access's provision to US-based licensed clinicians, we assessed the association between living farther from in-person care and NTMA use.

Despite reported NTMA benefits, telehealth may contribute to health inequities.[14,15] Telehealth usage for primary care services is higher for persons living 400% above than 100% below the federal poverty rate (42% vs 33%). Telehealth usage is also higher for privately insured patients and those with a graduate degree, compared with no or public health insurance and no graduate degree.[14,15] Among medication abortion telehealth users specifically, they tend to be older, have more education, and have been pregnant in the past compared with individuals seeking in-clinic care.[16] Alternatively, recent NTMA studies suggest its use is increased for persons with financial hardship or living below the federal poverty level.[6,9] The sociodemographics of individuals receiving NTMA is not fully understood.

In June 2022, the US Supreme Court decision in *Dobbs v Jackson Women's Health Organization* (*Dobbs*) struck down federal protections for abortion access. This study covers NTMA services meeting US state and federal regulations in the 2-year period before *Dobbs*, in which US-based Aid Access clinicians grew in number and expanded their licensures to 21 states and the District of Columbia. This analysis expands on our initial assessment of NTMA provided by US-based clinicians within the first 7 months to over the 2 years.[8] Using fulfilled NTMA requests as our primary outcome, we evaluated the association between distance from closest brick-and-mortar abortion clinic and number of fulfilled requests. We hypothesized greater fulfillments for individuals living farther from nearest abortion facility.

To better understand the socioeconomic status of NTMA users being served under state and federal regulations, we used Centers for Disease Control and Prevention (CDC) Social Vulnerability Index (SVI) as a proxy, and report percentage of fulfilled requests within SVI subcategories. The SVI comprises 15 social factors including poverty, lack of access to transportation, and adequate housing, where higher scores mean underresourced communities.[17] Although SVI was developed to prepare for emergency events, it is increasingly being used to better understand associations between social determinants of health and health care access.[18] Tracking geospatial shifts and the communities that utilize NTMA that are within state and federal regulations is important, especially as state abortion regulations are in flux following the *Dobbs* decision.

METHODS

In this study, we used intake form data between June 2020 and May 2022 from all individuals requesting NTMA via the Aid Access telehealth platform whose abortion medications ("fulfilled requests") were shipped to 21 states and Washington, DC. Services were provided by clinicians who were licensed to practice in the states served and, therefore, followed the abortion laws of each individual state. In states with parental notification or consent laws, Aid Access clinicians complied with these laws, fulfilling requests only to individuals aged 18 years and older. Follow-up data are not included in this analysis.

Participants

Study participants included pregnant individuals up to 11 weeks gestation who completed an online consultation form on the Aid Access platform, were determined to be appropriate candidates for NTMA by a licensed clinician, and were shipped FDA-approved mifepristone and misoprostol medications to end their pregnancies. The consultation form includes questions related to medical eligibility such as presence of intrauterine device, current health conditions, medications, age, state of residence, number of children, ability to get to a hospital in 60 minutes or less, last menstrual period, pregnancy test result, whether gestational duration was assessed by ultrasound, history of ectopic pregnancy or sexually transmitted infection, and allergy to abortion medications. Additional questions included comfort with decision to end their pregnancy, having a support person who can help during the abortion, and reasons for choosing telehealth services. Individuals completing the consultation were made aware that their deidentified responses may be used for research purposes and were allowed to decline questions unrelated to determining medical eligibility. The cost to receive an abortion through Aid Access is US $150, although a sliding-scale fee based on financial need is available.

Variables

To obtain our outcome of interest of county-level number of fulfilled NTMA requests, we matched zip code from the initial Aid Access request with county Federal Information Processing Standards (FIPS) codes using the Housing and Urban Development US Postal Services zip code crosswalk file (downloaded 4th quarter 2021).[19] For zip codes that matched to multiple counties, we used the county FIPS code for the county with the highest percentage of residential addresses from the zip code.[19]

Our primary predictor of interest included county-level distance to the nearest abortion facility. We used the Myers Abortion Facility Database to obtain time-varying distance to the nearest abortion facility. Using operation dates for each abortion facility, we created county abortion facility location data sets by study month and then used the county population centroid data from the 2020 US Census to calculate distance, in miles using the WGS84 ellipsoid, from the population centroid of each county to the nearest operating abortion facility for each month of the study with the GEOSPHERE package in R version 4.3.1 (R Foundation for Statistical Research, Vienna, Austria).[20]

We included 5 proxy measures for factors associated with barriers to travel for abortion care as controls in the Poisson regression analysis[21]:

1. Social vulnerability: people of color and persons from underresourced communities encounter the greatest barriers to abortion care.[22] Thus, we evaluated the association between county social vulnerability, using 2020 CDC SVI and fulfilled NTMA requests for each county included in this study.[17] One zip code in Alaska initially matched with the Valdez-Cordova Census Area but did not match with the county FIPS codes supplied in the 2020 CDC SVI data because it was split into 2 counties (Chugach Census Area and Copper River Census Area) in 2019. As the zip code resides fully in 1 of the Chugach Census Area, it was attributed to that county FIPS code.
2. Population of female persons of reproductive age: we controlled for persons at greatest risk for unwanted pregnancy by using age- and sex-based population estimates from the 2020 American Community Survey (5-year estimate). We used ages 15 to 49 years for all states, except parental consent or notification law states (CO, IL, ME, MI, MN, NH, RI, VA) in which we used 18 to 49 years.
3. Broadband access: access to NTMA may be dependent on having broadband access.[14,15] We used 2020 American Community Survey (5-year estimate) percentage of the population with broadband access.
4. Primary care access: we used primary care access as a proxy to control for contraceptive care access, which is essential for reducing unwanted pregnancy.[23] We used 2020–2021 Area Health Resource Files to obtain the number of primary care physicians by county. Because the data relied on 2019 FIPS codes, primary care physicians were allocated to the (now split) Valdez-Cordova Census Area. As such, we used population weighting (from the 2020 ACS 5-year estimate) to split the number of primary care physicians across the Chugach Census Area and the Copper River Census Area.
5. Republican vote share: we used Republican vote share as a proxy to control for persons living in counties that may be more hostile to abortion rights, which may impact where individuals obtain services.[24] We used proportion of Republican votes for the 2016 presidential election from the MIT Election Data and Science Lab 2000–2020 as a proxy for county-level politics.[25]

State Eligibility

Between 2020 and 2022, clinicians provided services in 3 states (NY, VT, WA) for the entire study period and in 17 states (AK, CA, CO, DC, ID, IL, MA, MD, ME, MI, MN, NJ, NM, NV, OR, RI, VA) for part of the study period. Because of changes in state laws, NTMA was interrupted in 2 states (CT, NH) for part of the study period (Appendix A, available as a supplement to the online version of this article at https://ajph.org).

County–Month Database Creation

We aggregated the number of completed requests by county and month, so that each observation (row in the data set) represents a county in a specific month during the 2-year study period, totaling 11 005 county-months. If a state was eligible for inclusion (clinicians were able to provide NTMA) during a specific month, but had no fulfilled requests, the aggregated count was 0 for that month (Appendix B, available as a supplement to the online version of this article at https://ajph.org). However, if a state was ineligible for NTMA during a specific month, the county-month was not included in the data set.

Statistical Methods

We use descriptive statistics to examine Aid Access user characteristics, vulnerability of counties in which these users lived, and trends in fulfilled requests by state. We applied Poisson models with a quadratic specification of distance to flexibly estimate the association between per-capita county-level Aid Access fulfilled requests (n = 11 005 county-months with 8170 total completed requests) and distance to the nearest brick-and-mortar facility. We excluded Alaska and Michigan because Alaska lacks road networks across much of the state, making it difficult or impossible to calculate driving distance and rendering the effects of distance incomparable to the rest of the country, and Michigan provided only 1 month of data. The model takes the following form:

$$(1)\quad E[FulfilledRequests_{c,s,t} | d_{c,s,t}, \beta X_{c,t}, pop_{c,t}] = exp(\alpha_1 d_{c,t} + \alpha_2 d^2_{c,t} + \beta X_{c,t} + \upsilon_s + \upsilon_t + ln(pop_{c,t}))$$

where $FulfilledRequests_{c,s,t}$ is the number of fulfilled Aid Access requests in county c in state s in monthly date t. Following a standard empirical method for studying the spatial distribution of the incidence of health outcomes, we modeled fulfilled requests using a Poisson regression with a population exposure.[26] This approach implicitly relies on the assumption that, conditional on the covariates, the number of expected requests in each county is proportional to its population of women of childbearing age, and the results were interpreted as changes in the relative rates of fulfilled requests per capita.

The explanatory variable of interest, $d_{c,t}$, measures the WGS84 ellipsoid distance from county c to the nearest abortion facility operating in month t. This was entered as a quadratic function to flexibly allow for a potential nonlinear relationship between distance and fulfilled requests in keeping with evidence from the existing literature on the effects of distance on travel to brick-and-mortar abortion facilities.[12,13] Because the estimated model is a Poisson with a population exposure, we interpreted the results as the relationship between increasing distance and the relative (percentage) change in fulfilled requests per capita.

All models additionally included state fixed effects υ_s to control for time-invariant state characteristics influencing fulfilled requests and monthly date fixed effects υ_t that controlled for spatially invariant temporal shocks to Aid Access requests. With these fixed effects included, the model estimated the relationship between distance to brick-and-mortar abortion facilities and demand for Aid Access NTMA, controlling for nationwide shocks to demand and state variation requests. Standard errors were clustered on counties to account for correlation of repeated observations of counties.

The vector $X_{c,t}$ includes an intercept and controls for county factors associated with challenges accessing abortion care, including SVI, broadband access, primary care access, and Republican vote shares, as noted under "Variables" previously. We estimated models both with and without these controls using the Stata version 18 (StataCorp LP, College Station, TX). We conducted data management using R version 4.3.1 with the MAPS and GGPLOT2 packages to provide and visualize geospatial information.[27] Estimates of alternative model specifications are presented in Appendix C (available as a supplement to the online version of this article at https://ajph.org) and were not meaningfully different than those presented here.

RESULTS

Between June 2020 and May 2022, 8411 individuals requested and received abortion medications from 8 US-based clinicians staffing the Aid Access Web-based platform for 21 states and DC. Aid Access users aged 14 to 49 years received fulfilled NTMA requests, with the highest percentage representing ages 20 to 24 years (29%; n = 2458) and 25 to 29 years (25%; n = 2077). The majority were nulliparous (57%; n = 4824) and sought abortion at less than 6 weeks gestation (62%; n = 5224). The top 3 reasons for choosing NTMA included cost (51%), responsibilities with work or school (36%), and keeping the abortion a secret (33%). About 90% (n = 7464) did not have an ultrasound before NTMA. Very few individuals reported feeling troubled about their decision to terminate their pregnancy (1.4%; n = 114). Almost half (49%) lived in counties with high social vulnerability (Table 1).

Monthly fulfilled medication abortion requests increased steadily over the study period as US clinicians became licensed in and served additional states, with May 2022 (n = 1009 shipments) having nearly more than 2.5 times the number of shipments as in May 2021 (n = 371 shipments) and 13 times the number of shipments as in June 2020 (n = 75; Figure 1). More than half of the total number of fulfilled requests went to individuals located in 4 states: 2 in the Western region (California: 21%; n = 1742 and Nevada: 10%; n = 802) and 2 in the Northeastern region (New York: 17%; n = 1389 and New Jersey: 10%; n = 833).

Counties with high or medium social vulnerability had more than twice the median number of Aid Access users per 100 000 reproductive-age females who requested NTMA than low social vulnerability counties. The median number of users from high vulnerability counties was 23 (interquartile range [IQR] = 6–52); from medium vulnerability counties was 20 (IQR = 0–41); and from low vulnerability counties was 10 (IQR = 0–31). States with highest proportion of fulfilled requests from high vulnerability counties included Nevada: 93.0% (n = 746), New Mexico: 92% (n = 236), and

TABLE 1— Characteristics of Individuals Who Requested and Received Abortion Medications From US-Based Clinicians Staffing Aid Access Platform: 2020–2022

Characteristic	No. (%)
Age, y	
<20	1093 (13.0)
20–24	2458 (29.2)
25–29	2077 (24.7)
30–34	1524 (18.1)
35–39	925 (10.9)
40–49	321 (3.8)
Missing	13 (0.2)
No. of children	
0	4824 (57.4)
1–2	2720 (32.3)
≥3	867 (10.3)
Weeks since last menstrual period	
<6	5224 (62.3)
6–7	2373 (28.2)
8–10	804 (9.6)
>10	8 (<0.1)
Missing	2 (<0.1)
Felt troubled about this decision	114 (1.4)
Had a hospital within 60 min	8106 (96.4)
Had somebody to help during the treatment	8187 (97.3)
Did not have an ultrasound	7464 (88.7)
Reason for Web-based abortion[a]	
Cost	4320 (51.4)
Work or school	2814 (33.5)
Secret	2805 (33.3)
COVID-19	2117 (25.2)
Stigma	2101 (25.0)
Distance	1894 (22.5)
Protesters	1813 (21.6)
Childcare	1337 (15.9)
Legal restrictions	415 (4.9)
Risk of abuse	291 (3.5)
Missing	590 (7.0)
Social vulnerability category	
Low	1395 (16.6)
Medium	2862 (34.0)
High	4152 (49.4)
Missing	2 (<0.1)

Note. The sample size was n = 8411.
[a]Question asked as "check all that apply."

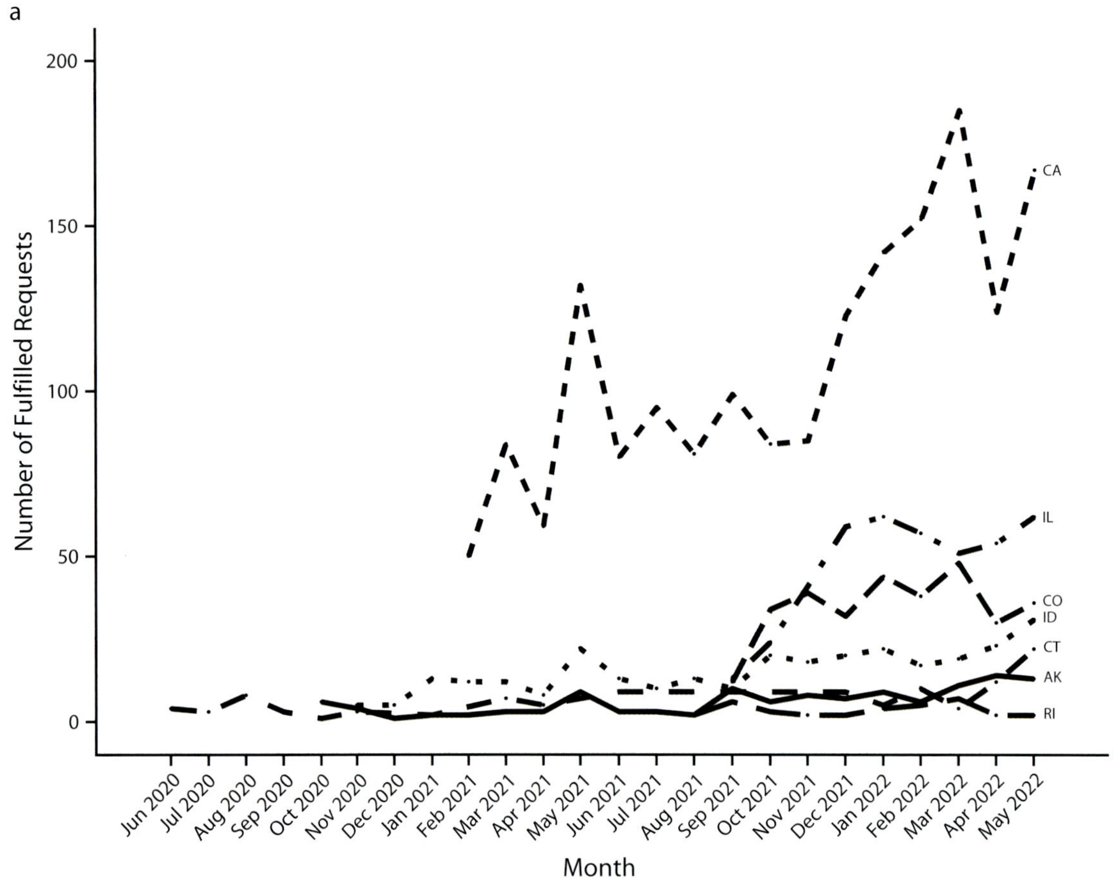

FIGURE 1— Monthly Fulfilled Medication Abortion Requests as US Clinicians Became Licensed in and Served in Additional States: United States 2020–2022

Note. Solid and dotted lines represent the corresponding state, as abbreviated on right side of graph. Michigan has a dot to represent only 1 month of data at the end of the 2-year period.

California: 73% (n = 1267). Conversely, states with highest proportions of fulfilled requests from low social vulnerability counties included Vermont: 100% (n = 45), New Hampshire: 96% (n = 49), and Maine: 63% (n = 20; Figure 2).

Aid Access clinicians served 8411 individuals in 788 counties within 21 states and DC totaling 11 005 county-months over the 2-year study period (Appendix B). Figure 3 shows, starting from a base of 0 miles, a 100-mile increase in distance to an abortion facility increased per-capita NTMA fulfillments by 60.9% (SE = 12.9; 95% confidence interval [CI] = 35.7%, 86.1%). When we controlled for county factors, per-capita NTMA fulfillments increased 30.3% (SE = 12.8; 95% CI = 5.2%, 55.4%). We found the estimated relationship was similar using a generalized estimating equation approach (55%; 95% CI = 31%, 78%), linear specification of distance (56%; 95% CI = 36%, 77%), or a cubic specification of distance (47%; 95% CI = 21%, 74%; Appendix C, available as a supplement to the online version of this article at https://ajph.org).

DISCUSSION

Our study shows that residing farther from brick-and-mortar abortion facilities was associated with increased requests for NTMA. For every 100-mile increase in distance to the nearest abortion facility, fulfilled NTMA requests increased more than 60%. Our findings are consistent with other studies evaluating similar NTMA models.[9,10] A recent study found that this model of care can avert substantial driving distance for persons living in rural areas and significantly facilitated timeliness to care for persons living 100 miles or more from the closest abortion facility.[10] Another study found that a 47-mile increase in distance to nearest abortion clinic is associated with 41% increase in requests.[9] Hybrid telehealth models have noted similar findings.[16] As

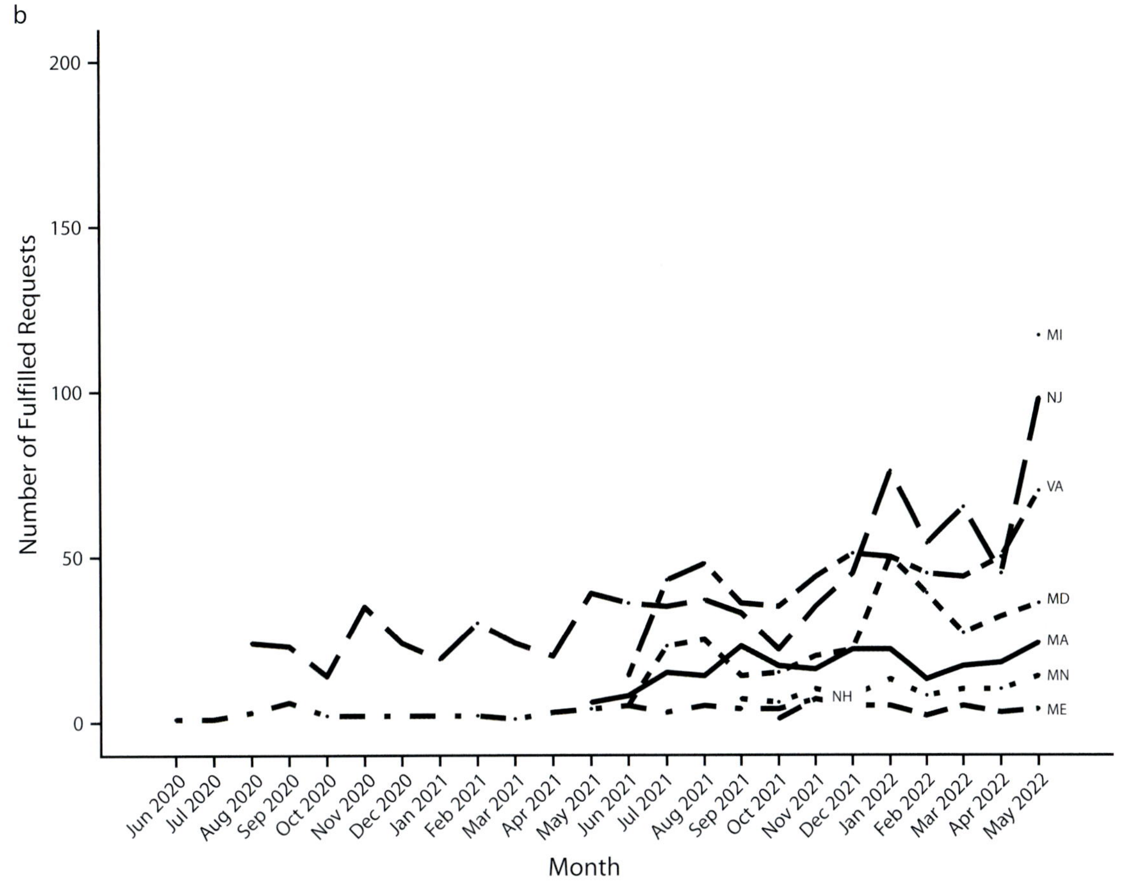

FIGURE 1— Continued

abortion facilities close in record numbers because of abortion bans, this study further supports existing literature that NTMA provides an essential service to individuals living in rural and remote areas who are far from in-person abortion services.[28]

Our findings also show how NTMA meets the needs of diverse individuals throughout the nation. A higher percentage of younger persons or persons residing in underresourced counties sought out Aid Access services, suggesting NTMA addresses an important care gap for marginalized people. In addition, as most individuals requesting NTMA were less than 6 weeks' gestation and had not opted for premedication ultrasound, we substantiate the existing literature showing that NTMA is timely and reduces unnecessary clinical testing.[10] Timely and affordable access to abortion is critically important to reduce pregnancy-related complications that increase each week when abortion services are delayed beyond the eighth week of pregnancy.[29]

Another unique study finding includes the remarkable speed with which US-based primary care clinicians stepped in to provide NTMA services when there was a brief window of opportunity to do so under state and federal regulations during COVID-19 Public Health Emergency. Within the 2-year study period, fulfilled NTMA requests by Aid Access clinicians increased by almost 15 times to more than 1000 NTMA requests monthly, representing almost a third of all virtual abortions in the United States just before the *Dobbs* decision.[1] The 2 years in which US-based clinicians provided this care were formidable, as clinicians participating in this study continue to serve individuals after the *Dobbs* decision under shield laws that protect abortion providers in states where abortion remains legal.[30] As of March 2024, US licensed clinicians are fulfilling close to 10 000 NTMA requests monthly in states with abortion bans or telehealth restrictions under their state shield laws.[1]

It is also important to point out that US-based clinicians' dramatic increase in NTMA occurred in response to the

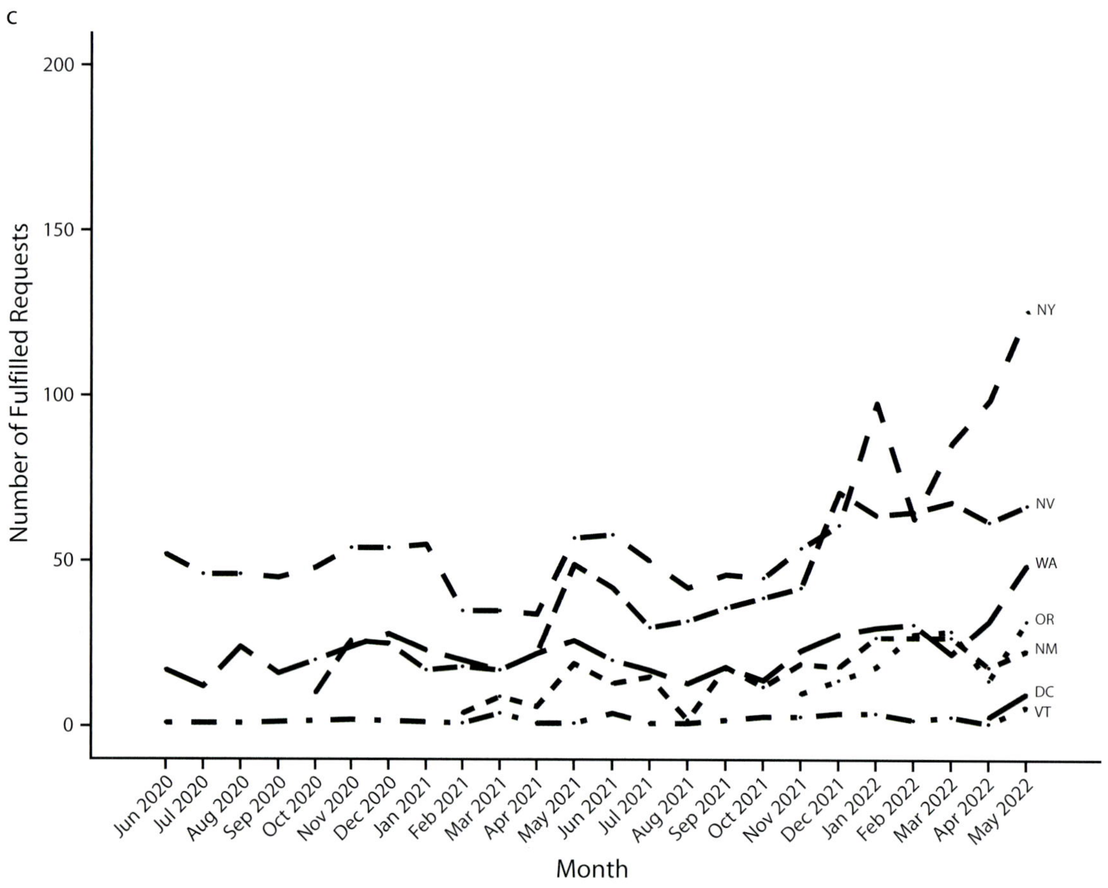

FIGURE 1— Continued

initial temporary, and now permanent, removal of FDA REMS in-person mifepristone requirement and the ability to provide telehealth across state lines. Although mifepristone has been available in the United States for prescription since 2000, the FDA REMS Program has historically impeded widespread provision of mifepristone by generalist clinicians, even though evidence suggests US primary care can routinely provide safe and effective early abortion care.[31,32] While the FDA removed the REMS in-person dispensing requirement, prescribers must comply with other burdensome REMS program requirements. Professional organizations continue to call on the FDA to remove mifepristone entirely from the REMS program because of its long-standing proven safety record.[33] This study shows that even with the removal of 1 of the REMS requirements, clinicians can reach individuals living large distances from in-person care in a timely manner.

The limitations of this study included a single telehealth provider site, which may not be generalizable to other models of telemedicine abortion provision. The demographics reported in this study were limited by self-reported data that could not be verified elsewhere and did not include race or ethnicity data. We did not collect information about medication shipment or receipt dates. We did not analyze number of overall requests made to Aid Access and whether a portion of those requests were referred to clinic-based services because of gestational age, concern for ectopic pregnancy, or another reason. It is possible addresses provided by individuals requesting NTMA did not necessarily represent their residence, because US-based clinicians do not require proof of home address. Approaches such as mail forwarding, general delivery, or driving across state borders allow persons seeking abortion to appear that their residence is where telehealth abortion is permissible.[34]

The absence of US federal protection for abortion has caused significant uncertainty and disruption in the traditional in-clinic abortion care model. Before the *Dobbs* decision, most abortion services occurred in facilities that required individuals to physically travel to receive care.[35] Alternative

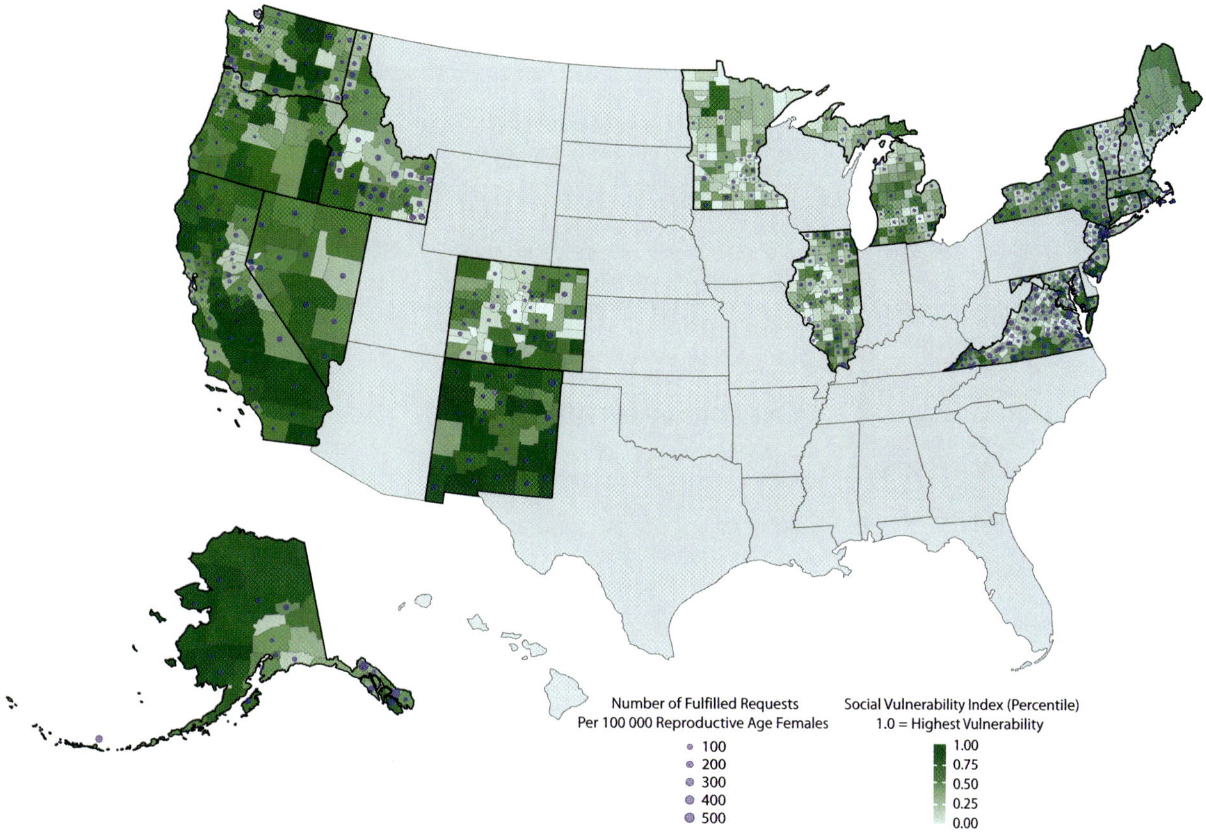

FIGURE 2— **Fulfilled Medication Abortion Requests by County Social Vulnerability: United States, 2020–2022**

Note. Purple dots represent medication abortion requests. Dark green indicates most-underresourced counties.

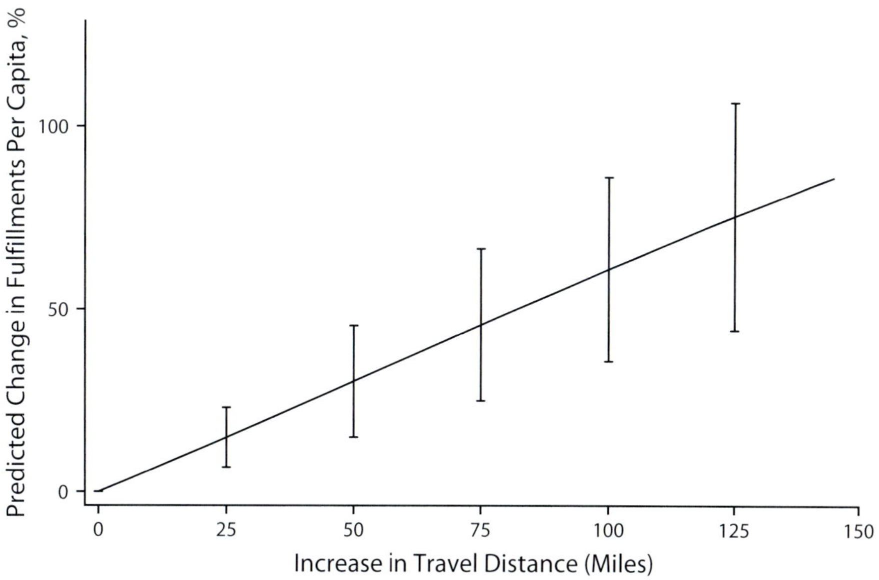

FIGURE 3— **Estimated Change in Fulfilled Requests as a Function of Increased Distance From the Nearest Brick-and-Mortar Abortion Facility: United States, 2020–2022**

Note. Distance was measured from a baseline of 0 miles. This gradient was estimated using the Poisson specification described in Equation 1. Whiskers indicate 95% confidence intervals.

approaches such as NTMA help ensure abortion access. Our findings show that persons living in underresourced counties are accessing NTMA services and that persons living far from abortion care facilities are even more reliant on telehealth access. AJPH

ABOUT THE AUTHORS

Emily M. Godfrey and Anna E. Fiastro are with the School of Medicine, Department of Family Medicine, University of Washington, Seattle. Erin K. Thayer is with the Department of Family Medicine, Keck School of Medicine of the University of Southern California, Los Angeles. Rebecca Gomperts is with Aid Access, Amsterdam, the Netherlands. Sophia M. Orlando is a student at the University of Washington School of Medicine. Caitlin K. Myers is with Middlebury College, Middlebury, VT.

CORRESPONDENCE

Correspondence should be sent to Emily M. Godfrey, MD, MPH, Box 354982, 4311 11th Ave NE, Seattle, WA 98105 (e-mail: godfreye@uw.edu). Reprints can be ordered at https://www.ajph.org by clicking the "Reprints" link.

PUBLICATION INFORMATION

Full Citation: Godfrey EM, Fiastro AE, Thayer EK, Gomperts R, Orlando SM, Myers CK. No-test telehealth medication abortion services provided by US-based clinicians in 21 states and the District of Columbia, 2020–2022. *Am J Public Health*. 2025;115(2):221–231.

Acceptance Date: September 30, 2024.

DOI: https://doi.org/10.2105/AJPH.2024.307892

ORCID iDs:

Emily M. Godfrey https://orcid.org/0000-0003-2408-7828

Anna E. Fiastro https://orcid.org/0000-0003-2901-7474

Erin K. Thayer https://orcid.org/0000-0002-3235-0748

Caitlin K. Myers https://orcid.org/0000-0002-3065-5521

CONTRIBUTORS

E. M. Godfrey and A. E. Fiastro conceptualized the data analysis plan and secured the funding for this project. R. Gomperts provided data access and supervised general research activities. A. E. Fiastro, E. K. Thayer, and C. K. Myers formalized the methods. E. K. Thayer and C. K. Myers performed the data analysis. E. M. Godfrey wrote the first draft of the article with the assistance of E. K. Thayer and S. M Orlando. All authors participated in review and editing of previous drafts of this article. All authors approved the final draft of the article.

ACKNOWLEDGMENTS

This study was supported in part by an anonymous gift through the University of Washington Foundation.

This study was previously published in abstract form in the *Annals of Family Medicine*, (2023;21 [suppl 3]:5335).

The authors would like to thank Aid Access and individuals who used the site for the use of their data to conduct this study and Azelea Sayavong for her editorial assistance.

Note. The content is solely the responsibility of the authors and does not necessarily represent the official views of the University of Washington.

CONFLICTS OF INTEREST

E. M. Godfrey receives honoraria from Organon outside the submitted work. In the previous 3 years, E. M. Godfrey and A. E. Fiastro have received funding from the Society of Family Planning to support collection of data on abortion access outside the submitted work. In the previous 3 years, C. K. Myers has received a grant from the Society of Family Planning to support the collection of data on abortion access. She also serves in an unpaid position on the Power to Decide Research Advisory Group. She also has served as a paid consultant for Planned Parenthood Federation of America on matters concerning the effects of abortion policy and access. This article is the authors' independent research, and none of these parties has a right to review this before its circulation.

HUMAN PARTICIPANT PROTECTION

The University of Washington Human Subjects Division determined this study does not involve human participants (IRB ID 00011880).

REFERENCES

1. Society of Family Planning. #WeCount report April 2022 to March 2024. August 7, 2024. Available at: https://doi.org/10.46621/878086iuzegt. Accessed August 30, 2024.
2. Fok WK, Mark A. Abortion through telemedicine. *Curr Opin Obstet Gynecol*. 2018;30(6):394–399. https://doi.org/10.1097/GCO.0000000000000498
3. Grossman D, Grindlay K. Safety of medical abortion provided through telemedicine compared with in person. *Obstet Gynecol*. 2017;130(4):778–782. https://doi.org/10.1097/AOG.0000000000002212
4. Raymond E, Chong E, Winikoff B, et al. TelAbortion: evaluation of a direct to patient telemedicine abortion service in the United States. *Contraception*. 2019;100(3):173–177. https://doi.org/10.1016/j.contraception.2019.05.013
5. Ralph LJ, Baba CF, Biggs MA, McNicholas C, Hagstrom Miller A, Grossman D. Comparison of no-test telehealth and in-person medication abortion. *JAMA*. 2024;332(11):898–905. https://doi.org/10.1001/jama.2024.10680
6. Koenig LR, Ko J, Valladares ES, et al. Patient acceptability of telehealth medication abortion care in the United States, 2021–2022: a cohort study. *Am J Public Health*. 2024;114(2):241–250. https://doi.org/10.2105/AJPH.2023.307437
7. Raymond EG, Grossman D, Mark A, et al. Commentary: no-test medication abortion: a sample protocol for increasing access during a pandemic and beyond. *Contraception*. 2020;101(6):361–366. https://doi.org/10.1016/j.contraception.2020.04.005
8. Godfrey EM, Thayer EK, Fiastro AE, Aiken ARA, Gomperts R. Family medicine provision of online medication abortion in three US states during COVID-19. *Contraception*. 2021;104(1):54–60. https://doi.org/10.1016/j.contraception.2021.04.026
9. Aiken ARA, Starling JE, Gomperts R. Factors associated with use of an online telemedicine service to access self-managed medical abortion in the US. *JAMA Netw Open*. 2021;4(5):e2111852. https://doi.org/10.1001/jamanetworkopen.2021.11852
10. Koenig LR, Becker A, Ko J, Upadhyay UD. The role of telehealth in promoting equitable abortion access in the United States: spatial analysis. *JMIR Public Health Surveill*. 2023;9:e45671. https://doi.org/10.2196/45671
11. Seymour JW, Thompson TA, Milechin D, Wise LA, Rudolph AE. Potential impact of telemedicine for medication abortion policy and programming changes on abortion accessibility in the United States. *Am J Public Health*. 2022;112(8):1202–1211. https://doi.org/10.2105/AJPH.2022.306876
12. Lindo J, Myers C, Schlosser A, Cunningham S. How far is too far? New evidence on abortion clinic closures, access, and abortions. *J Hum Resour*. 2020;55(4):1137–1160. https://doi.org/10.3368/jhr.55.4.1217-9254R3
13. Myers C. Forecasts for a post-Roe America: the effects of increased travel distance on abortions and births. *J Policy Anal Manage*. 2024;43(1):39–62. https://doi.org/10.1002/pam.22524
14. Anawade PA, Sharma D, Gahane S. A comprehensive review on exploring the impact of telemedicine on healthcare accessibility. *Cureus*. 2024;16(3):e55996. https://doi.org/10.7759/cureus.55996
15. Badr J, Motulsky A, Denis JL. Digital health technologies and inequalities: a scoping review of potential impacts and policy recommendations. *Health Policy*. 2024;146:105122. https://doi.org/10.1016/j.healthpol.2024.105122
16. Brown C, Neerland CE, Weinfurter EV, Saftner MA. The provision of abortion care via telehealth in the United States: a rapid review. *J Midwifery Womens Health*. 2023;68(6):744–758. https://doi.org/10.1111/jmwh.13586
17. Agency for Toxic Substances and Disease Registry. CDC/ATSDR Social Vulnerability Index (CDC/ATSDR SVI): overview. Centers for Disease Control and Prevention. Available at: https://www.atsdr.cdc.gov/place-health/php/svi/index.html. Accessed August 30, 2024.
18. Tran T, Rousseau MA, Farris DP, Bauer C, Nelson KC, Doan HQ. The social vulnerability index as a risk stratification tool for health disparity research in cancer patients: a scoping review. *Cancer Causes Control*. 2023;34(5):407–420. https://doi.org/10.1007/s10552-023-01683-1
19. Office of Policy Development and Research. HUD USPS zip code crosswalk files. Washington, DC: US Department of Housing and Urban Development; 2021.
20. US Census Bureau. Centers of Population. 2020. Available at: https://www.census.gov/geographies/reference-files/time-series/geo/centers-population.html. Accessed July 12, 2023.

21. Jerman J, Frohwirth L, Kavanaugh ML, Blades N. Barriers to abortion care and their consequences for patients traveling for services: qualitative findings from two states. *Perspect Sex Reprod Health*. 2017; 49(2):95–102. https://doi.org/10.1363/psrh.12024
22. Jones RK, Chiu DW, Kohn JE. Characteristics of people obtaining medication vs procedural abortions in clinical settings in the United States: findings from the 2021–2022 abortion patient survey. *Contraception*. 2023;128:110137. https://doi.org/10.1016/j.contraception.2023.110137
23. Gossett DR, Kiley JW, Hammond C. Contraception is a fundamental primary care service. *JAMA*. 2013;309(19):1997–1998. https://doi.org/10.1001/jama.2013.4262
24. Boonstra HD, Nash E. A surge of state abortion restrictions puts providers—and the women they serve—in the crosshairs. *Guttmacher Policy Rev*. 2014;17(1):9–15.
25. MIT Election Data and Science Lab. County presidential election returns 2000–2020. Cambridge, MA: Harvard Dataverse; 2021.
26. Selvin S. *Statistical Analysis of Epidemiologic Data*. 3rd ed. New York, NY: Oxford University Press; 2004. https://doi.org/10.1093/acprof:oso/9780195172805.001.0001
27. R Core Team. *R: A Language and Environment for Statistical Computing*. R Foundation for Statistical Computing. 2022. Available at: https://www.R-project.org. Accessed December 4, 2024.
28. Jones RK, Gibson C, Philbin J. The number of brick-and-mortar abortion clinics drops, as US abortion rate rises: new data underscore the need for policies that support providers. Guttmacher Institute. June 2024. Available at: https://www.guttmacher.org/report/abortion-clinics-united-states-2020-2024. Accessed August 30, 2024.
29. Bartlett LA, Berg CJ, Shulman HB, et al. Risk factors for legal induced abortion-related mortality in the United States. *Obstet Gynecol*. 2004;103(4):729–737. https://doi.org/10.1097/01.AOG.0000116260.81570.60
30. Cohen DS, Donley G, Rebouché R. Abortion shield laws. *NEJM Evid*. 2023;2(4):EVIDra2200280. https://doi.org/10.1056/EVIDra2200280
31. Razon N, Wulf S, Perez C, et al. Exploring the impact of mifepristone's risk evaluation and mitigation strategy (REMS) on the integration of medication abortion into US family medicine primary care clinics. *Contraception*. 2022;109:19–24. https://doi.org/10.1016/j.contraception.2022.01.017
32. National Academies of Sciences, Engineering, and Medicine. *The Safety and Quality of Abortion Care in the United States*. Washington, DC: National Academies Press; 2018.
33. The American College of Obstetricians and Gynecologists. ACOG relieved by Supreme Court decision allowing continued access to mifepristone, calls for removal of REMS. June 13, 2024. Available at: https://www.acog.org/news/news-releases/2024/06/acog-relieved-by-supreme-court-decision-allowing-continued-access-to-mifepristone-calls-for-removal-of-rems. Accessed August 30, 2024.
34. Plan C. Mail forwarding and other options. Available at: https://www.plancpills.org/mail-forwarding. Accessed August 30, 2024.
35. Jones RK, Kirstein M, Philbin J. Abortion incidence and service availability in the United States, 2020. *Perspect Sex Reprod Health*. 2022;54(4):128–141. https://doi.org/10.1363/psrh.12215

From Taboo to Teaching: Transforming Menstrual Health in Schools

Morgan Stein, RN, BSN

ABOUT THE AUTHOR

Morgan Stein is a registered nurse currently pursuing an MSN-FNP degree at Ohio University, Athens.

I am writing in response to the September 2024 article titled "The History of US Menstrual Health, School Nurses, and the Future of Menstrual Equity."[1] The article written by Sadie Bergen and her team was a wonderful contribution highlighting the need for consistent, robust menstrual health education in schools. Although menstruation has been part of life since the beginning of time, menstrual health remains significantly under addressed. Menstruation will at some point affect nearly half of the student population, and nearly 90% of menstruating females will suffer from some type of negative menstrual symptom.[2] With those staggering statistics, I wholeheartedly agree that schools should incorporate menstrual health education. After all, there are policies in place for other conditions such as nosebleeds and headaches, which affect a much smaller population.

However, I believe the responsibility for menstrual health education should not fall solely on school nurses. They play a crucial role, but an effective approach requires taking a different look and incorporating the multidisciplinary team. Teachers, nurses, primary care physicians, and school administrators should work together to develop and implement a standard menstrual health curriculum. Perhaps the information could be presented during normal instruction and not expected to come from the school nurse. Future studies could investigate the impact of pilot programs that integrate menstrual health education into their health curriculum.

In conclusion, the article makes a compelling case for the need to improve menstrual health education and support in schools. AJPH

CORRESPONDENCE

Correspondence should be sent to Morgan Stein, Ohio University School of Nursing, Grove Center E317, 1 Ohio University, Athens, OH 45701 (e-mail: ms710922@ohio.edu). Reprints can be ordered at https://www.ajph.org by clicking the "Reprints" link.

PUBLICATION INFORMATION

Full Citation: Stein M. From taboo to teaching: transforming menstrual health in schools. *Am J Public Health*. 2025;115(2):232.

Acceptance Date: November 16, 2024.

DOI: https://doi.org/10.2105/AJPH.2024.307941

ORCID iD:
Morgan Stein https://orcid.org/0009-0009-7343-0443

CONFLICTS OF INTEREST

The author has no conflicts of interest to disclose.

REFERENCES

1. Bergen S, Maughan ED, Johnson KE, Cogan R, Secor M, Sommer M. The history of US menstrual health, school nurses, and the future of menstrual health equity. *Am J Public Health*. 2024;114(9):903–908. https://doi.org/10.2105/AJPH.2024.307705
2. Brown N, Forrest LJ, Williams R, Piasecki J, Bruinvels G. "Everyone needs to be educated": pupils' voices on menstrual education. *Reprod Health*. 2024;21(1):121. https://doi.org/10.1186/s12978-024-01862-6

A School Nurse Perspective of Menstrual Health Equity

Sara L. Brown, RN, BSN

ABOUT THE AUTHOR

Sara L. Brown is a public health nurse and school nurse in a small, rural public health district in northwest Ohio. She is currently pursuing her master's degree in nursing at Ohio University.

I wish to bring further perspective to the crucial article "The History of US Menstrual Health, School Nurses, and the Future of Menstrual Health Equity" by Bergen et al. in your esteemed publication.[1] I have a unique perspective as a rural Ohio public health nurse and school nurse. The recent Ohio law mandating public schools to provide free menstrual products to students is a significant step forward.[2] However, there is still much to be done to enhance health literacy for menstruating students.

Rural areas face the challenges of period poverty, lack of health literacy, and the inability to afford menstrual supplies, which are all significant public health concerns. While school puberty education typically includes menstrual education, it is often inadequate.[3] School nurses are at the forefront of health education but face obstacles in providing vital menstrual health education. Significant issues include the lack of specific menstrual education and the shortage of resources for school nurses who wish to give this education. I concur with Bergen et al. on the complex medical needs of students. In my practice as a school nurse, I have witnessed an increase in diabetes, asthma, attention-deficit/hyperactivity disorder, anxiety, and depression. As a result, my school days are often filled with passing medications, monitoring children with diabetes, and seeing 50 to 60 students in the nurse clinic. Unfortunately, these needs take precedence over menstrual health education.

The American College of Obstetricians and Gynecologists believes that menstrual health is necessary for students' overall well-being and should be classified as a vital sign that every health care provider should assess.[4] This level of importance demands access to menstrual products and education to reduce stigma and the increased financial burden of having a period. Should these measures be universally implemented, student well-being and school attendance will also improve.[3] School nurses must advocate menstrual health and equity in schools by working with school administrators, health care providers, and parents. As health complexity in the student population grows, health education and support must be a priority in every school. AJPH

CORRESPONDENCE

Correspondence should be sent to Sara L. Brown, BSN, RN, 5997 N County Rd 5, Fostoria, OH 44830 (e-mail: sb343120@ohio.edu). Reprints can be ordered at https://www.ajph.org by clicking the "Reprints" link.

PUBLICATION INFORMATION

Full Citation: Brown SL. A school nurse perspective of menstrual health equity. *Am J Public Health*. 2025;115(2):233.

Acceptance Date: November 16, 2024.

DOI: https://doi.org/10.2105/AJPH.2024.307944

CONFLICTS OF INTEREST

There are no conflicts of interest to disclose.

REFERENCES

1. Bergen S, Maughan ED, Johnson KE, Cogan R, Secor M, Sommer M. The history of US menstrual health, school nurses, and the future of menstrual health equity. *Am J Public Health*. 2024;114(9):903–908. https://doi.org/10.2105/AJPH.2024.307705
2. Ohio Department of Education and Workforce. Menstrual products in schools. Available at: https://education.ohio.gov/Topics/Student-Supports/School-Wellness/Student-Health-and-Medication-Supports/Promoting-Student-Health/Menstrual-Products. Accessed September 18, 2024.
3. Miller TA, Farley M, Reji J, Obeidi Y, Kelley V, Herbert M. Understanding period poverty and stigma: highlighting the need for improved public health initiatives and provider awareness. *J Am Pharm Assoc (2003)*. 2024;64(1):218–221. https://doi.org/10.1016/j.japh.2023.10.015
4. Ramaiyer M, Lulseged B, Michel R, Ali F, Liang J, Borahay MA. Menstruation in the USA. *Curr Epidemiol Rep*. 2023;10(4):186–195. https://doi.org/10.1007/s40471-023-00333-z

Bergen et al. Respond

Sadie Bergen, MA, Erin D. Maughan, RN, PhD, MS, Karen E. Johnson, RN, PhD, Robin Cogan, RN, MEd, NCSN, Molly Secor, RN, PhD, MS, and Marni Sommer, RN, DrPH

ABOUT THE AUTHOR

Sadie Bergen and Marni Sommer are with the Department of Sociomedical Sciences, Columbia University Mailman School of Public Health, New York, NY. Erin D. Maughan is with the College of Public Health, George Mason University, Fairfax, VA. Karen E. Johnson is with the School of Nursing, University of Texas, Austin. Robin Cogan is with School of Nursing, Rutgers University, Camden, NJ. Molly Secor is with the Mark and Robyn Jones College of Nursing, Montana State University, Bozeman.

As the authors of "The History of US Menstrual Health, School Nurses, and the Future of Menstrual Health Equity,"[1] we wish to sincerely thank Brown and Stein for their thoughtful responses to our work. We entirely agree with Stein that menstrual health education would be best tackled by a multidisciplinary collaboration. We also concur with Stein that menstrual health education should be incorporated into regular classroom instruction rather than being siloed as the sole responsibility of a school nurse. We would add that school nurses can act as leaders in multidisciplinary teams of the kind Stein describes. The school nurse's scope of practice goes beyond direct education and care, extending to spaces where school curricula and policy are being set.

As a public health nurse and school nurse in rural Ohio, Brown has observed firsthand the overlapping issues of low health literacy and period poverty. These threats to menstrual equity are exacerbated when underresourced school nurses cannot be involved in shaping and delivering menstrual health education because they are responsible for the care of a student population with increasingly complex health conditions. Requiring that menstrual products be stocked in school bathrooms as well as nurses' offices might alleviate some of the immediate pressure on school nurses in this regard.

We are grateful to Brown for highlighting the geographic disparities in school nursing that exacerbate inequities in menstrual health. Children and adolescents in rural areas face intersecting health challenges, including higher rates of poverty, limited transportation, and fewer health care providers. They are more likely to rely on school health services to meet their basic health needs—including access to menstrual products and the full spectrum of menstrual care. Yet rural schools are also less likely to have any nursing support. Among schools that do have a nurse, fewer rural schools (56.2%) have full-time nurses than do urban schools (70.3%).[2] These statistics point to systematic underinvestment in rural school health and inevitable consequences for geographic and socioeconomic disparities in menstrual health. In both Brown's and Stein's responses, we see an implicit argument for improving school nursing capacity through adequate school nurse staffing that follows National Association of School Nurses guidelines.[3] We encourage advocates to make the case for investing in school nurses as a menstrual equity intervention. AJPH

CORRESPONDENCE

Correspondence should be sent to Sadie Bergen, PhD, Department of Sociomedical Sciences, Mailman School of Public Health, 722 W 168th St, New York, NY 10032 (e-mail: srb2161@columbia.edu). Reprints can be ordered at https://www.ajph.org by clicking the "Reprints" link.

PUBLICATION INFORMATION

Full Citation: Bergen S, Maughan ED, Johnson KE, Cogan Robin, Secor Molly, Sommer Marni. Bergen et al. respond. *Am J Public Health*. 2025;115(2):234.

Acceptance Date: November 16, 2024.

DOI: https://doi.org/10.2105/AJPH.2024.307942

ORCID iD:

Sadie Bergen https://orcid.org/0000-0002-3939-7645

CONTRIBUTORS

The authors contributed equally to this letter.

CONFLICTS OF INTEREST

The authors have no conflicts of interest to declare.

REFERENCES

1. Bergen S, Maughan ED, Johnson KE, Cogan R, Secor M, Sommer M. The history of US menstrual health, school nurses, and the future of menstrual health equity. *Am J Public Health*. 2024;114(9): 903–908. https://doi.org/10.2105/AJPH.2024.307705
2. Willgerodt MA, Tanner A, McCabe E, Jameson B, Brock D. Public school nurses in the United States: National School Nurse Workforce Study 2.0. *J Sch Nurs*. 2024;40(5):468–481. https://doi.org/10.1177/10598405241253565
3. National Association of School Nurses. Position statement: school nurse workload: staffing for safe care. 2020. Available at: https://www.nasn.org/nasn-resources/professional-practice-documents/position-statements/ps-workload. Accessed November 11, 2024.

Erratum In: "Health Care Delivery Site– and Patient-Level Factors Associated With COVID-19 Primary Vaccine Series Completion in a National Network of Community Health Centers"

In: Gold R, Steeves-Reece A, Ochoa A, et al. Health care delivery site– and patient-level factors associated with COVID-19 primary vaccine series completion in a national network of community health centers. *Am J Public Health*. 2024;114(11): 1242–1251.

When originally published, a funding statement was left out of the Acknowledgments section. The article's Acknowledgments section should read:

This research was funded by the National Institutes of Health (NIH; agreement OT2HL158287).

This work was also conducted with the Accelerating Data Value Across a National Community Health Center Network (ADVANCE) Clinical Research Network. ADVANCE is led by Oregon Community Health Information Network (OCHIN) in partnership with Health Choice Network, Fenway Health, and Oregon Health & Science University. ADVANCE is funded through the Patient-Centered Outcomes Research Institute (contract RI-OCHIN 01-MC).

We would like to thank Brenda McGrath, Teresa Schmidt, and Fran Biel from OCHIN, and Peter Thomas Baltrus from the Morehouse School of Medicine for providing editorial feedback and edits.

Note. The views and conclusions contained in this document are those of the authors and should not be interpreted as representing the official policies, either expressed or implied, of the NIH. AJPH

https://doi.org/10.2105/AJPH.2024.307773e

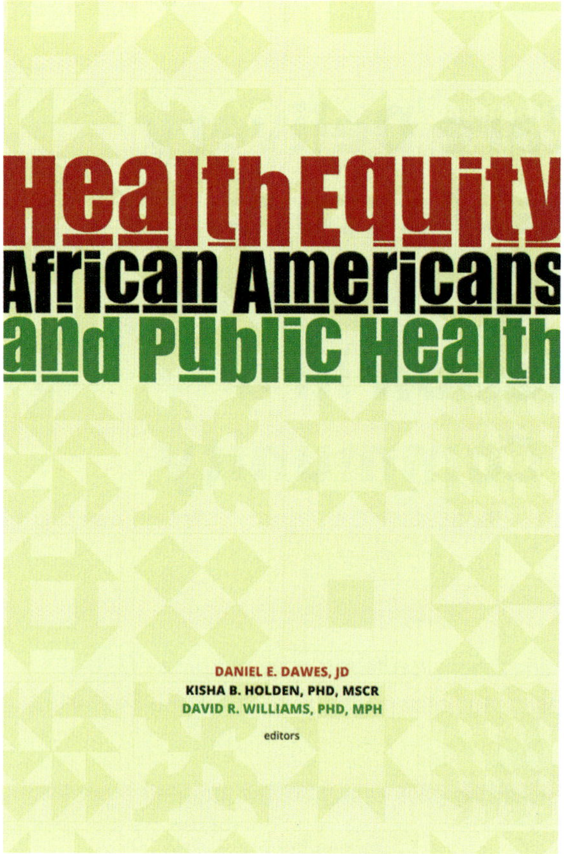

978-097553-3285, 2023, 650 PP, SOFTCOVER

Health Equity: African Americans and Public Health

Edited by: Daniel E. Dawes, JD, Kisha B. Holden, PhD, MSCR, and David R. Williams, PhD, MPH

Health Equity: African Americans and Public Health offers a unique perspective into the complex dimensions of health inequities as these pertain to African Americans. This book aims to help advance health equity by providing a critical examination of the factors that create, perpetuate, and exacerbate health inequities for African Americans. These findings may serve as catalysts for transforming health outcomes in the United States.

APHABOOKSTORE.ORG

APHA PRESS

AN IMPRINT OF AMERICAN PUBLIC HEALTH ASSOCIATION